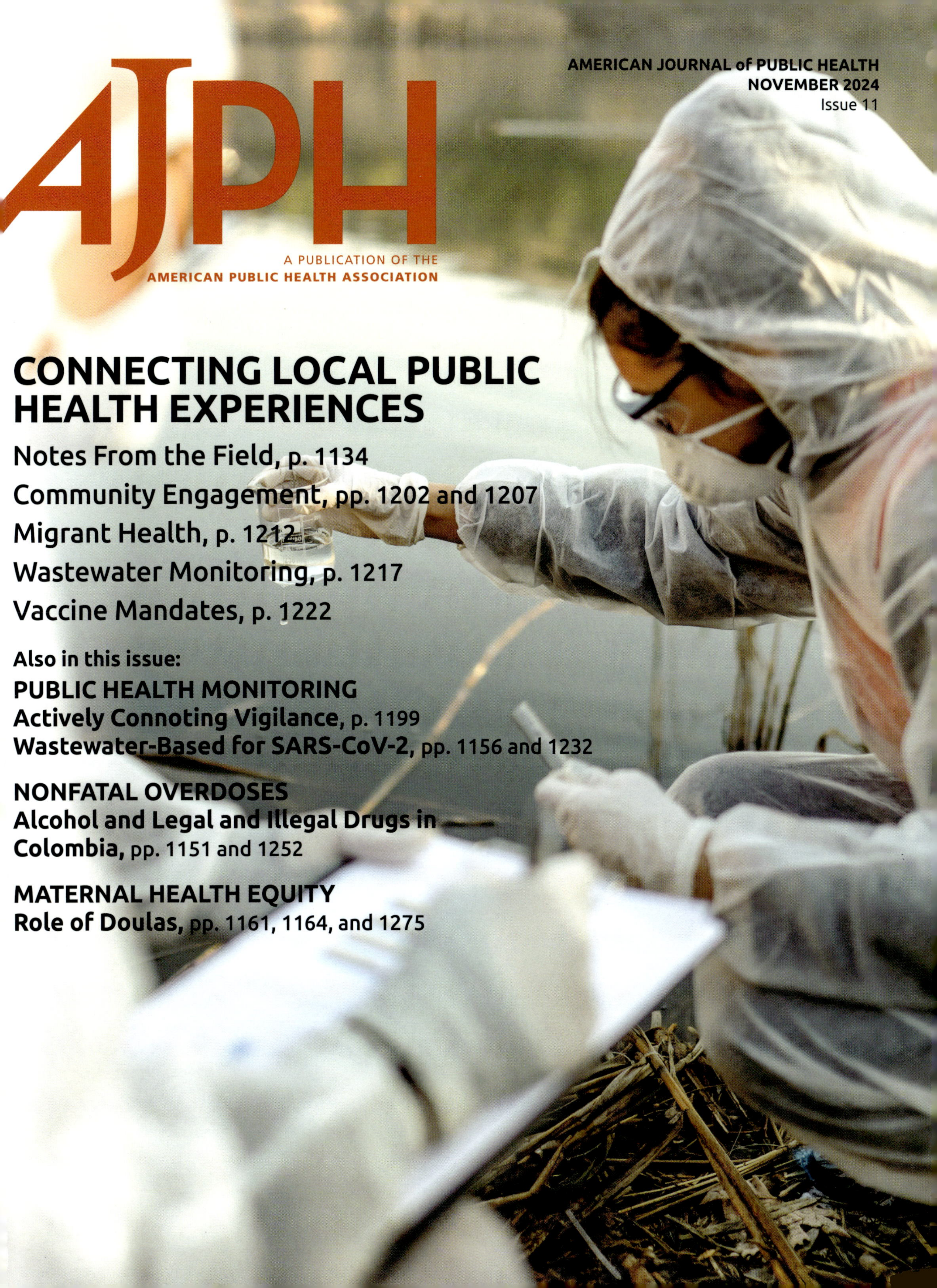

AJPH

A PUBLICATION OF THE
AMERICAN PUBLIC HEALTH ASSOCIATION

AMERICAN JOURNAL of PUBLIC HEALTH
NOVEMBER 2024
Issue 11

CONNECTING LOCAL PUBLIC HEALTH EXPERIENCES

Notes From the Field, p. 1134
Community Engagement, pp. 1202 and 1207
Migrant Health, p. 1212
Wastewater Monitoring, p. 1217
Vaccine Mandates, p. 1222

Also in this issue:

PUBLIC HEALTH MONITORING
Actively Connoting Vigilance, p. 1199
Wastewater-Based for SARS-CoV-2, pp. 1156 and 1232

NONFATAL OVERDOSES
Alcohol and Legal and Illegal Drugs in Colombia, pp. 1151 and 1252

MATERNAL HEALTH EQUITY
Role of Doulas, pp. 1161, 1164, and 1275

AJPH®, published monthly, is the official Journal of the American Public Health Association®, 800 I St NW, Washington, DC 20001-3710; (202) 777- APHA; TDD (202) 777-2500. APHA is a nongovernmental professional society founded in 1872, representing all disciplines and specialties in public health.

The *American Journal of Public Health*® (*AJPH*) (print ISSN: 0090-0036; electronic ISSN: 1541- 0048), first published in 1911, is the official journal of the American Public Health Association® (APHA). The oldest and largest organization of public health professionals in the world, APHA represents approximately 30 000 members from more than 50 occupations of public health.

Submissions: Visit www.editorialmanager.com/ajph or ajph.edmgr.com for online manuscript preparation and submission guidelines. Contributions of original unpublished research, social science analyses, scholarly essays, critical commentaries, departments, and letters to the editor are welcome. Questions? Write ajph.submissions@apha.org or call APHA at (202) 777-2469.

Print plus online subscriptions: Institutional price (print copy with online access for a single institution and all authorized users, regardless of geographic location) varies by size of organization and ranges from $993–$1445 for US organizations, and $1073–$1526 for international organizations (air delivery); multiple campuses not permitted without special arrangement. Details of the tiered pricing system at https://subscriptionoffice.com/pages/apha-landing-page. To order, write apha.subscriptions@apha.org.

Online-only subscriptions: Institutional price for one institution and its authorized users (regardless of geographic location) is $878–$1307. To order, write apha.subscriptions@apha.org. For academic consortia or multisite corporate subscriptions, contact apha.subscriptions@apha.org.

Print-only subscriptions: Institutional price is US $701, $782 international.

Back print issues: A limited number of print issues are for sale. Single copies are US $49, $55 international (air delivery). Shipping included; prepay only. To order, write apha.subscriptions@apha.org.

Reprints: For prices and ordering information on 50 or more reprints, check the Reprints section at www.ajph.org. To order smaller quantities of reprints (rush delivery), use the "Purchase Article" link on the article site itself.

Electronic access: Online articles more than 10 years old are available free for personal use at www.ajph.org. Recent articles are available through pay-per-view: single PDF article for $24, single issue access for 24 hours for $33, or entire site access for 24 hours for $38.

Postal information: Periodicals postage paid at Washington, DC, and additional mailing offices. Postmaster: Send address changes to American Journal of Public Health, 800 I St NW, Washington, DC 20001-3710.

Address changes: Send to AJPH, Membership Department (members) or AJPH Subscriptions (subscribers), APHA, 800 I St NW, Washington, DC 20001-3710. Or write to membership.mail@apha. org (members) or apha.subscriptions@apha.org (subscribers).

Advertising: For pricing and other information, see www.ajph.org. Please write to brian.selzer@ apha.org or call (202) 777-2470 for other advertising opportunities. Ask about special exhibit packages and sponsorships. Acceptance of advertising by the *Journal* does not imply endorsement of products.

Indexes: Publications that index or abstract articles from *AJPH* include the following: Ageline, Assia (Applied Social Science Index and Abstracts), Biological Abstracts, Chemical Abstracts, CINAHL, Criminal Justice Abstracts, EMBASE, EMCare, Environmental Abstracts, e-psyche, ERIC, ETOH (Alcohol and Alcohol Problems Science Database), Excerpta Medica, Food Science and Technology, General Science Index, Grateful Med, Hospital Literature Index, Human Resources Abstracts, International Pharmaceutical Abstracts (IPA), Medline, Physical Education Index, Pollution Abstracts, Psychological Abstracts, PsychINFO, Safety Science Abstracts, Sage Family Studies Abstracts, Sage Human Resources Abstracts, Science Citation Index, SCOPUS, SIIC Data Bases, Social Work Research and Abstracts, and Statistical Reference Index (SRI)/LexisNexis.

AJPH

A PUBLICATION OF THE
AMERICAN PUBLIC HEALTH ASSOCIATION

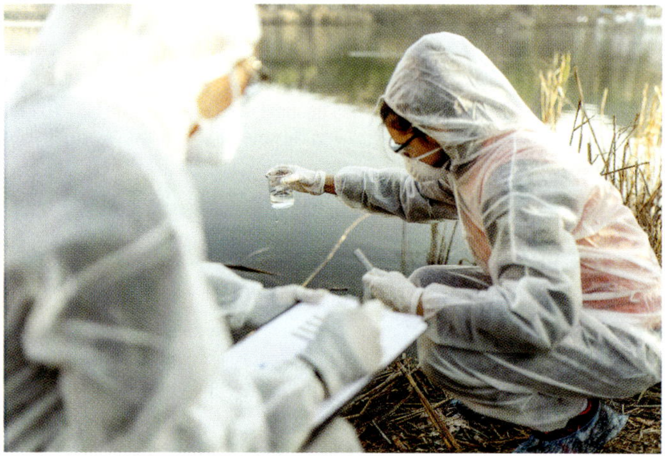

COVER: The cover depicts environmental scientists collecting wastewater samples at specific community sites. Such sampling can also be done at sewage treatment plants and in sewer networks. Wastewater analysis is increasingly used by local and federal agencies to enhance traditional public health monitoring, particularly for tracking infectious diseases. By analyzing concentration levels over time, trends in pathogen levels or chemical pollutants can be detected. These results are often compared with clinical and epidemiological data to gain insights into community health. For example, in Boston, MA, neighborhood-level monitoring of SARS-CoV-2 in wastewater revealed inequities that were missed at the treatment plant level.

Cover concept and selection by Aleisha Kropf. Photo by Phynart Studio/Getty. Printed with permission.

APHA
AMERICAN PUBLIC HEALTH ASSOCIATION
For science. For action. For health.

Promoting public health research, policy, practice, and education is the *AJPH* mission. As we widen our scope to embrace global issues, we also sharpen our focus to support the needs of public health practitioners. We invite contributions of original unpublished research, opinion and commentary, and letters to the editor.

The *Journal* is printed on acid-free recycled paper.

OPEN ACCESS ONLINE ONLY PODCAST DATA SUPPLEMENT AVAILABLE

EDITOR'S CHOICE

1134 Notes From the Field: Why They Are Important
A. Morabia

BOOKS & MEDIA

1136 Has Public Health Become Illiberal?
J. M. Samet

1139 A Crucial Book for Teaching Environmental, Sustainability, and Health Professions Students About the Health Consequences of Climate Change
L. R. Goldman

1143 The Making of the 1964 Surgeon General's Report on Smoking and Health
R. N. Proctor

OPINIONS, IDEAS, & PRACTICE

EDITORIALS

1146 Equitable Uptake of Life-Saving COVID-19 Primary Vaccine Series in Community Health Centers
R. C. Hechter

1148 On Race and Place in Substance Use Research
B. Ostrach and J. J. Carroll

1151 Mitigating Overdoses in Colombia
M. Diaz-Moreno and D. Rojas

1153 Tracking Drug Overdose in Latin America: The Epidemiological Potential of Prehospital and Emergency Department Data
J. R. Friedman

1156 Does Wastewater-Based Surveillance Protect the Health of Incarcerated Individuals?
R. H. Holm and T. Smith

1158 To Uncover Disparities, Collect and Disaggregate Self-Identification Data for Middle Eastern and North African Americans
A. Schachter, N. Maghbouleh, and R. D. Flores

1161 Doula Support as a Health Equity Strategy: Carving the Path Forward
H. L. Horan

1164 Progress on Doula Access, Persistent Challenges, and Next Steps for Birth Equity
C. Marshall and K. B. Kozhimannil

1167 Addressing Data Deficiencies to Prevent Pediatric Firearm Injuries: Insights From the American College of Surgeons (ACS) Firearm Study
D. C. Semenza

PERSPECTIVES

1170 An Agenda for Addressing Health-Harming Legal Needs in Indigenous Communities
M. Statz and B. Watters

1175 Beyond Stigma: The Case Against the Criminalization of Sex Work for HIV Prevention and Health Equity
T. Cochran, L. Smith, K. Ayers, and M. van Stone

1179 HIV Prevention in Foster Care Youths: Time for a Refocus
C. W. Adrian, S. L. Shipe, and K. Guastaferro

1184 The 2023 Maui Wildfires and the Mental Health Effects of Climate-Induced Relocation
A. Suresh, L. Tu, and F. C. Stanford

1188 Kratom Products Are Widely Available Throughout the United States
M. E. Rossheim, C. R. LoParco, K. K. Tillett, R. A. Yockey, H-C. Lin, and C. J. Berg

1191 Kids No Longer Smoke Cigarettes. Why Aren't We Celebrating?
K. E. Warner

1195 Rethinking Rankings in Public Health Graduate Education—Who Are They For?
J. P. Leider

1199 Public Health Monitoring: An Active Phrase for Vigilance, Warning, Guidance, and Accountability
N. Krieger

NOTES FROM THE FIELD: WHY ARE THEY IMPORTANT?

1202 Community Organizations, Local Health Equity Action Teams, and a Learning Collaborative to Address COVID-19 Disparities in Urban and Rural Communities
E. F. Ellerbeck, V. L. Collie-Akers, E. Ablah, S. Landry, A. Honn, S. Obermeier, M. Ramirez, Y. Chen, I. R. Knight, C. Y. Lumpkins, M. Ricketts, T. Carter, U. Wright, C. Watson, D. L. Kurz, S. McCrea-Robertson, S. Finocchario-Kessler, J. LeMaster, E. Corriveau, B. Crawford, J. He, and K. A. Greiner

1207 Reach and Engagement With Population Health Management Interventions to Address COVID-19 Among Safety-Net Health Care Systems
C. R. Schlechter, T. V. Kuzmenko, B. Orleans, J. Wirth, K. A. Kaphingst, B. Gibson, K. Kawamoto, T. Siaperas, A. Pruhs, C. P. Dinkins, T. Greene, Y. Zhang, J. J. Chipman, M. Friedrichs, C. Y. Lam, J. H. Pierce, E. P. Borsato, R. C. Cornia, L. Stevens, A. Martinez, R. L. Bradshaw, R. Hess, G. D. Fiol, and D. W. Wetter

1212 Reach, Adoption, Implementation, and Sustainability of the Mobile Health for Migrant Health (mHealth-4-Mhealth) Program: Nebraska, 2022–2023
R. J. McCulloh, E. Kerns, C. Abresch, M. Warren, F. Sanchez, G. Marfileno, L. Rivera, and M. J. Broadhurst

1217 Implementation of Neighborhood-Level Wastewater-Based Epidemiology to Measure and Mitigate Inequities in SARS-CoV-2 Infection in Boston, Massachusetts
T. L. Cowger, M. T. Sharp, J. D. Hart, B. O. Ojikutu, S. Nair, and K. T. Hall

1222 The Influence of a COVID-19 Vaccine Mandate on Vaccination Rates in a University Setting
E. B. Figueroa, B. Bohn, J. M. Oakes, and R. T. Demmer

1228 Automated Opt-Out Hepatitis C Testing to Reduce Missed Screening Opportunities in the Emergency Department
H. Sperring, G. Ruiz-Mercado, B.J. Yun, D. Twitchell, B. Shah, and E.M. Schechter-Perkins

RESEARCH & ANALYSIS

HEALTH MONITORING

1232 Four Models of Wastewater-Based Monitoring for SARS-CoV-2 Complementing Individual Screening in Jail Settings
S.S. Kennedy, L.B. Saber, V.M. Brown, R.A. Boehm, A.A. Olotu, J. Osei, J.A. Pluznik, L.R. Riback, E. Sidibeh, B. Jordan, E. O'Donovan, A. Mangla, C. Nzokou, T.L. Elam, J. Gubser, P.J. Koutoujian, K.A. Siddiqi, S. Wilensky, V.L. Phillips, A.G. Wurcel, C.J. Zawitz, M.J. Akiyama, and A.C. Spaulding

OPEN-THEMED RESEARCH

1242 Health Care Delivery Site- and Patient-Level Factors Associated With COVID-19 Primary Vaccine Series Completion in a National Network of Community Health Centers
R. Gold, A. Steeves-Reece, A. Ochoa, J. Oakley, R. Gunn, S. Liu, B.A. Hatch, S.T. O'Leary, C.I. Spina, T. Allen, and E.K. Cottrell

1252 Trends in Nonfatal Overdose Rates Due to Alcohol and Prescription and Illegal Substances in Colombia, 2010–2021
J. Santaella-Tenorio, J.S. Zapata-López, T.M. Fidalgo, V.S. Tardelli, L.E. Segura, M. Cerda, and S.S. Martins

1261 Long COVID Among People With Preexisting Disabilities
J.P. Hall, N.K. Kurth, L. McCorkell, and K.S. Goddard

1265 Cognitive Difficulty in Middle Eastern and North African Adults Living in the United States Compared With Other Racial and Ethnic Categories, 2017–2021
T.B. Kindratt and A. Smith

1275 Role of Doulas in Improving Maternal Health and Health Equity Among Medicaid Enrollees, 2014–2023
A.M. Falconi, L. Ramirez, R. Cobb, C. Levin, M. Nguyen, and T. Inglis

BACKMATTER

ERRATA

1286 Erratum In: "Control of SARS-CoV-2 Infection Rates at a Spanish University With In-Person Class Attendance"

OTHER DEPARTMENTS

1288 Subscription Form

PEER REVIEWERS

e1 *AJPH* Peer Reviewers 2023–2024: Thank You for Your Services
M. Henry, B. Selzer, A. Ferguson, and K. Crocker

Notes From the Field: Why They Are Important

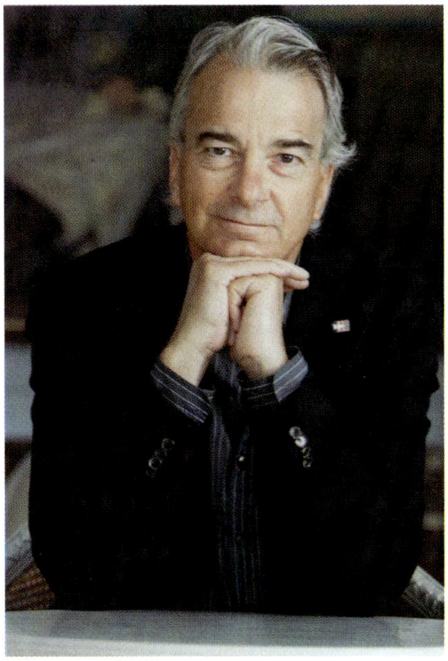

Alfredo Morabia, MD, PhD
Editor in Chief, *AJPH*

Notes From the Field (NFTF) has become a popular format for article submissions to *AJPH*. These articles are designed to share successful and impactful field experiences, typically at the local level. The format ensures that key information is presented clearly, making it possible for others to replicate these experiences in different contexts. Unlike research articles, NFTF pieces focus on describing processes in a reproducible way, rather than delving into methods, analysis, and findings. This emphasis on practical, actionable insights makes NFTF a valuable resource for public health practitioners and researchers alike.

These Notes have a maximum length of 1500 words, with an 80-word abstract, up to 15 references, and up to two tables, two figures, or one of each. The structure of the Notes includes the following subheadings:

1. Intervention and Implementation: Describe the goals, objectives, and practical implementation of the intervention.
2. Place, Time, and Persons: Specify the geographic location, the period during which the intervention was implemented, and the population targeted by the intervention.
3. Purpose: Explain the motivation and rationale behind the intervention.
4. Evaluation and Adverse Effects: Provide evidence on the effectiveness of the intervention and discuss any adverse or unintended consequences, if applicable. The "Evaluation and Adverse Effects" section is especially key, as Notes are intended to document interventions that have been fully implemented and evaluated, rather than those still in progress.
5. Sustainability: If ongoing continuation of the practice is desirable, describe the factors supporting its sustainability.
6. Public Health Significance: Highlight the importance of the program for public health, both locally and in broader contexts.

The six NFTF articles in this issue address a diverse array of public health challenges, including immigrant

Continued on page 1135...

HISTORY CORNER

47 YEARS AGO

The Importance of Direct Intervention

[T]here remain close at hand many problems available for and worthy of study which have the potential to lead to direct intervention that can result in clear cut contributions to the health of the public. Often these opportunities require but modest investment and the likelihood of success can be enhanced by following a corollary of Sutton's Law: Look for the causes of a problem where the cases occur. . . . Ten years [ago] . . . the Bureau of Health Statistics of the New York City Department of Health called attention to the frequent number of deaths due to falls from high places—primarily from windows—among young children. An epidemiologic analysis of existing data, cooperation with clinical colleagues, and a modest amount of field visiting to homes of non-fatal and fatal cases made it possible to identify the areas of highest risk and develop a direct preventive intervention. . . . While expanding its existing educational program—now targeted to the highest risk areas on the basis of additional data gathering—it moved to get satisfactory safety devices for the windows of apartments housing young children.

From *AJPH*, December 1977, p. 1135

populations, wastewater surveillance, COVID-19, hepatitis C screening, and postpartum opioid use for pain relief.

Ellerbeck et al. (p. 1202) describe how health equity action teams in Kansas engaged leaders from underresourced and marginalized communities during the pandemic to adapt COVID-19 testing and communication strategies to meet specific local needs.

Schlechter et al. (p. 1207) detail the SCALE-UP Utah initiative, a pragmatic clinical trial that promoted COVID-19 testing and vaccination through text messages sent to 107 898 patients across 28 clinics embedded in seven community health centers.

McCulloh et al. (p. 1212) used the Mobile Health for Migrant Health (mHealth-4-Mhealth) program to screen Nebraska households for health and sociomedical challenges, providing crucial linkages to community resources.

The Boston, Massachusetts, Public Health Commission (Cowger et al., p. 1217) demonstrated that neighborhood-level wastewater surveillance of SARS-CoV-2 (severe acute respiratory syndrome coronavirus 2) revealed inequities that were otherwise obscured by monitoring at the treatment plant level.

Figueroa et al. (p. 1222) conducted a rigorous survey of faculty and students across five university campuses in Rochester, Minnesota, regarding a vaccine mandate, illustrating both the benefits and challenges of implementing such mandates in educational settings.

Sperring et al. (p. 1228) report on the transition from an opt-in to an automated opt-out hepatitis C virus testing protocol, which significantly increased the identification of active hepatitis C virus infections in emergency departments.

A key strength of these Notes is their embodiment of balanced public health practice, ensuring that information and decision-making flow both ways—between professionals and the communities they serve.

The diverse institutional and geographical origins of the NFTFs demonstrate their relevance and appeal to a broad audience across the country. We prioritize rapid processing of these submissions to ensure timely dissemination on social media and other platforms.

The success of the NFTF format highlights its value in meeting a critical need in the public health community. We encourage public health departments, grassroots organizations, and frontline workers to continue using this platform to share their valuable experiences with *AJPH* readers. AJPH

DOI: https://doi.org/10.2105/AJPH.2024.307852

HISTORY CORNER

111 YEARS AGO

Health Department Reports and Notes

An interesting experiment for the purpose of creating immunity against tuberculosis is being tried in Pittsburgh under the direction of the Tuberculosis League of that city. Dr. William Charles White, Medical Director of the League, says it will probably take ten years before definite results of the work will be appreciated. The experiment is being conducted on the theory that much, if not all, tuberculosis infection begins in childhood. In view of this fact, the League is aiming to supervise the growth of every baby born for the next ten years in the South Side district of Pittsburgh. The babies and their mothers will be taken in charge at the birth of the infant, and everything possible will be done to increase the resisting power of the child to disease and to make it thereby immune to tuberculous infection. The theory is that by fortifying the body in the earliest period of a child's life, the infant will in most cases, become immune to the disease with which heredity and environment may threaten it.

From *AJPH*, July 1913, p. 717

Has Public Health Become Illiberal?

Jonathan M. Samet, MD, MS

ABOUT THE AUTHOR

Jonathan M. Samet is with the Colorado School of Public Health, Aurora, CO.

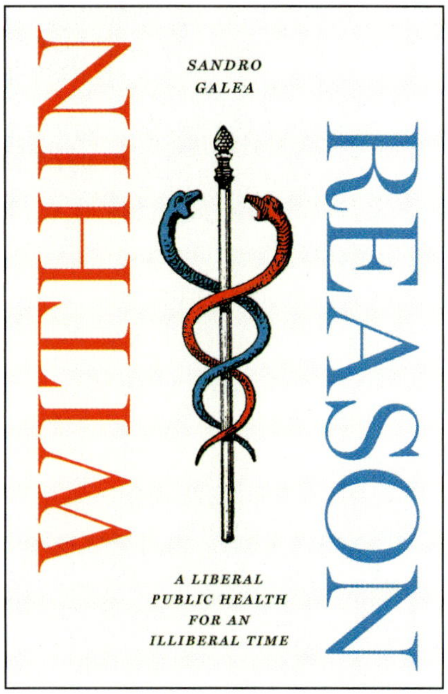

Within Reason: A Liberal Public Health for an Illiberal Time
By Sandro Galea
Chicago, IL: University of Chicago Press; 2023
304 pp; $22.50
ISBN-10: 0226822915
ISBN-13: 978-0226822914

Sandro Galea is one of the most productive and powerful voices in academic public health. His impact reaches broadly through his research contributions as a social epidemiologist; his thoughtful framing of how epidemiology can make a difference, labeled as an "epidemiology of consequence"; and his stream of commentary on public health and society. He is a thought leader.

WHAT IS ILLIBERAL?

In *Within Reason: A Liberal Public Health for an Illiberal Time*, Galea offers a series of essays reflecting on how the COVID-19 pandemic altered public health. The subtitle tells the story. In Galea's opinion, actions taken during the pandemic moved public health from being "liberal" to "illiberal," a storyline requiring readers to understand the distinction between these two seemingly opposing states. In *Within Reason*, liberal does not refer to its political connotations but to a set of core values from which public health has strayed, driven away from them by the exigencies of the pandemic: "forgetting our roots, becoming poor at weighing trade-offs, getting caught in media feedback loops, and cultivating influence rather than truth" (p263). For Galea, the roots of public health extend back to the European Enlightenment (17th and 18th centuries) and its scientific revolution and political liberalism. The "politicizing of science and public health institutions" also receives attention, but as a driver toward illiberalism, exemplified for Galea by reactions of the public health community to the Great Barrington Declaration, which set out a path toward herd immunity that was counter to mainstream public health opinion.[1]

Understanding illiberalism is central to appreciating the book. After struggling to find my own definition and criteria for illiberalism, I gave up. Galea himself is the decider in the pages of *Within Reason*, frustrating my reading of the book. And for me, it seems simplistic to create two strata—liberal or illiberal. Are there not different kinds and different extremes of illiberalism in Galea's formulation? Galea offers the example of China's effort to achieve "zero COVID" as an extreme of illiberalism. It is, but where is the demarcation between liberal and illiberal in the array of activities implemented to control the pandemic? Galea's bifurcation is convenient for these essays but simplifies too much.

He might have chosen another word than illiberalism for this proposed transformation of public health. In the introduction, he comments on the choice, referencing the illiberalism on the political right that came with the Trump era. His fundamental concern is that public health, generally, but not exclusively left-leaning, has become illiberal as well in response to the illiberalism of the right. He does not directly connect illiberalism as used in *Within Reason* to the wider use of the term. In today's era of emerging authoritarian regimes, illiberalism is a widely used term, referring to an antidemocratic political ideology. My response to the word conflated this general use of the term with Galea's specific formulation of illiberalism and likely biased my reading.

As I reviewed *Within Reason*, I was finishing Anne Applebaum's *Twilight of Democracy: The Seductive Lure of Authoritarianism* and starting *Fascism: A Warning* by Madeleine Albright. Both cover the rise of illiberal democracies and the move to fascism with examples such as Viktor Orbán in Hungary and Recep Erdoğan in Turkey. Per Albright, "An illiberal democracy is centered on the supposed needs of the community rather than the inalienable rights of the individual."[2(p172)] Extended to illiberal public health, this sentence captures one element of Galea's illiberalism, but has not public health always centered on the population? For example, in the 1905 *Jacobson v Massachusetts* decision, the Supreme Court upheld the state's authority to require smallpox vaccination. The global strategy for smallpox elimination, ring vaccination, would not have succeeded without mandatory vaccination.

Perhaps Galea's use of the illiberalism was influenced by this current geopolitical context. He does imply that some public health actions taken during the COVID-19 pandemic were authoritarian. Certainly, China's imprisonment of its citizens in their homes was authoritarian, and lockdowns in the United States were portrayed as antidemocratic ("small d" democracy) by some. In the United States, particularly as the pandemic played out, some public health measures were portrayed as infringing freedom and not justified by conservative politicians and pundits.

I am concerned by the retrospective way that Galea applies his concept of illiberalism. Public health actions taken during the pandemic reflected the perceived level of exigency at the time and the state of science, which was highly uncertain for many key issues. With hindsight, Galea finds illiberalism, perhaps with justification in his framing. Turning back to his five pillars of illiberalism, the pandemic was a time of media attention and influence for public health, and consideration of trade-offs gave much greater weight to curbing the pandemic than to the possible harms of public health measures. However, I do not think that the diverse elements of the public health community strayed too far from "our roots" in emphasizing pandemic control in decision-making.

TAKING ON BIG PROBLEMS

Another simplification troubled me: the treatment of public health as a monolith that can be captured using a collective "we." Although this lumping is a convenient artifice, public health is far too broad and heterogenous to be compressed into a single entity. It is not. The academic and practice sectors are not lumpable, and there is great heterogeneity across the thousands of agencies concerned with population health. Many others use this construct with such phrasings as "public health should do . . ." and, in my own field, "epidemiology should do. . . ." Since epidemiology is a scientific method, this anthropomorphization is off the mark. The commentaries would have been more nuanced with further splitting of public health into its relevant components.

Galea has always been willing to offer thoughts about big problems. In *Within Reason*, he continues to do so with essays such as "The Ongoing Challenge of Race" and "What Do We Want From Our Political System." With so many topics covered by five-page essays, he offers high-level thoughts, probing the systems underlying the issue. These system-based framings are informative, but go no deeper, and changing societal structures mostly lies outside of the scope of public health entities acting on their own.

For example, in "Borders in an Age of Pandemics," Galea addresses border closures and their consequences during the COVID-19 pandemic. Recall that the southern border of the United States has long been a hot political topic; at the pandemic's start, it became even hotter with border closures becoming a controversial issue, a modality not supported by the World Health Organization for pandemic control. Galea views border policy as within the purview of public health writ large, but is it? And his directive on the topic is at too a high level to set a path for the public health communities into terrain that is not theirs: quoting the chapter, "It is likewise true that public health can pursue a world without borders while at the same time allowing ourselves the freedom to act pragmatically, when crisis strikes"[(p50)]. The reminder of the public health significance of border policies is useful and timely, but the complexities of border policies themselves do not fit within the ambit of agencies concerned with public health. I see our task as informing about the public health consequences of border policies generally and specifically on such matters as border closure and pandemic control.

HOW TO READ THIS BOOK

Who should read *Within Reason* and how should they read it? Galea's target is the broad array of people in public health, and his hope is that the book will contribute to a shift back to a liberal public health. His audience is all of us. As to how to read *Within Reason*,

I approached the book in two ways: I read the first section, "Foundations," straight through and then hop-scotched through the essays of the second and third sections—"Heresies" and "Hopes." The second approach was more successful for me, as each essay stands alone, and, across the book, the essays are loosely stitched together. There is not a clear flow from one to the other that would warrant starting at the beginning and reading to the end.

Galea has generously shared his thoughts about many topics through his blogs and books. *Within Reason* adds to his oeuvre. It provides a useful snapshot of the thoughts of one of our leading thinkers across the crisis years of the COVID-19 pandemic. Galea offers a rich menu for readers; pick what you want to read. The essays are all thought-provoking. AJPH

CORRESPONDENCE

Correspondence should be sent to Jonathan M. Samet, 13001 E 17th Place, Aurora CO 80045 (e-mail: jon.samet@cuanschutz.edu). Reprints can be ordered at https://www.ajph.org by clicking the "Reprints" link.

PUBLICATION INFORMATION

Full Citation: Samet JM. Has public health become illiberal? *Am J Public Health*. 2024;114(11): 1136–1138.

Acceptance Date: July 25, 2024.

DOI: https://doi.org/10.2105/AJPH.2024.307831

ORCID iD:

Jonathan M. Samet https://orcid.org/0000-0001-5676-9175

CONFLICTS OF INTEREST

The author has no conflicts of interest to disclose.

REFERENCES

1. Great Barrington Declaration. Available at: https://gbdeclaration.org. Accessed August 13, 2024.
2. Albright M. *Fascism: A Warning*. New York, NY: Harper Perennial; 2018.

A Crucial Book for Teaching Environmental, Sustainability, and Health Professions Students About the Health Consequences of Climate Change

Lynn R. Goldman, MD, MS, MPH

ABOUT THE AUTHORS

Lynn R. Goldman is dean and professor of environmental and occupational health with the Milken Institute School of Public Health at the George Washington University, Washington, DC.

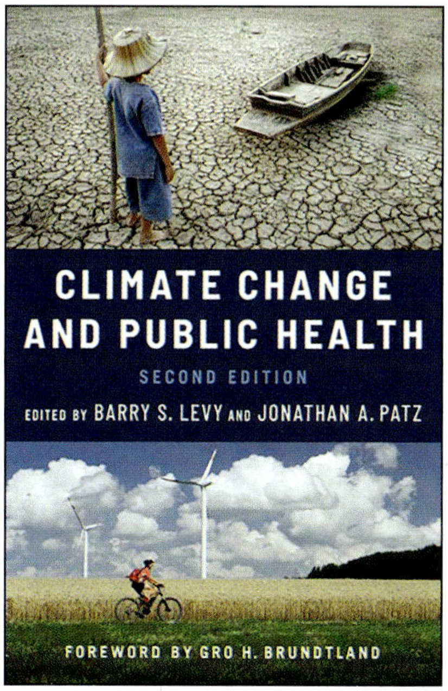

Climate Change and Public Health, 2nd Edition
By Barry S. Levy and Jonathan A. Patz
New York, NY: Oxford University Press; 2024
480 pp.; $74.95
Online ISBN: 9780197683323
Print ISBN: 9780197683293

Calls to action for universities to address climate and health in their curricula, especially for health professions, are proliferating. In the United States, several professional health school associations—public health (Association of Schools and Programs of Public Health),[1] medicine (Association of American Medical Colleges),[2] nursing (American Association of Colleges of Nursing),[3] and psychology (American Psychological Association)[4]—have recently identified climate as a threat to health and are now recommending schools educate about health and climate. At the same time, scientists primarily concerned with the environmental aspects of climate change are becoming more aware of the significance of human health consequences and incorporating this perspective into policy actions. The formation within the American Geophysical Union of a geohealth section and their publication of a specialized multidisciplinary journal (*Geohealth*)[5] is an example of a new convergence that is occurring as new knowledge about climate and health is being brought forward by researchers. Educational resources are being developed, as demonstrated by those curated by Columbia University's Global Consortium on Climate and Health Education.[6]

INTRODUCTION

So, do we need a textbook on climate and health? Resoundingly, yes! Fortunately, *Climate Change and Public Health,* edited by Barry Levy and Jonathan Patz, can fit the bill for those searching for a comprehensive textbook in this field. Levy and Patz are well known for their prodigious contributions to environmental public health science and education, and this book is a logical outgrowth of their work. This logically organized volume is jam-packed with information. Its broad coverage includes health impacts, policy and implementation issues, and critical public and political engagement issues. With 55 contributors, the book is evidence-based and filled with nuggets that interest the reader. They include helpful case studies and summary tables. Each chapter concludes with an excellent summary that serves as a guide for instructors and students alike. Importantly, by design, this book addresses climate change and its adverse health consequences and consistently includes information on what can be done to mitigate climate change and its implications, adapt to climate change, address inequities, and promote climate justice.

The editors state that the book is "primarily designed for students and mid-career professionals in public health and environmental sciences" but note that "students and mid-career professionals in other fields will likely find the book to be informative and useful" (p. xiii). I agree that it serves this dual purpose. I appreciated the consistent approach that, by design, serves a broad array of audiences and allows any student to comprehend the material, regardless of whether they have prior knowledge in fields as disparate as pulmonary disease or climate scenarios modeling. In that regard, nothing else like this book is on the market today.

OVERVIEW OF CLIMATE CHANGE AND HEALTH

Part I, the introduction, presents the foundation for any course in climate and health. Chapter 1, written by coeditors Levy and Patz, provides an overview of the health hazards associated with climate change within the framework of public health, including consideration of social justice and regional inequities in the distribution of these hazards across populations. They frame climate policy setting as engaging two "categories of preventive measures to address climate change," namely, "mitigation (a form of primary prevention)" (p. 19) and involving measures to reduce the production of the greenhouse gases that are the primary cause of climate change, and "adaptation (a form of secondary prevention)" (p. 19) and involving measures to reduce the adverse impacts of climate change. Chapter 2, written by a team led by a climatologist Stephen J. Vavrus and Patz, is a general overview of climate science as it applies to climate change and weather, including complexities around the interpretation of global observational data, application of both simple and complex climate models, understanding scenario building that is fundamental to policy discussion, and the nuances around attribution of extreme weather events to climate change.

UNDERSTANDING KNOWN HEALTH EFFECTS

The health effects of climate change, probably still incompletely appreciated and described, span across broad areas in public health and medical science and occur in occupational settings, in the general environment, and at home. Part II of the book thoroughly reviews current evidence about the impressive array of health effects of climate change in eight well-written and referenced chapters. In so doing, it is far more approachable than the systematic reviews produced periodically by the World Health Organization or the US Global Climate Research Program. It contains citations to these and other seminal sources that can guide students who want to dig deeper. Heat-related health impacts and preventive measures are well-described for the work environment (Tord Kjellstrom is the lead author) and in communities (in a chapter authored by California Environmental Protection Agency scientists Rupa Basu and Xiangmei Wu). The next chapter (written by a team led by epidemiologist Kari Nadeau) thoroughly covers the agents (air pollutants, pollen, mold, and heat) that negatively impact respiratory health, the consequences, and how to prevent them. University of California, Davis, veterinary medicine professors Christopher M. Barker and William K. Reisen provide a thorough and One Health–informed view of how (and where) climate change is increasing risks to specific vector-borne diseases. In the next chapter, authored by Jennifer R. Bratburd and Sandra L. McLellan, you can learn about the myriad ways in which climate change is increasing the transmission of waterborne diseases. The next chapter, authored by Jessica Fanzo, Kate R. Schneider, and Stanley Wood, tackles the significant associations, direct and indirect, of climate change with food insecurity and malnutrition. Clinical mental health impacts are covered by Thomas J. Doherty and Amy D. Lykins. Finally, Levy provides an excellent framework for understanding how climate change may be related to many forms of human violence from the individual to the international level. Through this point, this is a textbook that would be useful for teaching climate and health anywhere in the world to health and environmental students alike.

POLICY IMPLICATIONS, CLIMATE ADAPTATION, AND PUBLIC SUPPORT

Part III covers policymaking for climate mitigation. Chapters are authored by an array of outstanding experts: Kathleen M. Rest (policymaking process), Gregory F. Nemet (lead author, energy policy), Kathryn A. Zyla (transportation policy), and Patz (lead author, agriculture policy). This section is mostly more useful in the United States than globally. The overview of the policymaking process and the chapter on transportation policy are written with wonderful clarity and organization. This information is a "must" for US students who will have even a passing engagement with policymaking but may be less relevant to those outside the United States. The chapter on energy policy, while somewhat US-centric, provides more of a global perspective. A historical perspective on energy development globally, as well as context for how different national economies have come to depend on coal, oil, natural gas, or biofuels, would help students understand how these historical choices impact the political economics of energy production and either enhance or hinder the achievement of commitments to reduce the production of carbon dioxide, methane, and other greenhouse gases. The relative efficacy (in reducing emissions) of "cap-and-trade" versus gas taxes is not clearly delineated. The justice implications of cap-and-trade are described, but not those for gasoline taxes, for which health and economic side effects also fall disproportionately on lower-income people who must (for example) drive for work; the means for mitigating the distributional consequences of either of these approaches are not described. The chapter on agriculture rightly focuses on the primary purpose of agriculture—providing people with nutritious and safe food. A fascinating discussion of biofuels is instructive but felt peripheral in the context of a time in which the idea of burning biofuels as a transition from burning fossil fuels has become less policy-relevant, as the attendant negative impacts have become clearer, and the prices of solar and wind energy generation have dropped significantly.

Part IV, on climate adaptation, is an essential introduction to the topic. How can health systems that are already overwhelmed with endemic public health problems (and, as we saw, completely knocked off their feet by a global pandemic) gear up to address the myriad climate and health impacts that are already manifesting? Rather than attempting to address these impacts one disease at a time, Kristie L. Ebi's chapter presents steps that can be taken to strengthen public health delivery services, tailored not only to current but also foreseeable health threats resulting from climate change. Chapters 16 and 17 tackle environmental interventions—in terms of the built environment (Jason Vargo) but also the natural environment (led by Howard Frumkin)—that can increase climate resilience and promote health and wellness. While many of the examples are from the United States, there are principles and many good ideas here that can be adapted almost anywhere.

The final section on public and political support is where this textbook most veers into advocacy. The chapter on communicating the health relevance of climate change is authored by Mona Sarfaty and Edward Maibach. It gives valuable guidance on how to frame climate and health discussions, guidance that would be useful to scientists in many complex areas that are relevant to public policy globally. Much of the chapter is focused on the politicization of climate science in the United States, as well as the polarization across our two major political parties; this is a framing that is essential to understand in the United States but not relevant internationally, where the political context is also important but very different. The final chapters on movement building (Teddie M. Potter, Julia Frost Nerbonne, and Vishnu Laalitha Surapaneni) and climate justice (Rohini J. Haar and Barry S. Levy) are advocacy oriented. Students will find these topics, which are likely to be career relevant, in many cases, very interesting.

CONCLUSION

Climate Change and Public Health will be most helpful to students familiar with basic concepts of environmental health and public health. It is an essential book for teaching public health, medical, and nursing students at the graduate and postgraduate levels worldwide. It is a crucial resource for teaching environmental and sustainability students about the health consequences of climate change. It would be helpful to any scientist who is interested in an overview of the field. Overall, it is a wonderful contribution to the field and a handy addition to the reference shelf. AJPH

CORRESPONDENCE

Correspondence should be sent to Lynn R. Goldman, MD, MS, MPH, George Washington University Milken Institute School of Public Health, 650 New Hampshire Ave NW, 7th Floor, Washington, DC 20052 (e-mail: goldmanl@gwu.edu). Reprints can be ordered at https://www.ajph.org by clicking the "Reprints" link.

PUBLICATION INFORMATION

Full Citation: Goldman LR. A crucial book for teaching environmental, sustainability, and health professions students about the health consequences of climate change. *Am J Public Health*. 2024;114(11):1139–1142.

Acceptance Date: July 18, 2024.

DOI: https://doi.org/10.2105/AJPH.2024.307818

ORCID iD:

Lynn R. Goldman https://orcid.org/0000-0002-1104-3407

CONFLICTS OF INTEREST

There are no conflicts of interest relevant to this effort.

REFERENCES

1. Task Force on Climate Change and Health. *Responding to the Climate Change and Health Crisis: A Framework for Academic Public Health.* Washington, DC: Association of Schools and Programs of Public Health; 2022.
2. Mallon W, Cox N. *Climate Action in Academic Medicine: An Overview of How Medical Schools and Teaching Hospitals and Health Systems Are Responding to Climate Change.* Washington, DC: Association of American Medical Colleges; 2022.
3. Demorest S, Cook C, Schenk E, Harris LW, Earley A. School of nursing climate commitment: nursing faculty bring climate to the classroom. *Int J Environ Res Public Health.* 2024;21(5):589. https://doi.org/10.3390/ijerph21050589
4. APA Task Force on Climate Change. *Addressing the Climate Crisis: An Action Plan for Psychologists, Report of the APA Task Force on Climate Change.* Washington, DC: American Psychological Association; 2022.
5. American Geophysical Union. Geohealth. 2024. Available at: https://connect.agu.org/geohealth/home. Accessed July 11, 2024.
6. Columbia University, Mailman School of Public Health. Global Consortium on Climate and Health Education. 2024. Available at: https://www.publichealth.columbia.edu/research/programs/global-consortium-climate-health-education. Accessed July 11, 2024.

The Making of the 1964 Surgeon General's Report on Smoking and Health

Robert N. Proctor, PhD

ABOUT THE AUTHOR

Robert N. Proctor is professor of the history of science and professor by courtesy of pulmonary medicine at Stanford University, Stanford, CA.

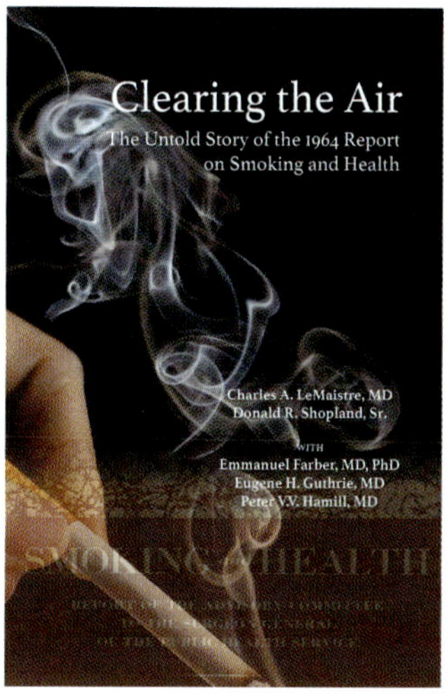

Clearing the Air: The Untold Story of the 1964 Report on Smoking and Health
By Charles A. LeMaistre and Donald R. Shopland, with Emmanuel Farber, Eugene H. Guthrie, and Peter V. V. Hamill
San Francisco, CA: University of California Health Humanities Press; 2024
385 pp; $29.95 or downloadable for free at: https://escholarship.org/uc/item/1f84x7hv.
ISBN: 979-8-9899229-2-5

The year 1964 was an important one for human health fortunes. On January 11, US Surgeon General Luther Terry released his much-anticipated report, concluding that cigarettes cause cancer, chronic bronchitis, and several other maladies. The event was held on a Saturday, to prevent a stock market collapse like that caused by the release of Wynder, Graham, and Croninger's mouse painting experiments in December 1953.

The report itself was not so much new science as a juried review of previous publications. Care was taken not to offend powerful interests: cigarette makers were allowed to veto anyone suggested to serve on the Advisory Committee responsible for drafting the report, and half of those chosen were smokers, half were nonsmokers. And no one was allowed to serve on the committee who had already stated publicly that cigarettes cause harm. The committee in this sense was more like a jury of innocents, or as Charles A. LeMaistre and Donald R. Shopland explain in *Clearing the Air: The Untold Story of the 1964 Report on Smoking and Health*, "*none* of the ten Committee members were experts in the field of smoking and health." Which is also why Michael Shimkin at the National Cancer Institute called it "the Flat Earth Committee." To put that in perspective, imagine if the authors of today's Intergovernmental Panel on Climate Change reports were barred from having ever recognized climate change as real!

There's much that is new in LeMaistre and Shopland's book. We learn that the Surgeon General's Committee was originally composed of 11 members, including Herman F. Kraybill from the National Cancer Institute. Kraybill had been named to serve as the committee's executive director, but in August of 1962 he made the fatal mistake of telling a journalist that the evidence "definitely suggests tobacco is a health hazard."[1] The industry's legal goons jumped on this and got Kraybill removed from the committee. It was not enough that he himself was a smoker, or even that his father grew eight acres of tobacco on his farm in Pennsylvania. Kraybill was fired for speaking truth to a hometown reporter.

As for truth, much of the controversy swirling around cigarettes at this time was being ginned up by the industry. The science linking cigarettes to cancer and heart disease had been nailed down by the mid-1950s, and even earlier in Germany and Argentina.[2] And cigarette makers admitted as much in their internal documents. An epidemiological study financed by Reynolds in the 1940s had shown that smoking causes mouth cancer, and Claude Teague's clandestine 1953 "Survey of Cancer Research" had noted the confluence of evidence from epidemiology, animal experiments, and chemistry. And in yet another report by the industry's main PR firm we find two of the companies' research directors assuming the reality of both cancer causation and addiction: one exclaimed, "Boy, wouldn't it be wonderful if *our* company was first to make a cancer-free cigarette"; another remarked on the money that could be made from compulsive smoking: "fortunately for us it's a habit they can't break."[3]

None of this was shared with the Surgeon General's Committee. Reynolds also kept secret its 1962 assessment that whereas the evidence linking cigarettes to cancer was "overwhelming," the evidence against was "scant." Cigarette makers also didn't provide the committee with documents from Project Ariel, a secret collaboration between Brown & Williamson in Louisville, BATCo in London, and Battelle Labs in Geneva. Project Ariel, named for Britain's first satellite, developed an effective nicotine inhaler, designed to deliver addiction without the "unattractive side effects" of cancer and emphysema.[4] Cigarette makers also concealed their secret Ecusta experiments, conducted by the world's largest producer of cigarette paper—and tax forms and Bible paper—which showed that it was the tobacco and not the paper that was making cigarettes so lethal.

The Surgeon General's Committee was called into being by President Kennedy, who on May 23, 1962, was asked at a press conference whether he agreed with reports linking smoking and cancer. Kennedy asked his surgeon general to form a committee to investigate the matter, and although the final report got a lot right, they also got some things wrong. A chapter on the "Beneficial Aspects" of tobacco, for example, concluded that smoking was a "habit" rather than an "addiction." The author of that chapter, Maurice Seevers, had previously worked for the industry; cigarette makers also appointed him (in 1964) head of the American Medical Association's Education and Research Foundation (AMA-ERF) with $18 million from the industry. Cigarette makers by this means forged a 15-year alliance with the AMA, during which time that august body refused to say that cigarettes cause cancer and denied there was any need for warnings. In 1986, when Don Shopland was asked about the AMA's cozying up to Big Tobacco, he quipped that the medical association "should be horsewhipped."[5]

The formation of the AMA-ERF is only one of several ways the industry tried to undermine the report. Most remarkable, perhaps—and new to me from reading this book—is that cigarette makers pressured their friends in Congress to remove the surgeon general as head of the US Public Health Service. The Public Health Service had been captained by the surgeon general for nearly a century, but cigarette makers successfully pressured President Johnson to demote and defang that office. The Office of the Surgeon General was "technically abolished" in 1967, and *Clearing the Air* tells how its eviscerated support staff—the National Clearinghouse for Smoking and Health—was moved from Washington, DC, to a former girl's dormitory at Emory University in Atlanta.

Cigarette makers accelerated their attacks in the 1970s, with the Tobacco Institute launching its "Truth Squad" and "College of Tobacco Knowledge"—and dozens of other bodies designed to deny or distract from cigarette harms. The industry by this time was riding high, with total consumption not peaking until 1981—when more than 630 billion cigarettes were smoked in the United States. *Clearing the Air* points out that President Nixon in 1973 fired Surgeon General Jesse Steinfeld for raising the secondhand smoke alarm, and for several years thereafter we didn't even have a surgeon general. Other courageous public servants eventually stepped up, like Joseph Califano, who revived the Office on Smoking and Health (in 1978) and became the first secretary of health to recognize smoking as "slow motion suicide" and the nation's "leading preventable cause of death."

Clearing the Air has had a long gestation. Charles LeMaistre, one of the 10 original members of the committee, proposed the volume more than 20 years ago but died before it could be brought to completion. Donald Shopland, the only surviving author, was only 18 when he started working as a staffer for the committee and would go on to have a long and courageous career in public health.

Much of the book reads as a day-by-day chronology, with fascinating observations on the sense of fear surrounding preparation of the report, and the enforcement of military-grade security. Readers will learn about a disturbing effort in May 1963 to force the report to a premature ending, causing a mini revolt within the committee to reassert its independence.

Rose-colored glasses have led many people to celebrate the report as the beginning of the end of tobacco, but the reality is that most cigarette deaths have occurred in the decades since. American cigarette makers in 1963 spent only about $250 million marketing cigarettes, but 40 years later they were spending more than 60 times that amount ($15.1 billion in 2003).[6] We still live in a world where the leading preventable cause of death is trivialized as a "personal" or "lifestyle" choice, a world where shark bites get more attention than the daily toll from smokes. If 1964 was a fruitful beginning, we still have a ways to go to understand the depths of

Big Nic's chicanery,[7] and how best to escape from its frightful clutches. This fine book will help us move in that direction. AJPH

CORRESPONDENCE

Correspondence should be sent to Robert N. Proctor, History Department, Stanford University, Stanford, CA 94305 (e-mail: rproctor@stanford.edu). Reprints can be ordered at https://www.ajph.org by clicking the "Reprints" link.

PUBLICATION INFORMATION

Full Citation: Proctor RN. The making of the 1964 Surgeon General's report on smoking and health. *Am J Public Health*. 2024;114(11):1143–1145.

Acceptance Date: July 22, 2024.

DOI: https://doi.org/10.2105/AJPH.2024.307825

ORCID iD:

Robert N. Proctor https://orcid.org/0000-0002-8910-5647

CONFLICTS OF INTEREST

R. N. Proctor has served as an expert witness in tobacco litigation.

REFERENCES

1. Teplitz B. Ex-Mariettan will lead smoking study. *Lancaster Intelligencer Journal*. August 27, 1962. Available at: https://www.industrydocuments.ucsf.edu/tobacco/docs/#id=gkxy0214. Accessed February 9, 2024.
2. Proctor RN. Angel H. Roffo: the forgotten father of experimental tobacco carcinogenesis. *Bull World Health Organ*. 2006;84(6):494–496. https://doi.org/10.2471/BLT.06.031682
3. Dakin EF. Forwarding memorandum. December 15, 1953:2. Available at: https://www.industrydocuments.ucsf.edu/tobacco/docs/#id=ymby0042. Accessed July 20, 2024.
4. Yeaman A. Implications of Battelle Hippo I and II and the Griffith Filter. July 17, 1963. Available at: https://industrydocuments.library.ucsf.edu/tobacco/docs/#id=hrwh0097. Accessed November 9, 2023.
5. Kenney C. Tobacco wars. *Boston Globe Magazine*. May 4, 1986. Available at: https://www.industrydocuments.ucsf.edu/tobacco/docs/#id=flnn0141. Accessed December 12, 2024.
6. Federal Trade Commission Cigarette Report for 2007 and 2008, Table 2C. 2011. Available at: https://www.industrydocuments.ucsf.edu/tobacco/docs/#id=xgvc0218. Accessed May 18, 2024.
7. Akselrad D, Proctor RN. Why did Philip Morris stop making cigarettes at Auschwitz? *Public Cult*. 2024;36(1):47–74. https://doi.org/10.1215/08992363-11121486.

Equitable Uptake of Life-Saving COVID-19 Primary Vaccine Series in Community Health Centers

Rulin C. Hechter, MD, PhD

ABOUT THE AUTHORS

Rulin C. Hechter is with the Department of Research and Evaluation, Kaiser Permanente Southern California, Pasadena, CA, and the Department of Health Systems Science, Kaiser Permanente Bernard J. Tyson School of Medicine, Pasadena, CA.

See also Gold et al., p. 1242.

AJPH November 2024, Vol. 114, No. 11

Rapid development of effective vaccines and efficient and equitable vaccination implementation are critical in responding to a public health crisis due to a new pandemic. The COVID-19 pandemic started in early 2020 in the United States. The COVID-19 vaccination program in the United States was launched on December 14, 2020, with an interim recommendation for two doses of an mRNA COVID-19 vaccine (i.e., the primary series).[1] The high vaccine efficacy against severe disease and mortality caused by COVID-19, as well as the population-level benefit afforded by mild protection against severe acute respiratory syndrome coronavirus 2 (SARS-CoV-2) infection (before the emergence of the omicron [B.1.1.529] variant) conferred by vaccination, has substantially altered the trajectory of the COVID-19 pandemic in the last few years. A mathematical modeling study estimated that vaccinations prevented 14.4 million deaths from COVID-19 globally between December 8, 2020 and December 8, 2021. This estimate rose to 19.8 million deaths from COVID-19 averted when excess deaths was used as an estimate of the true extent of the pandemic, representing a global reduction of 63% in total deaths (19.8 million of 31.4 million) during the first year of COVID-19 vaccination.[2]

However, there are many social, geographic, political, economic, and environmental factors that create challenges to COVID-19 vaccination access and acceptance and contribute to inequity of COVID-19 vaccination. Recent data from the Centers for Disease Control and Prevention (CDC) show relatively low vaccine uptake of updated 2023–2024 COVID-19 vaccine and disparities in vaccination by race and ethnicity,[3] with much lower vaccination rates seen among non-Hispanic Black adults (8%) and Hispanic adults (8%), nearly half that of White adults (15%). Adults without health insurance were much less likely to report vaccination (4%) than people with insurance (15%).[3] Today, COVID-19 remains an important cause of hospitalization and death, especially for older adults and people with certain underlying medical conditions. Ensuring vaccination equity and addressing barriers to vaccination are critical to the national vaccination effort and the overall COVID-19 response.

In this issue of *AJPH*, Gold et al. (p. 1242) evaluated multilevel factors, including health care delivery site–level factors, associated with variation in COVID-19 vaccination rate between January 1, 2022, and December 31, 2022 in health care settings that serve patients regardless of ability to pay. The authors used Epic electronic health record data of a national network of community health centers (CHCs) located in 34 states, including Federally Qualified Health Centers, rural health centers, and similar care delivery sites serving low-income populations who are at elevated risk of developing severe illness from COVID-19. They examined the completion of the COVID-19 primary vaccine series, and found that the majority of patients (72%) completed the series by the end of 2022. The higher vaccination rate among new patients suggests that CHCs may have played a critical role in increasing vaccine access. However, there were disparities identified. For example, health care delivery site located in a non-Medicaid expansion state was associated with lower likelihood of COVID-19 primary vaccine series completion for both new and established patients. In addition, sites in isolated communities and rural communities had significantly lower primary series completion than sites in urban communities. In contrast to the national COVID-19 vaccination data, the authors found that Hispanic/Latino patients had a higher likelihood of COVID-19 vaccination than non-Hispanic/Latino patients receiving care in CHCs. Furthermore, even in these care settings with relatively equal access to care, Medicaid beneficiaries and uninsured patients were less likely to complete the primary series than those with private insurance. This finding is in concordance with studies conducted in other large integrated health care organizations of completion rates of primary series,[4,5] and studies of bivalent mRNA COVID-19 vaccines.[6] It is concerning that patients with certain conditions associated with severe COVID-19 disease, such as overweight, obesity, and smoking, were less likely to have completed a primary series.

Given the current low uptake of the updated 2023–2024 COVID-19 vaccines, the findings of this study remind us that adequate access to vaccines in low-income, high-risk populations, especially in rural communities, remains a challenge to achieving a high national COVID-19 vaccine coverage. Additional resources to develop and implement effective interventions and policies at the health care delivery site, state, and national levels are warranted. AJPH

CORRESPONDENCE

Correspondence should be sent to Rulin C. Hechter, MD, PhD, 100 S. Los Robles Ave, 2nd Floor, Pasadena, CA 91101 (e-mail: Rulin.C.Hechter@kp.org). Reprints can be ordered at https://www.ajph.org by clicking the "Reprints" link.

PUBLICATION INFORMATION

Full Citation: Hechter RC. Equitable uptake of life-saving COVID-19 primary vaccine series in community health centers. *Am J Public Health.* 2024;114(11):1146–1147.

Acceptance Date: July 21, 2024.

DOI: https://doi.org/10.2105/AJPH.2024.307822

ORCID iD:
Rulin C. Hechter https://orcid.org/0000-0001-8684-6506

CONFLICTS OF INTEREST

The author claims no conflicts of interest related to this article.

REFERENCES

1. Dooling K, McClung N, Chamberland M, et al. The Advisory Committee on Immunization Practices' interim recommendation for allocating initial supplies of COVID-19 vaccine—United States, 2020. *MMWR Morb Mortal Wkly Rep.* 2020;69(49):1857–1859. https://doi.org/10.15585/mmwr.mm6949e1
2. Watson OJ, Barnsley G, Toor J, Hogan AB, Winskill P, Ghani AC. Global impact of the first year of COVID-19 vaccination: a mathematical modelling study [erratum in *Lancet Infect Dis.* 2023;23(10):e400]. *Lancet Infect Dis.* 2022;22(9):1293–1302. https://doi.org/10.1016/S1473-3099(22)00320-6
3. Centers for Disease Control and Prevention. COVID-19 vaccine uptake and CDC's commitment to vaccine equity. 2023. Available at: https://www.cdc.gov/ncird/whats-new/vaccine-equity.html. Accessed July 18, 2024.
4. Hechter RC, Qian L, Liu IA, et al. COVID-19 vaccination coverage and factors associated with vaccine uptake among people with HIV. *JAMA Netw Open.* 2024l;7(6):e2415220. https://doi.org/10.1001/jamanetworkopen.2024.15220
5. Xu S, Hong V, Sy LS, et al. Risk factors for not completing a 2-dose primary series of messenger RNA COVID-19 vaccination in a large health care system in southern California: retrospective cohort study. *JMIR Public Health Surveill.* 2023;9:e46318. https://doi.org/10.2196/46318
6. Bruxvoort KJ, Sy LS, Hong V, et al. Factors associated with uptake of bivalent mRNA COVID-19 vaccines in a large US health care system. *Vaccine.* 2023;41(49):7460–7468. https://doi.org/10.1016/j.vaccine.2023.11.012

On Race and Place in Substance Use Research

Bayla Ostrach, PhD, MA, CIP, and Jennifer J. Carroll, PhD, MPH, MA

ABOUT THE AUTHORS

Bayla Ostrach is with Fruit of Labor Action Research & Technical Assistance, LLC, Marshall, NC, and Boston University School of Medicine, Boston, MA. Jennifer J. Carroll is with North Carolina State University, Raleigh, NC.

In "The War on Drugs, Racialized Capitalism, and Health Care Utilization Among White People Who Use Drugs in 22 Rural Appalachian Counties," Cooper et al.[1] examine certain forms of systemic oppression in the United States as these affect people who use drugs (PWUD). Joining the concepts of racialized capitalism and critical Whiteness studies to analyze survey data collected in 22 Appalachian counties across four states, Cooper et al. ask whether the impacts of the War on Drugs commonly observed among urban, primarily Black and Hispanic PWUD persist among White, largely rural PWUD.

As medical anthropologists who collaborate with harm reduction organizations in both rural and urban areas of southern Appalachia, we welcome Cooper et al.'s focus on the lived experiences of Appalachian PWUD as well as the important questions they raise about the impacts of the War on Drugs on more rural, predominantly (though certainly not exclusively) White populations. We particularly find their research questions—whether stop and searches, arrest, incarceration, and community supervision are correlated with (possibly by acting as barriers that escalate) unmet health care needs—a valuable inquiry.

Yet we are puzzled by their appeal to White supremacy, in a seemingly broad sense, to explain the survival of their null hypothesis and the tacit assumption within that appeal that a direct comparison can be made between class-, place-, and race-based experiences with health care and law enforcement systems in urban versus rural areas, as they suggest their data can (with limitations) do. In particular, they frame their discussion around this comparison without first asking whether law enforcement interactions and unmet health care needs are themselves the same phenomena in and across these regions. A significant body of peer-reviewed research suggests they are not.

Garriott's 2011 ethnography on methamphetamine use in rural West Virginia described in stark terms how the policing power of the state extends well beyond the criminal–legal system, making community members complicit in criminalization and rendering ordinary interactions with friends, neighbors, and kin as dangerous as law enforcement interactions.[2] Buer's 2020 ethnography of women who use opioids in Appalachian Kentucky illuminates how the health care and criminal–legal systems are functionally the same, with health care professionals regularly triggering criminal–legal responses and the criminal–legal system largely controlling treatment access.[3] In a study coauthored with syringe service program staff, one of us found that urban PWUD in Appalachian North Carolina perceived health care and criminal–legal systems to be equivalent, reducing health care seeking even when direly needed.[4]

Similarly, in the public health literature, scholars have published evidence that Appalachian residents' desire to avoid law enforcement interaction curtails uptake of harm reduction services[5]; that fear of law enforcement response in Appalachia reduces willingness to carry or administer naloxone during an overdose[6]; and that Appalachian PWUD are stopped and searched by law enforcement significantly more often if they obtained syringes from a syringe service program or another PWUD.[7] In a statewide survey of 414 PWUD in North Carolina, we and our coauthors found that law enforcement interactions in the Appalachian region of the study drove statistical trends completely.[8] Put succinctly, White Appalachians were abused by local law enforcement so regularly and severely that our data implied that, across the state, Black North Carolinians were treated significantly better by law enforcement than White North Carolinians; in actuality, White Appalachian North Carolinians received significantly worse treatment than all other participants, including non-Appalachian Black residents.[8] In light of this body of research, scholars assume the equivalence of law enforcement or health care–related phenomena across urban–rural and even regional Appalachian divides at their own methodological risk.

Although we agree with Cooper et al.'s assertion that the pathway linking race-based harm and discrimination to reduced health care access among Black PWUD is "unlikely to operate among White Appalachian PWUD," it does not logically follow that White

Appalachian PWUD enjoy "freedom from such saturating and persistent criminal–legal control" often experienced by Black and Hispanic urban counterparts, or that such freedom, if it did exist, could be a "persistent hallmark of Appalachian Whiteness."[1(p1093–1094)] Although it is appropriate for the authors to hypothesize social processes that might have shaped their findings, this hypothesis elides the nuance inherent in such processes. Existing research suggests the opposite: White Appalachian PWUD are overpoliced and subject to different—but not necessarily less severe—law enforcement surveillance and abuse than their urban, Black, and Hispanic counterparts.

We do not claim possession of—or even access to—the "right" answers to the questions Cooper et al. raise. However, in light of challenges posed by existing literature to the suggestion that White supremacy explains their findings, we offer two suggestions. First, we encourage deeper theoretical engagement with critical Whiteness studies. This means acknowledging the contributions of foundational scholars like Baldwin[9] and Du Bois[10] as well as more contemporary scholars like Crenshaw.[11] These contributions include the following: White experience is not simply life in the absence of anti-Black or anti-Hispanic discrimination; class and gender intersect differently with different racial identities; and White supremacy operates in service of Whiteness as an institution, not in service of individual White people. A recent noteworthy addition to this literature is *Whiteout: How Racial Capitalism Changed the Color of Opioids in America* by Hansen et al.,[12] which effectively engages critical race theory and Whiteness studies to illustrate how White supremacy—in service of Whiteness—conspired with a shifting regulatory environment to ensure that Whites were disproportionately vulnerable to harm in the first wave of prescription opioid overdose.

Second, we encourage recognition of the necessity of in-depth qualitative research to inform human participant research. Cooper et al. measured "unmet need for medical care" through a dozen indicators of why that need wasn't met.[1(p1088)] Would White, rural participants perceive "unmet health care needs" comparably to Black and Hispanic urban residents?[1(p1086)] Would investigators and participants agree on what constitutes unmet need? Did the reasons listed possess the same salience, coherence, or distinctiveness across survey takers? In other words, were these the right questions to ask in the first place? Exploratory, qualitative research can address these questions—and help identify previously undiscovered causal mechanisms that might better explain Cooper et al.'s findings and establish a more nuanced picture of the racialization of Drug War policies in Appalachia.

Above all, we advocate for a deeper integration of public health principles and practices with the social sciences—disciplines that have long explored and refined theories of human interaction that public health scholars increasingly observe in epidemiological terms. We are medical anthropologists who proactively seek out intersections of multiple frameworks and methodologies; it is our bias and prerogative to claim multidisciplinary approaches as indispensable. Cooper et al.'s contribution is itself a testament to the utility some of our best public health scholars find in sociological and anthropological theories. We commend these authors for engaging with social constructs of race, racism, and Whiteness, just as we commend this journal for valuing such application of critical theories to quantitative data. We hope this is a harbinger of more such scholarship to come. The complex interplay of myriad social systems is essential for understanding how the harms of substance use emerge and how they can be interrupted. On this point, we and Cooper et al. are in complete and enthusiastic agreement. AJPH

CORRESPONDENCE

Correspondence should be sent to Bayla Ostrach, 1685 NC 213 #4, Marshall, NC 28753 (e-mail: hrresearchappalachia@gmail.com). Reprints can be ordered at https://www.ajph.org by clicking the "Reprints" link.

PUBLICATION INFORMATION

Full Citation: Ostrach B, Carroll JJ. On race and place in substance use research. *Am J Public Health*. 2024;114(11):1148–1150.

Acceptance Date: August 3, 2024.

DOI: https://doi.org/10.2105/AJPH.2024.307840

ORCID iDs:

Bayla Ostrach https://orcid.org/0000-0003-2803-3747

Jennifer J. Carroll https://orcid.org/0000-0001-5711-7419

CONTRIBUTORS

B. Ostrach and J. J. Carroll conceptualized, drafted, and finalized the manuscript.

ACKNOWLEDGMENTS

We express appreciation to Brittany Price for proofreading.

CONFLICTS OF INTEREST

The authors have no conflicts of interest to disclose.

REFERENCES

1. Cooper HLF, Livingston MD, Crawford ND, et al. The war on drugs, racialized capitalism, and health care utilization among White people who use drugs in 22 rural Appalachian counties. *Am J Public Health*. 2024;114(10):1086–1096. https://doi.org/10.2105/AJPH.2024.307744
2. Garriott W. *Policing Methamphetamine: Narcopolitics in Rural America*. New York, NY: New York University Press; 2011.
3. Buer LM. *Rx Appalachia: Stories of Treatment and Survival in Rural Kentucky*. Chicago, IL: Haymarket Books; 2020.

4. Ostrach B, Hixon V, Bryce A. "When people who use drugs can't differentiate between medical care and cops, it's a problem." Compounding risks of law enforcement harassment & punitive healthcare policies [erratum in *Health Justice*. 2024;12(1):19]. *Health Justice*. 2024;12(1):3. https://doi.org/10.1186/s40352-023-00256-3

5. Davis SM, Kristjansson AL, Davidov D, Zullig K, Baus A, Fisher M. Barriers to using new needles encountered by rural Appalachian people who inject drugs: implications for needle exchange. *Harm Reduct J*. 2019;16(1):23. https://doi.org/10.1186/s12954-019-0295-5

6. Garcia V, McCann L, Lauber E, Vaccaro C, Swauger M, Heckert AD. High-risk individuals and naloxone use: implications for THN programs in rural Appalachian communities. *J Appalach Health*. 2023;5(3):9–21. https://doi.org/10.13023/jah.0503.02

7. Carpenter DM, Zule WA, Hennessy CM, Evon DM, Hurt CB, Ostrach B. Factors associated with perceived ease of access to syringes in Appalachian North Carolina. *J Rural Health*. 2023;39(1):212–222. https://doi.org/10.1111/jrh.12698

8. Morrissey B, Hughes T, Ostrach B, et al. "They don't go by the law around here": law enforcement interactions after the legalization of syringe services programs in North Carolina. *Harm Reduct J*. 2022;19(1):106. https://doi.org/10.1186/s12954-022-00690-w

9. Baldwin J. The fire next time. In: *James Baldwin: Collected Essays*. New York, NY: Library of America; 1998.

10. Du Bois WEB. *Darkwater: Voices From Within the Veil*. Oxford, UK: Oxford University Press; 2014.

11. Crenshaw K. *On Intersectionality: Essential Writings*. New York, NY: New Press; 2017.

12. Hansen H, Netherland J, Herzberg D. *Whiteout: How Racial Capitalism Changed the Color of Opioids in America*. Berkeley, CA: University of California Press; 2023.

Mitigating Overdoses in Colombia

Mauro Diaz-Moreno, MSc, and Daniel Rojas, BS

ABOUT THE AUTHORS

Mauro Diaz-Moreno and Daniel Rojas are with Corporación Acción Técnica Social, Bogotá, Colombia.

See also Friedman, p. 1153, and Santaella-Tenorio et al., p. 1252.

In their article, Santaella-Tenorio et al. (p. 1252) examined data from the Colombian public health surveillance system (SIVIGILA) to calculate overdose rates regarding variables such as gender, age groups, and substance type. Despite the limitations of the data, the authors clearly showed their findings. However, there are some topics involving drug use in Colombia and social context that are important to consider.

First, the studies about drug use in Colombia performed by governmental agencies, such as the National Survey on Psychoactive Substance Use conducted in 2019 and the Survey on Psychoactive Substance Use in Bogotá undertaken in 2022,[1,2] are the primary information sources nowadays. Both studies showed that cannabis and cocaine are the first and second most consumed illicit substances, respectively. On the other hand, other drugs, such as amphetamine-type stimulants, synthetic drugs, and opioids, are not representative of the Colombian population. However, the data on some substances may be underreported because the surveys do not focus on people who use drugs. For example, the Bogotá study reported zero annual prevalence of heroin use,[2] which is far from the reality.

Santaella-Tenorio et al.'s article shows an increase in overdoses involving the use of cannabis from 2010 to 2017 and a decrease from 2018 to 2021. Nevertheless, the methodology SIVIGILA used to define cannabis overdose is not fully understood. Cannabis is known for not producing signals of overdose, such as serotonin syndrome or respiratory depression. Even fatal cases are rare. For this reason, it is difficult to understand what cannabis overdose means in the surveillance data. In the same way, according to the Mortality Associated With Drug Use 2013–2020 Study performed by the Colombian National Institute of Legal Medicine and Forensic Sciences (INMLCF),[3] cannabis was detected in 1813 deceased individuals. Although the INMLCF study emphasizes that the presence of the substances does not prove cause of death, the information could be misinterpreted.

According to the 2019 Colombian drug use survey, there was a decrease in cannabis use compared with 2013.[1] However, this information contrasts with the popularity of cannabis in society and the increases in cannabis users' associations across the country. During the first stage of lockdowns in 2020, cannabis was the most used illegal substance, and 19% of people reported cannabis first use.[4] In addition, long-period lockdowns motivated people to grow their own (cultivation of up to 20 cannabis plants is allowed in Colombia). Although recent bills about the recreational use of cannabis have failed in Congress, they are gaining more support year by year. We do not consider it appropriate to correlate the reduction in cannabis overdoses with consumption trends reported because the data seem unrealistic. As the authors explained, changes in consumption patterns could have influenced the overdose trend after 2018.

Second, one of the most remarkable of the article's findings is the trend of intentional and unintentional overdose with tranquilizers and sedatives after 2018, especially in young women. The authors related that trend to higher levels of distress and other mental health issues during the COVID-19 pandemic. It is well-known the pandemic caused economic problems worldwide and exacerbated income inequality, but Colombia's situation was unique. In 2021, there were massive strikes in Colombia related to an unpopular tax reform and social inequality.[5] The protest resulted in police brutality and an increase in violence in urban areas that could have affected the mental health of the population. However, some issues directly affected women more than men, such as the gender pay gap, fewer job opportunities, domestic violence, sexual abuse, and unintended pregnancy. According to the Colombian Women's Observatory, there was a 142% increase in calls to emergency hotlines in 2020 compared with 2019, and more than 90% of the calls were made by women.[6] On the other hand, The National Statistical System reported an increase in births among girls aged younger than 14 years (22.2%) and among women aged 14 to 19 years (6.3%) in the second quarter of 2021 compared with the same period in 2020.[7]

Third, the authors attributed an increase in overdose trends to the maturation of the surveillance system and improvement in case collection.

AJPH November 2024, Vol. 114, No. 11

However, data on overdoses from people living in rural areas, extreme poverty, and homelessness may be underestimated. Colombia has been distinguished in its implementation of the war on drugs and has invested millions of dollars to confront organized crime, specifically cocaine trafficking. Regarding the long-lasting violence that has multidimensional causes, the rural population has suffered extreme violence for decades. Moreover, rural areas' lack of infrastructure for health attention could affect epidemiological data.

Finally, although the article shows an increasing trend of opioid overdose after 2018, the number is low compared with overdoses related to other substances. Colombian studies show a preference for cannabis and stimulants over opioids. Furthermore, the article reveals that only 0.3% of all overdoses were fatal. Despite the limitations of the studies discussed, the Colombian data contradict the mediatic narrative about fentanyl's presence in the illegal market in our country.

In conclusion, we found Santaella-Tenorio et al.'s work valuable because they examined data that are not widely known. We highlight the integration of outcomes from several studies that are needed to understand drug use in Colombia. The early detection of novel psychoactive substances, more investment in the health system, and the enhancement of protocols could improve data collection and mitigate overdoses. AJPH

CORRESPONDENCE

Correspondence should be sent to Mauro Diaz-Moreno, Calle 33 19-60, Bogotá, Colombia (e-mail: maurodiazmoreno@gmail.com). Reprints can be ordered at https://www.ajph.org by clicking the "Reprints" link.

PUBLICATION INFORMATION

Full Citation: Diaz-Moreno M, Rojas D. Mitigating overdoses in Colombia. *Am J Public Health*. 2024;114(11):1151–1152.

Acceptance Date: August 11, 2024.

DOI: https://doi.org/10.2105/AJPH.2024.307851

ORCID iDs:

Mauro Diaz-Moreno https://orcid.org/0000-0001-8583-2874

Daniel Rojas https://orcid.org/0000-0002-4021-9993

CONTRIBUTORS

Both authors contributed equally to this editorial.

CONFLICTS OF INTEREST

Both authors declare that they have no conflicts of interest.

REFERENCES

1. Ministerio de Justicia y del Derecho, Observatorio de Drogas de Colombia. Estudio nacional de consumo de sustancias psicoactivas en Colombia 2019. 2019. Available at: https://www.minjusticia.gov.co/programas-co/ODC/Documents/Publicaciones/Consumo/Estudios/estudio%20Nacional%20de%20consumo%202019v2.pdf?csf=1&e=iV5Ih3. Accessed June 31, 2024.
2. Mayor de Bogotá A. Secretaría Distrital de Salud de Bogotá; Oficina de las Naciones Unidas contra la Droga y el Delito (UNODC). Estudio de consumo de sustancias psicoactivas en Bogotá D.C. 2022. 2022. Available at: https://www.unodc.org/documents/colombia/2023/septiembre-9/estudio_de_consumo_de_sustancias_psicoactivas_bogota_2022.pdf. Accessed June 31, 2024.
3. Ministerio de Justicia y del Derecho, Observatorio de Drogas de Colombia; Instituto Nacional de Medicina Legal y Ciencias Forenses. Estudio de mortalidad asociada al consumo de sustancias psicoactivas 2013-2020. 2022. Available at: https://www.minjusticia.gov.co/programas-co/ODC/Documents/Publicaciones/Consumo/Estudios/Nacionales/informe%20de%20resultados.pdf. Accessed June 31, 2024.
4. Échele Cabeza. Informe sobre el consumo de drogas en cuarentena. Available at: https://www.echelecabeza.com/informe-sobre-el-consumo-de-drogas-en-cuarentena. Accessed June 31, 2024.
5. International Crisis Group. The pandemic strikes: responding to Colombia's mass protests. 2021. Available at: https://www.crisisgroup.org/latin-america-caribbean/andes/colombia/090-pandemic-strikes-responding-colombias-mass-protests. Accessed June 31, 2024.
6. Instituto Nacional de Medicina Legal y Ciencias Forenses. Violencia intrafamiliar durante la pandemia por COVID-19. 2022. Available at: https://www.medicinalegal.gov.co/blog/-/blogs/violencia-intrafamiliar-durante-la-pandemia-por-covid-19. Accessed June 31, 2024.
7. Barradas S, Guarín Á, Solyszko I, Varela N. Es esencial prevenir el embarazo temprano en Colombia. 2022. Available at: https://uniandes.edu.co/es/noticias/psicologia/se-debe-prevenir-el-embarazo-temprano-en-colombia. Accessed June 31, 2024.

Tracking Drug Overdose in Latin America: The Epidemiological Potential of Prehospital and Emergency Department Data

Joseph R. Friedman, MD, PhD, MPH

ABOUT THE AUTHOR

Joseph R. Friedman is with the Department of Psychiatry, University of California, San Diego.

See also Diaz-Moreno and Rojas, p. 1151, and Santaella-Tenorio et al., p. 1252.

Latin America has a particular relationship with the overdose crisis unfolding among its northern neighbors. Substances produced in Latin America—especially fentanyl analogs and methamphetamine produced in Mexico and cocaine produced in South America—are implicated in a drug crisis of profound magnitude occurring in the United States and Canada. Yet overdose death rates in Latin America remain quite low, at least in official statistics. According to the Global Burden of Disease Study, in 2021 the drug-related death rate in Latin America and the Caribbean was 0.52 per 100 000, compared with 1.74 globally and 21.31 in the United States.[1]

However, there are troubling signs that this may be changing as synthetic drug production ramps up globally. For instance, in Colombia, fentanyl has appeared in combination with other psychoactive drugs, leading to overdoses.[2,3] Seizures of fentanyl analogs—either illicitly manufactured or diverted pharmaceuticals—have also risen in Costa Rica, Brazil, Peru, Chile, and Argentina, where cocaine cut with carfentanil caused a 24-death outbreak in Buenos Aires in 2022.[3–5] In the midst of these emerging signs, the capacity of Latin America's monitoring systems to quickly and accurately detect a synthetic drug crisis deserves consideration.

Mortality registries are often poorly equipped to quickly detect overdose outbreaks, even in high-resource settings. Autopsy investigations rely on toxicological analysis that can be expensive and time intensive. After aggregation and dissemination, statistics are often several years out-of-date when released. Furthermore, given the expenses involved in toxicological testing, probable overdose fatalities are often not investigated as such or are recorded as "drug overdose" with no information on the specific drugs involved.

The arrival of fentanyl to Mexico exemplifies some of these challenges. Although numerous media sources, frontline harm reduction agencies, and independent research reports have documented an emerging overdose crisis on Mexico's northern border from illicitly manufactured fentanyl,[6,7] official statistics have yet to reflect this. In 2020 official sources stated that an improbably low 19 deaths occurred from opioid overdoses in Mexico.[8] Yet when the medical examiner's office in a northern border city began using point-of-care fentanyl test strips, they discovered that 23% of all deceased individuals tested positive, suggesting a massive underregistration of fentanyl-involved deaths.[8] Nevertheless, even recently published academic articles, using mortality registries, continue to reflect low death rates (e.g., 12 opioid-involved overdose deaths in 2019[9]), as most overdoses are recorded without specific drug information, and many likely go unrecorded entirely.[10]

In this context of sparse and often inaccurate official mortality data, prehospital and emergency department (ED) records offer many advantages. They reflect a valuable set of routinely collected variables, such as sociodemographic information, precise geographic markers, diagnostic and treatment codes, and information about mortality and other outcomes.[11] These data are generally available immediately, and they can be aggregated and disseminated rapidly.

The US experience with the National Emergency Medical Services (EMS) Information System (NEMSIS) is instructive. NEMSIS aggregates records from more than 90% of US ambulance activations, making summary statistics available rapidly, with an estimated 75% of clinical encounters centrally recorded within approximately one week.[11] This system proved highly valuable during the early months of the COVID-19 pandemic, when there was great interest in shifting overdose rates but no updated official data source. NEMSIS provided an early signal of rising overdose death trends, available just a few weeks into the pandemic, which later proved to be highly correlated with subsequently released official mortality statistics.[11]

Considering the prospect of a possible synthetic drug crisis in Latin America, a linked system of data from prehospital systems and EDs offers tremendous potential. In this issue of *AJPH*, Santaella-Tenorio et al. (p. 1252) highlight such a system in Colombia, where ED records were aggregated through a mandatory reporting system (called SIVIGILA: Sistema Nacional de Vigilancia en Salud Pública/ National Public Health Surveillance System) to describe all fatal and nonfatal overdoses observed in EDs between 2010 and 2021. They note a rising rate of nonfatal overdoses from tranquilizers, sedatives, antidepressants, or a combination of these, which deserve further study and policy attention.

Another key advantage of prehospital and ED data is that they allow the tracking of nonfatal drug-related outcomes such as soft tissue infections and drug-induced psychosis. The nonfatal sequalae of illicit drug use, such as those of stimulant intoxication, greatly outnumber fatal outcomes and are arguably of greater on-the-ground importance in numerous local contexts across Latin America. Although not reflected in overdose death data, these trends can be tracked rapidly via prehospital and ED records.

For optimal epidemiological utility, EMS-based overdose detection systems should do the following:

1. be centrally aggregated,
2. provide rapidly available public summary statistics,
3. show a breakdown by key dimensions relevant to health equity for each local context (e.g., race/ ethnicity, indigenous identity, language group, gender),
4. use at least point-of-care toxicology testing, and
5. ensure validity with subsequently released official measures of population-level outcomes.

The SIVIGILA system performs very well on some of these dimensions even as challenges remain. As Santaella-Tenorio et al. note, toxicological testing was rarely used in the clinical encounters described, and data largely reflect patient and family self-report regarding substances implicated in overdoses. Although gold standard toxicological screening using mass spectrometry can be costly and time intensive, implementing standardized rapid toxicological testing with point-of-care urine drug screening would be a low-cost method of improving the capacity of the system to detect shifting overdose patterns. Commendably, microdata from the SIVIGILA system are publicly available, albeit with a considerable lag, with records through 2022 currently ready for download.

Using EMS records for surveillance also entails methodological challenges. During the initial implementation period, as well as any subsequent system scale-up periods when additional facilities or jurisdictions are added to the system, the number of observed overdoses is expected to rise. This is a function of greater clinical volume in the system rather than a true increase in the underlying overdose rate in the population. A frequently used work-around to deal with this issue is using overdose encounters as a rate per clinical encounter, rather than per population.[11]

An EMS-based early detection network is likely to be just one of several complementary strategies for detecting emerging drug-related harms. Existing drug alert systems—such as SATA (the Early Alert System for the Americas), which is managed by the Organization of American States—often use data from law enforcement seizures.[3] Such data should not be relied on for public health monitoring, as they often do not reflect population-level health trends and are usually not made available to community organizations, researchers, or the public in a timely fashion. Their use for public health purposes is also ethically fraught, as they are generated as part of processes that deprive people of liberty, and not explicitly for the promotion of health.

Alternatively, community-engaged drug-checking programs can empower people who use drugs to immediately assess the contents of their substances via spectroscopy or immunoassay-based strips. These results can also inform health care providers and public health authorities which substances should be routinely tested for in clinical overdose encounters. Implementing routine, comprehensive toxicological testing during fatal overdose autopsy investigations is a critical step for ensuring that official mortality statistics are accurate and, if done quickly, can also inform rapid public health response.

In the context of these distinct resources that can be used to triangulate information about emerging overdose trends, the unique strengths of ED and EMS data lie in their rapid, clinically derived nature, which allows them to be quickly aggregated and made available to the public. AJPH

CORRESPONDENCE

Correspondence should be sent to Joseph R. Friedman, Department of Psychiatry, University of California San Diego, 200 W. Arbor Dr, MC #8218, San Diego, CA 92103 (e-mail: joseph.robert.friedman@gmail.com).

PUBLICATION INFORMATION

Full Citation: Friedman JR. Tracking drug overdose in Latin America: the epidemiological potential of prehospital and emergency department data. *Am J Public Health*. 2024;114(11):1153–1155.

Acceptance Date: August 28, 2024.

DOI: https://doi.org/10.2105/AJPH.2024.307862

CONFLICTS OF INTEREST

The author reports no conflicts of interest.

REFERENCES

1. Naghavi M, Ong KL, Aali A, et al. Global burden of 288 causes of death and life expectancy decomposition in 204 countries and territories and 811 subnational locations, 1990–2021: a systematic analysis for the Global Burden of Disease Study 2021. *Lancet*. 2024;403(10440):2100–2132. [Erratum in: *Lancet*. 2024;403(10440):1988. https://doi.org/10.1016/S0140-6736(24)00824-9.] https://doi.org/10.1016/S0140-6736(24)00367-2
2. Colombian Ministry of Justice. Ministry of Justice and Law inspects the current situation with fentanyl in Colombia. 2024. Available at: https://www.minjusticia.gov.co/Sala-de-prensa/Paginas/Minjusticia-puso-la-lupa-sobre-la-situacion-actual-del-fentanilo-en-Colombia.aspx. Accessed August 29, 2024.
3. Organización de los Estados Americanos. Early alert system for the Americas. Available at: https://www.oas.org/ext/es/principal/oea/nuestra-estructura/sg/ssm/cicad/observatorio-interamericano-drogas/sata-documentos-paises. Accessed August 5, 2024.
4. Bastos FI, Krawczyk N. Reports of rising use of fentanyl in contemporary Brazil is of concern, but a US-like crisis may still be averted. *Lancet Reg Health Am*. 2023;23:100507. https://doi.org/10.1016/j.lana.2023.100507
5. BBC World News. Carfentanilo, el medicamento para dormir elefantes que encontraron en la cocaína adulterada que mató a 24 personas en Argentina. Available at: https://www.bbc.com/mundo/noticias-america-latina-60328501. Accessed August 29, 2024.
6. Friedman J, Bourgois P, Godvin M, et al. The introduction of fentanyl on the US–Mexico border: an ethnographic account triangulated with drug checking data from Tijuana. *Int J Drug Policy*. 2022;104:103678. https://doi.org/10.1016/j.drugpo.2022.103678
7. Fleiz C, Arredondo J, Chavez A, et al. Fentanyl is used in Mexico's northern border: current challenges for drug health policies. *Addiction*. 2020;115(4):778–781. https://doi.org/10.1111/add.14934
8. Linthicum K, Blakinger K, Sheets C. Mexico says it doesn't have a fentanyl problem. New data reveal a hidden epidemic. *Los Angeles Times*. Available at: https://www.latimes.com/world-nation/story/2023-07-07/mexico-fentanyl-meth-epidemic-data-shows. Accessed August 29, 2024.
9. Ospina-Escobar A, Cervantes CAD. Trends in drug overdose deaths in Mexico (1999–2019). A national descriptive analysis and interstate comparison. *Int J Drug Policy*. 2024;129:104464. https://doi.org/10.1016/j.drugpo.2024.104464
10. Henson RM, Mullachery PH, Sánchez-Pájaro A, et al. Spatial heterogeneity in fatal overdose rate trends in Mexican cities: 2005–2021. *Am J Public Health*. 2024;114(7):705–713. https://doi.org/10.2105/AJPH.2024.307650
11. Friedman J, Mann NC, Hansen H, et al. Racial/ethnic, social, and geographic trends in overdose-associated cardiac arrests observed by US emergency medical services during the COVID-19 pandemic. *JAMA Psychiatry*. 2021;78(8):886–895. https://doi.org/10.1001/jamapsychiatry.2021.0967

Does Wastewater-Based Surveillance Protect the Health of Incarcerated Individuals?

Rochelle H. Holm, PhD, and Ted Smith, PhD

ABOUT THE AUTHORS

Rochelle H. Holm and Ted Smith are with the Christina Lee Brown Envirome Institute, School of Medicine, University of Louisville, Louisville, KY.

See also Kennedy et al., p. 1232.

AJPH November 2024, Vol. 114, No. 11

Where should we do wastewater-based surveillance (WBS), when should we start, how should we do it, and what health risks should we monitor are likely ongoing policy questions for carceral facilities. The US criminal justice system incarcerates individuals for both short and long durations, which has implications for health management. Of particular concern is employing protocols to control infectious diseases. Jails typically have transient populations and hold individuals for short-term pretrial detention, which creates a dynamic scenario for infectious disease identification. By contrast, prisons house individuals for longer periods, thus offering more certainty about the population represented in environmental screening tools such as WBS.[1] In this issue of *AJPH*, Kennedy et al. (p. 1232) consider WBS across four different jail populations, architectural designs, sewer system configurations, and funding levels to test its potential for public health surveillance improvement.

WBS, when paired with existing clinical testing programs, may uniquely offer a complementary infectious disease surveillance approach for carceral facilities. Obtaining the health status of incarcerated individuals and facility staff and comparing that with the combined environmental samples from both groups can provide a more comprehensive view. Kennedy et al. found the most informative applications in larger jails with multiple sewer collection points. WBS has also been used in prisons with only a single campus-wide sewer collection point, where a severe acute respiratory syndrome coronavirus 2 (SARS-CoV-2) wastewater threshold was calculated to estimate the presence of at least one case of infection in a correctional facility.[2] Paired clinical data are still required. Although regular screening of a facility's entire population would ensure the greatest protection, the operational burden and financial cost are prohibitive.

Narrower screening (e.g., testing only the symptomatic) introduces the risk of underreporting. Other work has shown that conducting asymptomatic testing in jails was not common during the pandemic.[3] We know that community public health agencies throughout the pandemic underestimated the incidence of COVID-19,[4,5] and this can be assumed to also apply to carceral facilities. Before considering full census clinical screening, we suggest that WBS be a prerequisite indicator. Facilities may not need to initiate broad-based individual testing if the pathogen is not present in the wastewater, there have been no recent infections, and there have been no transfers of incarcerated individuals within and between facilities over a one-week period. This may result in smarter resource allocation and cost savings for carceral leadership.

From a policy standpoint, there are several practical challenges regarding the timing and frequency of wastewater testing and the choice of sampling method. The findings by Kennedy et al.—that WBS can be used across a range of facilities (i.e., cells vs dorms) and wastewater sample types (i.e., Moore swab or grab sample)—are consistent with those of the Water Environment Federation.[6] Because of differences in detention duration, the sampling design in jails may require more frequent wastewater testing than that in prisons. Moreover, once a jail or prison is set up for WBS, it is not automated and requires continual labor-intensive facility sampling and laboratory services. However, these facilities can use external laboratories to analyze the samples: private service contracts, government public health laboratories, or academic partners. For these, cost, turnaround time, and overall feasibility should dictate the course. Kennedy et al. also detail issues, such as the lack of historical sewer diagrams, that cause start-up problems. Investment in aging carceral facility sewer infrastructure is needed to enable easier wastewater sampling.

Before the COVID-19 pandemic, limited WBS in carceral facilities predominantly focused on illicit drug or prescription misuse surveillance, in some cases being paired with random individual drug testing.[7–9] The COVID-19 pandemic presented an opportunity for infectious disease management because the SARS-CoV-2 virus is shed in feces.[10] Other pathogens may not be present in feces or urine, and therefore WBS may not be as useful for detecting them. Effective treatment options for COVID-19 and vaccination prevent severe disease. Some diseases present acute symptoms quickly and may not benefit from environmental sampling and its associated turnaround times.

As COVID-19 cases have continued at low levels, the authors' work suggests that when the wastewater concentration is below the detection limit, less comprehensive protocols can be enacted (e.g., only testing the symptomatic). This demonstrates that at least some degree of clinical testing burden can be replaced by wastewater testing, providing a cost savings for the jails in their study. Periodic scope and schedule adjustments based on disease spread and severity should be anticipated and done in collaboration with carceral facility leadership. Curiously, the National Institute of Corrections is not advocating that states do more wastewater testing. In the study by Kennedy et al., jail leadership voluntarily and proactively used wastewater data as another source of information for lowering the level of health risk.

Key health policy recommendations on the utility of WBS in prisons and jails for the protection of incarcerated individuals during the next outbreak include the following:

- Approach WBS sampling design and data use in prisons versus jails differently.
- Use WBS data as complementary information; clinical case data are still required.
- Target wastewater testing where the disease can be clinically managed to limit facility spread.
- Have high confidence in negative wastewater concentration to guide less comprehensive individual testing protocols.
- Consider WBS across a range of facilities, sampling types, and laboratory analysis models.
- Plan periodic sampling design adjustments.
- View future carceral facility sewer infrastructure and health investment jointly.

Kennedy et al. provide a real-world demonstration of the role of WBS in jails to guide health policy across a range of population sizes, architectural designs, sewer system configurations, and funding levels. Ultimately, for policy experts across carceral facilities seeking direction, getting better data on vulnerable populations is hard, but WBS provides an opportunity. AJPH

CORRESPONDENCE

Correspondence should be sent to Rochelle H. Holm, Christina Lee Brown Envirome Institute, School of Medicine, University of Louisville, 302 E Muhammad Ali Blvd, Louisville, KY 40202 (e-mail: rochelle.holm@louisville.edu). Reprints can be ordered at https://www.ajph.org by clicking the "Reprints" link.

PUBLICATION INFORMATION

Full Citation: Holm RH, Smith T. Does wastewater-based surveillance protect the health of incarcerated individuals? *Am J Public Health*. 2024;114(11): 1156–1157.

Acceptance Date: August 16, 2024.

DOI: https://doi.org/10.2105/AJPH.2024.307857

ORCID iDs:

Rochelle H. Holm https://orcid.org/0000-0001-8849-1390

Ted Smith https://orcid.org/0000-0003-2804-4294

CONTRIBUTORS

Both authors conceptualized, drafted, and revised the editorial.

ACKNOWLEDGMENTS

The authors received research funding from the Commonwealth of Kentucky Department of Corrections (contracts PON2 527 2200001913 1; PON2 527 2100001185).

CONFLICTS OF INTEREST

The authors report no potential or actual conflicts of interest from funding or affiliation-related activities pertinent to this editorial.

REFERENCES

1. Hassard F, Smith TR, Boehm AB, et al. Wastewater surveillance for rapid identification of infectious diseases in prisons. *Lancet Microbe*. 2022;3(8): e556–e557. https://doi.org/10.1016/S2666-5247(22)00154-9
2. Han D, Linares P, Holm RH, Chandran K, Smith T. Wastewater threshold as an indicator of COVID-19 cases in correctional facilities for public health response: a modeling study. *Water Res*. 2024;260: 121934. https://doi.org/10.1016/j.watres.2024.121934
3. Levintow SN, DiRosa E, Carda-Auten J, et al. SARS-CoV-2 mitigation strategies, testing, and cases at 254 jails in the US Southeast, October 2020 to May 2021. *Am J Public Health*. 2022; 112(11):1589–1598. https://doi.org/10.2105/AJPH.2022.307012
4. Albani V, Loria J, Massad E, Zubelli J. COVID-19 underreporting and its impact on vaccination strategies. *BMC Infect Dis*. 2021;21(1):1111. https://doi.org/10.1186/s12879-021-06780-7
5. Keith RJ, Holm RH, Amraotkar AR, et al. Stratified simple random sampling versus volunteer community-wide sampling for estimates of COVID-19 prevalence. *Am J Public Health*. 2023;113(7):768–777. https://doi.org/10.2105/AJPH.2023.307303
6. Water Environment Federation. Pilot program for onsite testing of SARS-CoV-2 in correctional facility wastewater. 2022. Available at: https://www.accesswater.org/publications/-10086386/summary-report-for-pilot-program-for-onsite-testing-of-sars-cov-2-in-correctional-facility-wastewater. Accessed September 3, 2024.
7. Postigo C, de Alda ML, Barceló D. Evaluation of drugs of abuse use and trends in a prison through wastewater analysis. *Environ Int*. 2011;37(1):49–55. https://doi.org/10.1016/j.envint.2010.06.012
8. Brewer AJ, Banta-Green CJ, Ort C, Robel AE, Field J. Wastewater testing compared with random urinalyses for the surveillance of illicit drug use in prisons. *Drug Alcohol Rev*. 2016;35(2):133–137. https://doi.org/10.1111/dar.12185
9. Van Dyken E, Lai FY, Thai PKO, et al. Challenges and opportunities in using wastewater analysis to measure drug use in a small prison facility. *Drug Alcohol Rev*. 2016;35(2):138–147. https://doi.org/10.1111/dar.12156
10. Hoffmann T, Alsing J. Faecal shedding models for SARS-CoV-2 RNA among hospitalised patients and implications for wastewater-based epidemiology. *JR Stat Soc Ser C Appl Stat*. 2023;72(2):330–345. https://doi.org/10.1093/jrsssc/qlad011

To Uncover Disparities, Collect and Disaggregate Self-Identification Data for Middle Eastern and North African Americans

Ariela Schachter, PhD, Neda Maghbouleh, PhD, and René D. Flores, PhD

ABOUT THE AUTHORS

Ariela Schachter is with the Department of Sociology, Washington University, Saint Louis, MO. Neda Maghbouleh is with the Department of Sociology, University of British Columbia, Vancouver. René D. Flores is with the Department of Sociology, University of Chicago, Chicago, IL.

See also Kindratt and Smith, p. 1265.

Middle Eastern and North African (MENA) Americans are largely invisible in federal data and surveys, as they usually lack a distinct category for self-identification.[1] This data gap obscures whether MENA Americans experience adverse life circumstances more than other groups.[2] We argue that researchers should immediately begin designing research instruments that offer a MENA category for self-identification in race/ethnicity questions and should analyze the significant heterogeneity in MENA populations. This approach will provide crucial insights into the health and well-being of this diverse, understudied group.

Because of the lack of self-reported race/ethnicity data, researchers have used creative methods to identify likely MENA Americans and explore possible health disparities.[3,4] In this issue of *AJPH*, Kindratt and Smith (p. 1265) use the ancestry and country of birth measures in the American Community Survey (ACS) to identify MENA adults and compare their odds of cognitive difficulties with those of self-identified White, Black, Hispanic/Latino, Asian, American Indian or Alaska Native, and Native Hawaiian/other Pacific Islander adults aged 45 years and older. They found that MENA adults reported higher rates of cognitive difficulties than did all other tested groups except Native Hawaiian/other Pacific Islander adults, after adjusting for education and nativity status.

Other research similarly identifies health disparities both between MENA and non-MENA individuals and within the MENA category based on country of origin, nativity, and arrival cohort.[5–7] The literature suggests that these difficulties may stem from the stress of lifetime discrimination, a central social determinant of health. A thorough comparison of MENA Americans' health, both with other US groups and within the MENA category, is crucial.[5]

Although insightful, research based on the ACS ancestry variable has potential limitations. Individuals who report MENA ancestries may be a select group, which can affect the measurement of life outcomes, as those reporting a certain ethnic ancestry may not identify with or be perceived as belonging to that group. For example, individuals with Hispanic ancestry who do not identify as Hispanic tend to have a higher socioeconomic status than those who do.[8] Thus, collecting self-reported racial/ethnic data on MENA Americans is critical. Self-identification is the most common measure for studying demographic changes, vital statistics, and disease rates.[9] Self-reported race/ethnicity respects individuals' perceptions of their identity and would enable researchers to compare health indicators of self-identified MENA Americans with those of other ethnoracial groups, resulting in more comparable and standardized estimates.

A MENA category was originally planned for the 2020 US Census but was canceled at the last minute. In March 2024 the US Office of Management and Budget (OMB) finally approved revisions to its Statistical Policy Directive 15, including a MENA check box in all federally collected data. This decision follows extensive research showing that many MENA Americans do not identify as White and that, when given the option, most choose the MENA category.[1,10] Furthermore, most non-MENA White Americans perceive MENA individuals as distinctly non-White based on ancestry, appearance, and cultural cues.[1,11]

There is no reason to delay implementing the OMB revisions. Depending on federal changes can be risky, as seen when the MENA check box was last considered but ultimately excluded at the 11th hour. Researchers developing new health surveys should ensure that they include a MENA option in identity questions to properly capture this in the resulting data set.

Yet, there is a risk of treating the newly visible MENA population as homogeneous, which could obscure significant internal differences. It is crucial that new data sets capture detailed self-reported race/ethnicity measures, including national origin, to reflect the diversity in the MENA community. Disaggregated data are essential for examining the varied experiences in the MENA community and their health implications. As Ford and Sharif noted in *AJPH,* this research must be expansive enough to encompass a broad spectrum of individuals, while also clarifying intragroup and intersectional inequalities.[12] Detailed MENA data can be reaggregated to comply with OMB guidelines, ensuring fresh data insulated from political uncertainties.

To highlight the substantial heterogeneity among MENA Americans, Figure 1 illustrates differences in health insurance coverage and college degree attainment—critical factors that can influence health outcomes—across various MENA ancestry groups. We use the same data from the 2017–2021 five-year ACS as Kindratt and Smith. Figure 1 shows that, compared with Lebanese Americans—a relatively advantaged group—nearly all other major MENA ethnic groups are less likely to have health insurance ($P < .05$). These gaps range from relatively small, at less than 2 percentage points (Iranians, Syrians, and Israelis), to a full 9 to 10 percentage point gap (Algerians and Sudanese) in coverage relative to Lebanese Americans. Furthermore, Figure 1 shows even greater disparities in education levels, but with several groups being significantly more educated than Lebanese Americans. These differences underscore the likely large health disparities among MENA Americans and suggest that their origins are complex.

In light of the recent Statistical Policy Directive 15 announcement and the importance of self-reported data, we recommend that researchers do the following:

1. Immediately offer a MENA category in all self-reported race/ethnicity data-collection tools. For too long, the health disparities that MENA Americans face have been hidden because of the absence of a distinct race/ethnicity category, masking the potential effects of structural racism on this group. This invisibility also complicates, if not entirely hinders, the delivery of culturally sensitive and relevant public health services to the MENA community. Public health scholars should not wait

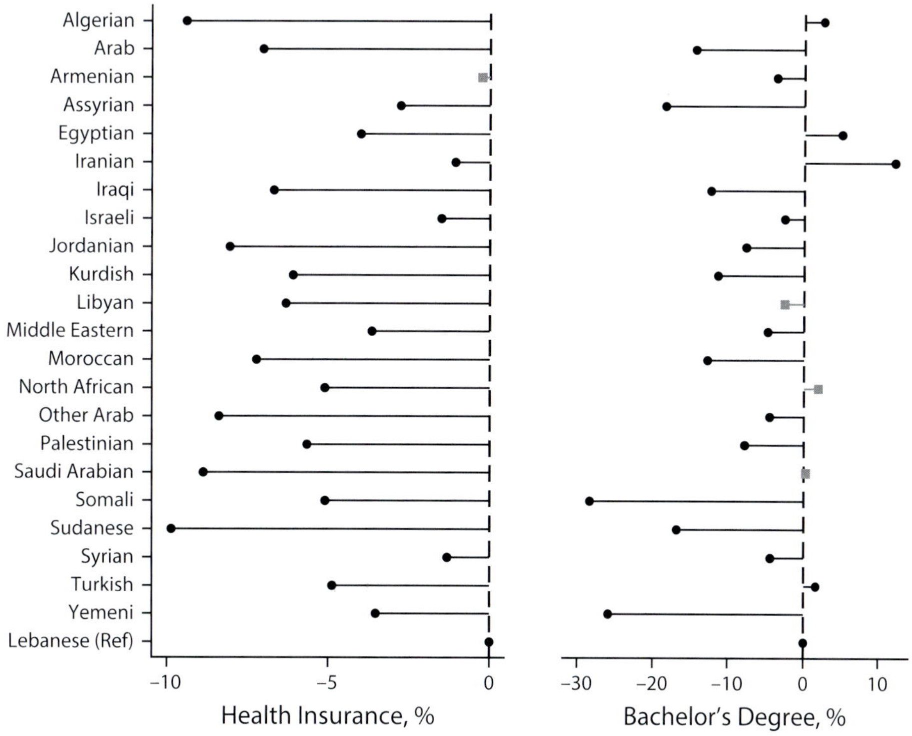

FIGURE 1— Weighted Health Insurance Status and College Degree Attainment Differences by MENA Ancestry: American Community Survey, 2017–2021

Note. MENA = Middle Eastern and North African. Squares denote $P > .05$.

AJPH November 2024, Vol. 114, No. 11

for the OMB deadline to begin offering a MENA category in all data-collection efforts.

2. Avoid treating the MENA community as a monolith by ensuring data disaggregation. Although we urge scholars to recognize the distinct experiences of MENA Americans compared with non-Hispanic Whites, we also caution against treating MENA Americans as a monolithic group. Like Asian Americans, the MENA population includes subgroups that are socioeconomically advantaged and those that are disadvantaged relative to White Americans; these subgroups likely face differential morbidity risks.[13] Only with disaggregated data in the MENA population can population health scholars begin to understand these disparities.

In summary, introducing a MENA category in federal surveys is a positive step beyond the limitations of the currently available ancestry and nativity data, but it is just the beginning. Expanding this category across all data sets and acknowledging the diversity in the MENA community will provide a clearer understanding of their unique health challenges. Our data need to reflect real-life experiences to accurately measure health disparities and guide effective public health practices. This comprehensive approach will enhance research accuracy and ensure that MENA Americans are no longer invisible in medical and social data. AJPH

CORRESPONDENCE

Correspondence should be sent to Ariela Schachter, PhD, Associate Professor, Washington University in St Louis, Sociology, 1 Brookings Dr, Saint Louis, MO 63130-4862 (e-mail: ariela@wustl.edu). Reprints can be ordered at https://www.ajph.org by clicking the "Reprints" link.

PUBLICATION INFORMATION

Full Citation: Schachter A, Maghbouleh N, Flores RD. To uncover disparities, collect and disaggregate self-identification data for Middle Eastern and North African Americans. *Am J Public Health*. 2024;114(11):1158–1160.

Acceptance Date: August 29, 2024.

DOI: https://doi.org/10.2105/AJPH.2024.307864

ORCID iDs:

Ariela Schachter https://orcid.org/0000-0002-7404-4140

Neda Maghbouleh https://orcid.org/0000-0001-8541-2079

René D. Flores https://orcid.org/0000-0002-9137-3261

CONTRIBUTORS

The authors contributed equally to this editorial.

ACKNOWLEDGMENTS

The authors thank Armin Sauermann for his research assistance and Hedwig Lee for her generous feedback.

Note. The opinions expressed in this editorial are solely the authors' and do not necessarily reflect the official policy or position of the 2030 Census Advisory Committee, US Census Bureau, or US government.

CONFLICTS OF INTEREST

The authors have no conflicts of interest to declare.

REFERENCES

1. Maghbouleh N, Schachter A, Flores RD. Middle Eastern and North African Americans may not be perceived, nor perceive themselves, to be White. *Proc Natl Acad Sci U S A*. 2022;119(7):e2117940119. https://doi.org/10.1073/pnas.2117940119
2. Sharif MZ, Maghbouleh N, Baback Boozary AS. COVID-19 disparities among Arab, Middle Eastern, and West Asian populations in Toronto: implications for improving health equity among Middle Eastern and North African communities in the United States. *Health Promot Pract*. 2024;25(4):531–536. https://doi.org/10.1177/15248399221142898
3. Al-Rousan T, Kamalyan L, Bernstein Sideman A, et al. Migration and cognitive health disparities: the Arab American and refugee case. *J Gerontol B Psychol Sci Soc Sci*. 2023;78(1):111–123. https://doi.org/10.1093/geronb/gbac129
4. Kindratt TB, Dallo FJ, Zahodne LB. Cognitive disability among Arab Americans by nativity status and arrival year: lack of evidence for the healthy migrant effect. *J Racial Ethn Health Disparities*. 2022;9(5):2056–2062. https://doi.org/10.1007/s40615-021-01144-y
5. Awad GH, Kia-Keating M, Amer MM. A model of cumulative racial–ethnic trauma among Americans of Middle Eastern and North African (MENA) descent. *Am Psychol*. 2019;74(1):76–87. https://doi.org/10.1037/amp0000344
6. Read JG, Ajrouch KJ, West JS. Disparities in functional disability among Arab Americans by nativity, immigrant arrival cohort, and country of birth. *SSM Popul Health*. 2019;7:100325. [Erratum in: Erratum regarding missing declaration of competing interest statements in previously published articles. *SSM Popul Health*. 2020;12:100715. https://doi.org/10.1016/j.ssmph.2020.100715]. https://doi.org/10.1016/j.ssmph.2018.100325
7. Abuelezam NN, El-Sayed A, Galea S, Gordon NP. Understanding differences within ethnic group designation: comparing risk factors and health indicators between Iranian and Arab Americans in Northern California. *BMC Public Health*. 2021;21(1):1074. https://doi.org/10.1186/s12889-021-11121-z
8. Duncan B, Trejo SJ. Tracking intergenerational progress for immigrant groups: the problem of ethnic attrition. *Am Econ Rev*. 2011;101(3):603–608. https://doi.org/10.1257/aer.101.3.603
9. Roth WD. The multiple dimensions of race. *Ethn Racial Stud*. 2016;39(8):1310–1338. https://doi.org/10.1080/01419870.2016.1140793
10. Ajrouch KJ, Jamal A. Assimilating to a White identity: the case of Arab Americans. *Int Migr Rev*. 2007;41(4):860–879. https://doi.org/10.1111/j.1747-7379.2007.00103.x
11. Schachter A, Flores RD, Maghbouleh N. Ancestry, color, or culture? How Whites racially classify others in the US. *Am J Sociol*. 2021;126(5):1220–1263. https://doi.org/10.1086/714215
12. Ford CL, Sharif MZ. Arabs, Whiteness, and health disparities: the need for critical race theory and data. *Am J Public Health*. 2020;110(8):e2–e3. https://doi.org/10.2105/AJPH.2020.305749
13. Đoàn LN, Chau MM, Ahmed N, Cao J, Chan SWC, Yi SS. Turning the health equity lens to diversity in Asian American health profiles. *Annu Rev Public Health*. 2024;45:169–193. https://doi.org/10.1146/annurev-publhealth-060222-023852

Doula Support as a Health Equity Strategy: Carving the Path Forward

Holly L. Horan, PhD

ABOUT THE AUTHOR

Holly L. Horan is with the Global and Rural Women's Health Program, Department of Obstetrics and Gynecology, Heersink School of Medicine, University of Alabama at Birmingham.

See also Marshall and Kozhimannil, p. 1164, and Falconi et al., p. 1275.

The *White House Blueprint for Addressing the Maternal Health Crisis*[1] indicates that doulas are part of a multipronged solution to mitigating the high rates of maternal morbidity and mortality in the United States: outcomes that disproportionately affect Black, Brown, Indigenous, and low-income people. The most recent data on maternal mortality serves as evidence of these inequities, with 49.5 maternal deaths per 100 000 live births for Black perinatal populations, a significantly higher rate when compared with Asian (13.2), Hispanic (16.9), and White (19.0) groups.[2] At least 70% of maternal deaths are attributed to nonclinical, social determinants, including racism and income level, leading to calls for research that can advance perinatal health care system improvements with a focus on equity.[3]

"Doula" is a Greek term for a woman caregiver who serves other women. Doulas are trained, nonclinical support professionals who provide education, resources, advocacy, and other physical, emotional, cultural, and spiritual supports to expecting individuals, new parents, and postpartum persons.[4,5] Doulas prioritize respectful support and center the expecting person and their loved ones by providing care and companionship. Their support services are linked to improved outcomes, including lower rates of cesarean birth, premature labor, and infant mortality; increased rates of breastfeeding initiation; and improved infant and maternal mental health outcomes. Doulas have also been shown to reduce racial disparities in health outcomes—especially for cesarean birth, which is associated with an elevated risk of postpartum complications.[6]

Doula support is also beneficial for clinically and socially higher-risk populations, such as Medicaid recipients. However, until recently, there was a lack of sufficient data to measure this effect at the population level. Doula support is largely believed to be an exclusive, financially privileged service because it is not covered by most state or commercial insurance plans. This means that most expecting families cannot afford to pay out of pocket for this care, with recent estimates of private practice doula fees ranging from $500 to $5000 or more.[7] This partially explains why only 6% of all perinatal persons have utilized doula support. In addition, there is a low number of doulas trained to provide support to clinically and socially higher-risk clients, and these doulas are at higher risk for financial insecurity because of the lack of effective reimbursement models for their services.[8,9]

Medicaid reimbursement for doula support is a critical strategy for increasing access to this service. This coverage is currently available in 13 states and Washington, DC. All but one US state has an initiative to increase access to doula support. These initiatives involve actively reimbursing for doula support, implementing a reimbursement model, and engaging in adjacent legislative or public health action. Community-based doula programs focus on training and supporting a diverse doula workforce, with the intention of increasing the number of perinatal people in a local area who can access and utilize racially and culturally congruent doula services. Medicaid reimbursement for doula services is typically lower than private practice reimbursement and ranges from $450 to $3500 per doula client depending on the state.[10] The continued increase in the implementation of Medicaid reimbursement in other US states will require additional research showing that doulas have a positive effect on perinatal outcomes and inequities. There is also a need to examine the growth and diversification of the doula workforce and the mechanisms for effectively supporting doulas to serve socially and clinically higher-risk clients.

The study by Falconi et al., reported in "Role of Doulas in Improving Maternal Health and Health Equity Among Medicaid Enrollees, 2014–2023" (p. 1275), is one of the first to examine the impact of doula support across nine US states. They used propensity score matching for 722 perinatal persons who received doula care (i.e., the control group) between 2014 and 2023; they then retrospectively analyzed medical and pharmacy claims data from the Healthcare Integrated Research Database. They also conducted subgroup analyses to examine the effect of race (Black vs White) and area-level infant mortality rate (IMR)—a proxy variable used to measure the social, economic, and environmental determinants associated with perinatal health outcomes.

The results of Falconi et al. showed that individuals in the control group were more likely to have a doula if they were older (28.0 vs 27.2 years), Black (43.7% vs 22.4%), lived in an urban setting (66.2% vs 52.5%), and were giving birth in a county with fewer hospital or obstetric services available (mean = 4.3 vs 6.6). Doula support was associated with a 47% lower risk of cesarean birth, a 29% lower risk of preterm birth, a 116% increased likelihood of having a vaginal birth after a previous cesarean, and a 46% increased likelihood that the client would attend their postpartum visit. Doula support was positively correlated with postpartum visit attendance for Black individuals—the only result that showed a significant difference between race, outcomes, and doula support status. Doula-supported individuals who lived in counties with a high area-level IMR had a lower likelihood of having a cesarean birth, and those living in counties with a low area-level IMR were more likely to attend their postpartum visit. Falconi et al. conclude that doula support could be an effective strategy for mitigating perinatal health disparities, especially in the intrapartum and postpartum periods.

Falconi et al. advance the research on the benefits of doula support for Medicaid clients. Their results and discussion also provide important guidance that should be elevated to continue to carve a path forward for future research on doula support as an effective health equity strategy. For example, existing research shows that IMRs are higher in rural areas. IMRs and excess infant deaths are highest in Black, Brown, and Indigenous populations living in rural communities. Risk factors associated with IMR, including smoking, obesity, and poverty, are common across all racial and ethnic groups.[11] Future research should examine the effect of doula support for Medicaid clients of color in rural areas. Their results also showed that the doula-supported sample had a higher frequency of individuals who were Black, lived in urban areas, and were less likely to have access to obstetric services. These results suggest that the intersection of race, geography, and access is an area for further investigation as Medicaid reimbursement is implemented in other states.

Doula support as a health equity strategy is not a new idea; however, the current increase in institutional support will generate more data that can be used to better understand the effects of this care. Future research should focus on examining racial and cultural congruence between doulas and their clients and its effect on outcomes.[6] These data could support the allocation of resources for public health programming, such as training, reimbursement, and identifying priority populations in a specific state or county. An additional line of research should examine the development of Medicaid reimbursement models and their effects on the doula workforce and how policymakers collaborate with local doulas and other allied professionals to do this work.[10] Robust research on the effects of doula support, the diversification of the doula profession, and the creation of doula policies and reimbursement models could be used to increase knowledge and acceptance of this profession among health care professionals and clinical leadership—relationships that are often tenuous in many hospital-based contexts, where the majority of birthing people receive their care.[12] AJPH

CORRESPONDENCE

Correspondence should be sent to Holly L. Horan, Women & Infants Center, 1700 6th Ave South, Birmingham, AL 35249-7333 (e-mail: hhoran@uabmc.edu). Reprints can be ordered at https://www.ajph.org by clicking the "Reprints" link.

PUBLICATION INFORMATION

Full Citation: Horan HL. Doula support as a health equity strategy: carving the path forward. *Am J Public Health*. 2024;114(11):1161–1163.

Acceptance Date: August 19, 2024.

DOI: https://doi.org/10.2105/AJPH.2024.307858

ACKNOWLEDGMENTS

I wish to thank the families, doulas, colleagues, and others who support and sustain this work.

CONFLICTS OF INTEREST

The author has no conflicts of interest to disclose.

REFERENCES

1. White House. White House blueprint for addressing the maternal health crisis. 2022. Available at: https://www.whitehouse.gov/wp-content/uploads/2022/06/Maternal-Health-Blueprint.pdf. Accessed September 2, 2024.
2. Hoyert DL. Maternal mortality rates in the United States, 2022. May 2024. Available at: https://www.cdc.gov/nchs/data/hestat/maternal-mortality/2022/maternal-mortality-rates-2022.pdf. Accessed September 2, 2024.
3. Joseph KS, Boutin A, Lisonkova S, et al. Maternal mortality in the United States: recent trends, current status, and future considerations. *Obstet Gynecol*. 2021;137(5):763–771. https://doi.org/10.1097/AOG.0000000000004361

4. Klaus MH, Kennell JH. The doula: an essential ingredient of childbirth rediscovered. *Acta Paediatr.* 1997;86(10):1034–1036. https://doi.org/10.1111/j.1651-2227.1997.tb14800.x
5. National Health Law Program. What is a doula? 2020. Available at: https://healthlaw.org/wp-content/uploads/2020/04/WhatIsADoula_4.16.2020.pdf. Accessed September 2, 2024.
6. Sobczak A, Taylor L, Solomon S, et al. The effect of doulas on maternal and birth outcomes: a scoping review. *Cureus.* 2023;15(5):e39451. https://doi.org/10.7759/cureus.39451
7. Harnish A. How to make working with a doula more affordable. 2023. Available at: https://www.whattoexpect.com/pregnancy/labor-and-delivery/how-much-do-doulas-cost. Accessed September 2, 2024.
8. Declerq E, Sakala C, Corry M, Applebaum S, Herrlich A. Listening to mothers III: pregnancy and childbirth. 2013. Available at: https://collective.coloradotrust.org/wp-content/uploads/sites/2/2020/02/listening-to-mothers-iii-pregnancy-and-birth-2013.pdf. Accessed September 2, 2024.
9. Spivey A, Barajas-Roman E. Prioritize doulas in Black and Brown communities. *Health Aff Forefront.* June 2, 2022. Available at: https://perma.cc/WXN9-PDGA. Accessed September 2, 2024. https://doi.org/10.1377/forefront.20220531.102507
10. National Health Law Program. Doula Medicaid project. Available at: https://healthlaw.org/doulamedicaidproject. Accessed September 2, 2024.
11. Womack LS, Rossen LM, Hirai AH. Urban–rural infant mortality disparities by race and ethnicity and cause of death. *Am J Prev Med.* 2020;58(2):254–260. https://doi.org/10.1016/j.amepre.2019.09.010
12. Neel K, Goldman R, Marte D, Bello G, Nothnagle MB. Hospital-based maternity care practitioners' perceptions of doulas. *Birth.* 2019;46(2):355–361. https://doi.org/10.1111/birt.12420

Progress on Doula Access, Persistent Challenges, and Next Steps for Birth Equity

Cassondra Marshall, DrPH, MPH, and Katy Backes Kozhimannil, PhD, MPA

ABOUT THE AUTHORS

Cassondra Marshall is with the Maternal, Child, and Adolescent Health Program, University of California, Berkeley, School of Public Health. Katy Backes Kozhimannil is with the Division of Health Policy and Management, University of Minnesota School of Public Health, Minneapolis.

See also Horan, p. 1161, and Falconi et al., p. 1275.

Ensuring access to doula support for pregnant and birthing people in the United States should be a policy priority. Having support from a doula—a trained nonclinical birth worker who provides emotional, physical, and informational support during the perinatal period and for other reproductive health experiences—has been associated with positive health outcomes and high patient satisfaction.[1] For decades, research has demonstrated that doula support during the perinatal period is associated with many desirable perinatal outcomes, including fewer unnecessary cesarean deliveries, fewer preterm births, better birth experiences, and reduced postpartum depression and anxiety.[1,2] In addition, especially for Black, Indigenous, and People of Color (BIPOC) who give birth, doula support is associated with more autonomy and respect.[3,4] Doula support has no documented harms and many potential benefits, yet, in a country grappling with a maternal health crisis, most birthing people do not have doula support.

STRONG EVIDENCE ON BENEFITS OF DOULA CARE

In this issue, Falconi et al. (p. 1275) assess the relationship between doula care and pregnancy-related health outcomes in a Medicaid-enrolled population. Noting that some of the previous research has been limited to data from a single hospital or state, the authors conducted analyses using health plan data from a geographically diverse population from nine states. Using propensity score matching with 722 matched pairs, the authors found that individuals who received doula support during pregnancy had 47% lower risk of cesarean delivery and 29% lower risk of preterm birth, compared with those without doula support. In addition, those with doula support were 46% more likely to have a postpartum visit, an important finding not previously reported.

Overall, the authors' findings are consistent with a large body of work demonstrating the benefits of doula support as well as the potential cost-effectiveness of insurance coverage of doula care, particularly for Medicaid enrollees. As Medicaid pays for nearly half of all US births, mostly via managed care, public payers and health plans play an essential role in facilitating financial access to evidence-based services like doula care.

IMPROVING HEALTH EQUITY VIA DOULA ACCESS

Falconi et al. state that health insurance coverage of doula care has gained traction as a "strategy for improving persistent challenges in maternal health," citing reports from the Surgeon General and the White House. Indeed, advocates, policymakers, and researchers have increasingly identified Medicaid coverage of doula support as an important policy strategy to improve maternal and infant health outcomes.

Notably, Medicaid covers a disproportionately greater share of births to individuals who are BIPOC and rural residents. Furthermore, risk of maternal morbidity and mortality is highest among those with multiple marginalized identities (e.g., BIPOC, rural, Medicaid enrollee).[5] As such, Medicaid coverage of doula care has the potential to address inequities and ensure access for those at highest risk,[6] if implemented with community-engaged and person-centered principles and in combination with broader protections and resources for reproductive health. In 2014, only two state Medicaid programs covered doula services.[7] Ten years later, 15 states and the District of Columbia cover doula care through Medicaid, and additional states have

AJPH November 2024, Vol. 114, No. 11

proposed or are developing doula coverage benefits.[8]

EQUITABLE IMPLEMENTATION OF MEDICAID COVERAGE

Medicaid coverage of doula support is likely to increase across the country, either through efforts at the state level or through federal programs or requirements. However, adding doula care as a covered benefit does not necessarily ensure access because of myriad implementation barriers. It is the support of a doula—not the passage of a law about Medicaid coverage—that confers benefits to pregnant and birthing people. Still, passing laws and implementing policies to increase access to doula care for Medicaid enrollees is an important first step, and attention to health equity should be at the core.[7]

State Medicaid programs should prioritize quality and equitable access when developing a doula benefit and can learn from other states that have already implemented doula policies. For example, Oregon and Minnesota, the first two states to cover doula services through Medicaid, faced implementation challenges including low reimbursement rates, limited racial/ethnic diversity and geographic distribution of the doula workforce, and lack of awareness or acceptance of doulas by maternity care clinicians in some settings. Doulas encountered challenges—from reimbursement to certification—while navigating the Medicaid system, and health plans and clinical sites faced logistical, informational, and financial roadblocks. Stakeholders have since identified lessons learned from these early adopter states and other localized doula pilot programs, including the importance of working in close partnership with doulas and community-based doula organizations when designing and implementing benefits, setting dignified and appropriate reimbursement rates, and providing technical assistance and support for doulas as they enroll as Medicaid providers and navigate contracting with health plans and billing.[6,9,10] However, when integrating doulas as Medicaid providers, it is important to ensure that their work, which is a nonclinical intervention, is not overly medicalized and is respected and supported within its scope.

One state that integrated many of these best practices is California, where doulas, health plans, clinicians, and other stakeholders have been engaged in designing and implementing their state's Medicaid benefit.[9,11] Meaningful collaboration requires patience, continual dialogue, and reimagining what is possible within state Medicaid programs. A collaborative approach may be the key to ensuring that pregnant, birthing, and postpartum Medicaid beneficiaries can equitably access and benefit from the support that doulas provide.[10]

A COMPREHENSIVE APPROACH THAT INCLUDES DOULA CARE

While doula support is rightly cited as one evidence-based intervention to address the US maternal mortality crisis broadly, and for marginalized groups specifically, it is critical to recognize that doulas are not the solution to this crisis. Doulas operate within a health care system that produces dismal and inequitable maternal health outcomes. Although increased access to doula care may enhance racial equity in maternal health, only a handful of states with doula access focus explicitly on racial equity.[7] The US maternal mortality crisis is a complex problem, with many contributing factors including restrictive reproductive health policies, interpersonal and structural racism, social determinants of health, intimate partner violence, economic inequality, and community and public health infrastructure. No single intervention can solve this crisis. Doula care is a necessary component of the comprehensive strategy needed to address the nation's deepening maternal health crisis, but no study of doula care to date—including Falconi et al.—has shown an association with reduced maternal mortality.[1] Future studies should endeavor to examine the roles doulas can play within a comprehensive policy strategy, and, as doula care expands, larger studies may be able to assess associations with social drivers and structural determinants of maternal morbidity and mortality and with these outcomes directly.

The fact is, despite a changing policy landscape and well-documented benefits, doula support remains largely inaccessible to pregnant and birthing people; it is not typically covered by insurance and is unaffordable to those who cannot afford the out-of-pocket cost. Doula care can offer humane support through life transitions, but it is out of reach for many. Efforts to expand Medicaid coverage of doula care are trying to change that. To improve maternal health equity, the United States needs a comprehensive strategy that incorporates, but does not solely rely on, doulas and the support they provide. AJPH

CORRESPONDENCE

Correspondence should be sent to Cassondra Marshall, DrPH, MPH, UC Berkeley School of Public Health, 2121 Berkeley Way #5127, Berkeley, CA 94720 (e-mail: cassiejm@berkeley.edu).

PUBLICATION INFORMATION

Full Citation: Marshall C, Kozhimannil KB. Progress on doula access, persistent challenges, and next steps for birth equity. *Am J Public Health*. 2024;114(11):1164–1166.

Acceptance Date: August 19, 2024.

DOI: https://doi.org/10.2105/AJPH.2024.307859

ORCID iDs:

Cassondra Marshall https://orcid.org/0000-0001-5299-9176

Katy Backes Kozhimannil https://orcid.org/0000-0002-5734-9049

CONTRIBUTORS

C. Marshall drafted the editorial. K. B. Kozhimannil conceptualized and revised the editorial.

ACKNOWLEDGMENTS

C. Marshall receives support from the National Institutes of Health/National Institute on Minority Health and Health Disparities (K01MD016169, PI: Marshall).

The authors are grateful to Alyssa Fritz, MPH, RD, CLC, and Ashley Nguyen, MPH, for helpful edits and suggestions.

Note. The information, conclusions, and opinions expressed in this article are those of the authors, and no endorsement by the funder is intended or should be inferred.

CONFLICTS OF INTEREST

C. Marshall receives funding from the California Department of Health Care Services, which implements the California Medicaid Program, Medi-Cal.

REFERENCES

1. Alvarado G, Schultz D, Malika N, Reed N. United States doula programs and their outcomes: a scoping review to inform state-level policies. *Womens Health Issues*. 2024;34(4):350–360. https://doi.org/10.1016/j.whi.2024.03.001
2. Kozhimannil KB, Hardeman RR, Attanasio LB, Blauer-Peterson C, O'Brien M. Doula care, birth outcomes, and costs among Medicaid beneficiaries. *Am J Public Health*. 2013;103(4):e113–e121. https://doi.org/10.2105/AJPH.2012.301201
3. Kozhimannil KB, Vogelsang CA, Hardeman RR, Prasad S. Disrupting the pathways of social determinants of health: doula support during pregnancy and childbirth. *J Am Board Fam Med*. 2016;29(3):308–317. https://doi.org/10.3122/jabfm.2016.03.150300
4. Mallick LM, Thoma ME, Shenassa ED. The role of doulas in respectful care for communities of color and Medicaid recipients. *Birth*. 2022;49(4):823–832. https://doi.org/10.1111/birt.12655
5. Interrante JD, Tuttle MS, Admon LK, Kozhimannil KB. Severe maternal morbidity and mortality risk at the intersection of rurality, race and ethnicity, and Medicaid. *Womens Health Issues*. 2022;32(6):540–549. https://doi.org/10.1016/j.whi.2022.05.003
6. Kozhimannil KB, Hardeman RR. Coverage for doula services: how state Medicaid programs can address concerns about maternity care costs and quality. *Birth*. 2016;43(2):97–99. https://doi.org/10.1111/birt.12213
7. Ogunwole SM, Karbeah J, Bozzi DG, et al. Health equity considerations in state bills related to doula care (2015–2020). *Womens Health Issues*. 2022;32(5):440–449. https://doi.org/10.1016/j.whi.2022.04.004
8. National Health Law Program. NHeLP's Doula Medicaid Project: current state efforts at expanding access to doula care. Available at: https://healthlaw.org/doulamedicaidproject. Accessed August 7, 2024.
9. Marshall C, Nguyen A, Yang CE, Gómez AM. Facilitators and barriers to Medicaid doula benefit implementation in California: perspectives from managed care plans and risk-bearing organizations. *Womens Health Issues*. 2024:S1049-3867(24)00047-1. https://doi.org/10.1016/j.whi.2024.05.006
10. Bey A, Brill A, Porchia-Albert C, Gradilla M, Strauss N. Advancing birth justice: community-based doula models as a standard of care for ending racial disparities. Every Mother Counts; 2019. Available at: https://everymothercounts.org/wp-content/uploads/2019/03/Advancing-Birth-Justice-CBD-Models-as-Std-of-Care-3-25-19.pdf. Accessed August 7, 2024.
11. Institute for Medicaid Innovation. Key learnings from the Doula and Perinatal Community Health Worker in Medicaid Learning Series. October 2023. Available at: https://medicaidinnovation.org/wp-content/uploads/2023/10/DCLS_Report_2023_FINAL.pdf. Accessed August 7, 2024.

Addressing Data Deficiencies to Prevent Pediatric Firearm Injuries: Insights From the American College of Surgeons (ACS) Firearm Study

Daniel C. Semenza, PhD

ABOUT THE AUTHOR

Daniel Semenza is an associate professor in the Department of Sociology, Anthropology, and Criminal Justice, Rutgers University—Camden and the Department of Urban-Global Public Health in the School of Public Health, Rutgers University, New Brunswick, NJ. He is the director of Interpersonal Violence Research at the New Jersey Gun Violence Research Center, Rutgers University.

Since 2020, firearm injury has been the leading cause of death among children and adolescents in the United States.[1] Flynn-O'Brien et al. analyzed data from nearly 3000 children injured with a firearm across 128 trauma centers collected from the Trauma Quality Improvement Project (TQIP) database.[2] The study, which covered the period from March 2021 through February 2022, found that roughly two thirds of the children were shot during an assault, and the remainder were injured unintentionally or by self-inflicted means. The authors analyzed how the context of pediatric firearm injury differs by intent and identified the factors that contribute to missing data across key contextual variables. The findings highlight clear demographic and racial disparities in risk for pediatric firearm injury, which echo prior studies.[3] The majority of youths in the study across injury intent were Black, male, non-Hispanic children living in urban areas characterized as distressed or at risk. Yet the results also shine a light onto crucial blind spots regarding the context of pediatric firearm injuries due to high levels of missing data in the TQIP database.

The national data infrastructure for nonfatal firearm injury is not currently comprehensive, accessible, or granular enough to provide the information necessary to inform policy and practice, despite the fact that gun violence is a leading national public health problem.[4] The TQIP database is designed to enhance data transparency and provide best-practice guidelines to improve trauma care, offering an opportunity to better understand nonfatal firearm injuries, particularly among children. Yet the data suffer from extensive missingness, which hinders these efforts. For example, using the TQIP data, Flynn-O'Brien et al. found that only about 19% of the injured children had an adverse childhood experience (ACE), despite emerging evidence that ACEs increase risk for firearms exposure.[5] However, most cases in the study (56%) were missing data regarding ACEs, making it difficult to confidently interpret the findings. Roughly half of all cases had missing data on experiences of prior trauma separate from ACEs, past violent assaults and injuries, and prior suicide attempt and self-harm. In cases of assault, the data showed that most children are shot by a stranger, although data were missing for more than one third of all cases. Data were also missing for more than half of all cases concerning the type of firearm used in the injury, largely because of missingness for assault-related injuries. Further, about 64% of the cases had missing data regarding firearm ownership and access in the home, whereas nearly 90% of the data were missing method of firearm storage.

The amount of missing data in the article by Flynn-O'Brien et al. is concerning and makes it challenging to draw strong conclusions about how preinjury and event context influence pediatric firearm injury. Similar problems with missing data have been documented in TQIP data for firearm injuries among adults.[6] As the authors note, "Missingness imposes significant challenges to data interpretability and generalizability, and hampers the ability of researchers to make meaningful and valid conclusions."[2(p1107)] Missingness in the data was found to differ by factors such as intent and designation of

AJPH November 2024, Vol. 114, No. 11

the trauma center reporting data. The authors interpreted their findings about these inconsistencies to reflect differences in available resources for data collection and a care team's level of comfort at asking questions, particularly in the case of assault, where those injured or their families may lack trust in the health care system or have concerns about information being used against them.

How can we fully address gun violence as the leading cause of death among children if we do not have a clear understanding of the problem in the first place? Data fidelity has been a long-standing issue in gun violence research, and this study helps us to know what we don't know.[7] The study underscores data deficiencies in health care settings that influence knowledge about pediatric firearm injury, but it is imperative to consider that incomplete data can also lead to less effective policymaking. For instance, the high level of missing data on ACEs and other contextual factors in the TQIP database could cause policymakers to underestimate the true prevalence of these risk factors among children injured by firearms. This could result in an insufficient allocation of resources for preventive measures to adequately address ACEs, thereby failing to mitigate a root cause of firearm injuries among children.

Collection of data on preinjury and event-level factors related to pediatric firearm injury must be improved to enhance knowledge about the ecological context and proximate firearm behaviors that heighten the risk of children being shot. The present data landscape remains insufficient and disjointed, even as dozens of children are shot with a firearm every day.[8] General surveillance of nonfatal firearm injuries in the United States only began in 2020 and remains limited to 12 states with coarse data granularity. In the absence of accessible public systems, some gun violence researchers who study nonfatal shootings have turned to databases created by nonprofit organizations such as the Gun Violence Archive and newsrooms like The Trace.[9] In light of the concerns highlighted by Flynn-O'Brien et al. about missing data in the trauma center database, researchers should continue to utilize valid data from alternative sources, such as interviews with parents who are firearm owners and national surveys.

However, concurrent efforts should also be made to reduce missingness in the TQIP database. Trauma centers can adopt standardized data collection protocols that include mandatory fields for key variables related to firearm injuries and automated data collection systems that prompt providers to complete missing fields before submission to enhance data completeness. Health care providers must also be trained on the importance of collecting detailed and accurate information, particularly in sensitive cases involving assault. Drawing upon successful models in active public health surveillance, such as the National Violent Death Reporting System, can provide insights into effective strategies for comprehensive data capture and monitoring.

Better data on the risk and protective factors for pediatric firearm injury can inform broader public health efforts to reduce these injuries. For example, child access prevention (CAP) or safe storage laws are designed to prevent children from accessing firearms in the home by requiring firearm owners to lock up their firearms, with penalties for failing to do so. Only 26 states have adopted some type of CAP law, despite strong evidence that they reduce firearm injuries among children.[10] Comprehensive data on the relationship between firearm storage methods and pediatric firearm injury by intent can provide additional evidence to support broadening CAP law coverage around the country. Additionally, recent research shows that people often store firearms insecurely but most are open to considering secure storage to prevent child access.[11] Continued research on why firearm owners store their firearms unsafely and their openness to alternative storage methods can inform tailored messaging and public outreach that reinforces safe storage as a critical means for saving children's lives and preventing injury.[12] The safety of our children should be the nation's top priority, and firearm injuries are preventable. It is our collective responsibility to implement the necessary systems, starting with high-quality data and effective research, to protect them. AJPH

CORRESPONDENCE

Correspondence should be sent to Daniel Semenza, 405-7 Cooper St, Camden, NJ 08102 (e-mail: Daniel.semenza@rutgers.edu). Reprints can be ordered at https://www.ajph.org by clicking the "Reprints" link.

PUBLICATION INFORMATION

Full Citation: Semenza DC. Addressing data deficiencies to prevent pediatric firearm injuries: insights from the American College of Surgeons (ACS) firearm study. *Am J Public Health*. 2024;114(11):1167–1169.

Acceptance Date: July 28, 2024.

DOI: https://doi.org/10.2105/AJPH.2024.307836

ORCID iD:

Daniel C. Semenza https://orcid.org/0000-0002-3843-9559

ACKNOWLEDGMENTS

Thank you to Flynn-O'Brien and colleagues for conducting the important study to which this essay responds.

CONFLICTS OF INTEREST

The author has no conflicts of interest to disclose.

REFERENCES

1. Goldstick JE, Cunningham RM, Carter PM. Current causes of death in children and adolescents in the United States. *N Engl J Med.* 2022;386(20):1955–1956. https://doi.org/10.1056/NEJMc2201761
2. Flynn-O'Brien KT, Sathya C, Kotagal M, et al. Pre-injury and event-related characteristics of pediatric firearm injuries: The American College of Surgeons Firearm Study, United States, March 2021–February 2022. *Am J Public Health.* 2024;114(10):1097–1109. https://doi.org/10.2105/AJPH.2024.307754
3. Andrews AL, Killings X, Oddo ER, Gastineau KA, Hink AB. Pediatric firearm injury mortality epidemiology. *Pediatrics.* 2022;149(3):e2021052739. https://doi.org/10.1542/peds.2021-052739
4. US Surgeon General. Firearm violence: a public health crisis in America. 2024. Available at: https://www.hhs.gov/sites/default/files/firearm-violence-advisory.pdf. Accessed July 8, 2024.
5. Novak A, Semenza D, Gutman C, Heard-Garris N, Testa A, Jackson DB. Adverse childhood experiences and trajectories of firearm exposure in childhood. *J Pediatr.* 2024;270:114008. https://doi.org/10.1016/j.jpeds.2024.114008
6. Rivara FP, Hink AB, Kuhls DA, et al. Firearm injuries treated at trauma centers in the United States. *J Trauma Acute Care Surg.* 2024;96(6):955–964. https://doi.org/10.1097/TA.0000000000004172
7. Roman JK, Cook P. *Improving Data Infrastructure to Reduce Firearms Violence.* Chicago, IL: NORC at the University of Chicago; 2021.
8. Lee LK, Douglas K, Hemenway D. Crossing lines—a change in the leading cause of death among US children. *N Engl J Med.* 2022;386(16):1485–1487. https://doi.org/10.1056/NEJMp2200169
9. Gobaud AN, Mehranbod CA, Kaufman E, et al. Assessing the gun violence archive as an epidemiologic data source for community firearm violence in 4 US cities. *JAMA Netw Open.* 2023;6(6):e2316545. https://doi.org/10.1001/jamanetworkopen.2023.16545
10. Azad HA, Monuteaux MC, Rees CA, et al. Child access prevention firearm laws and firearm fatalities among children aged 0 to 14 years, 1991–2016. *JAMA Pediatr.* 2020;174(5):463–469. https://doi.org/10.1001/jamapediatrics.2019.6227
11. Anestis MD, Moceri-Brooks J, Johnson RL, et al. Assessment of firearm storage practices in the US, 2022. *JAMA Netw Open.* 2023;6(3):e231447. https://doi.org/10.1001/jamanetworkopen.2023.1447
12. Beidas RS, Rivara F, Rowhani-Rahbar A. Safe firearm storage: a call for research informed by firearm stakeholders. *Pediatrics.* 2020;146(5):e20200716. https://doi.org/10.1542/peds.2020-0716

An Agenda for Addressing Health-Harming Legal Needs in Indigenous Communities

Michele Statz, PhD, and Brieanna Watters, MA

ABOUT THE AUTHORS

Michele Statz is with the Department of Family Medicine and Biobehavioral Health, University of Minnesota Medical School, Duluth, and the University of Minnesota Law School, Minneapolis. Brieanna Watters is with the Department of Sociology, University of Minnesota, Minneapolis.

AJPH November 2024, Vol. 114, No. 11

In the United States, unmet civil legal needs are increasingly characterized as "health-harming legal needs."[1] There is a good reason for this: when unresolved, common civil issues such as evictions, domestic violence, child custody, and access to medical benefits have devastating health consequences for individuals and families.[2] Also, research shows that low-income people and communities of color disproportionately experience civil legal problems and their concomitant health and mental health impacts, a reality that both reflects and sustains deep structural inequities in the United States.[3]

Although we might presume that low-income Indigenous people also experience high rates of civil legal needs, data on the civil issues of American Indians and Alaska Natives (AI/ANs) remain problematically limited. For instance, the Legal Services Corporation's Justice Gap report,[4] arguably the most referenced and comprehensive source of data on civil legal needs, fails to mention—let alone collect meaningful data on—AI/ANs. Other familiar sources of data, among them the Pew Charitable Trusts Civil Legal Survey[5] and the 2021 Justice Needs Report,[6] also entirely neglect Indigenous people. This is despite the undisputed correlation between income and legal problems and the fact that the poverty rate among US AI/AN populations (24%) is higher than that of all other racial or ethnic groups.

Although there are smaller entities that collect data on the civil legal needs of Indigenous people, these data are often state specific or pertain to discrete topic areas such as child welfare. As a result, we continue to lack robust, comprehensive data about how Indigenous people in the United States experience health-harming legal needs and, correspondingly, what barriers and opportunities exist to meaningfully address them.

Yet there is still more to this story: even if the aforementioned studies did collect data on Indigenous communities, the methods and structures of prevailing legal needs assessments are overwhelmingly designed by non-Native people with Anglo-adversarial systems in mind. As a result, the typical data collection tools likely do not, and cannot, make visible what is meaningful and logical in Indigenous understandings of justice and health.[7] This reality reflects broader structural inequities, among them the limited Indigenous presence in access to justice (A2J) scholarship and decision making, the "quantitative avoidance"[8] of Indigenous communities by colonizing methodologies, and, crucially, the many missed opportunities to innovate prevailing civil justice delivery models via the expertise and perspectives of Indigenous people.

This editorial emerges from the urgent recognition of the public health implications of continuing to neglect Indigenous A2J in the United States. In what follows, we describe the social and structural determinants of health that are widely associated with Indigenous communities and discuss how these phenomena reflect specific legal needs and research frameworks. Recognizing the consequential interplay of absent data, irrelevant measures, and insufficient A2J support, we look largely outside the United States to highlight Indigenous-driven A2J interventions that reflect the necessary synergy of emergent data, policy, and practice. Also, we put forth recommendations for implementing both system-level and local change to meaningfully expand A2J and address health inequities in AI/AN communities.

THE ACCESS TO JUSTICE CRISIS AND OTHER HEALTH DETERMINANTS

According to the recent Justice Gap report, 74% of all low-income US households experience at least one civil legal need per year, with individuals not receiving any or enough legal help for 92% of these problems. This A2J crisis (i.e., the inability of individuals to obtain the knowledge, tools, and advocacy needed to enforce their rights) is caused by a variety of complex factors. Among them are the cost of legal representation, the limited capacity of free legal aid, negative perceptions of the legal system, and the absence of a right to counsel in civil matters. As a result of these factors, a host of legal issues not only remain unaddressed but are often compounded, further jeopardizing access to shelter, food, safety, family stability, and critical services.

The A2J crisis arguably affects the health of all low-income Americans in some way, including Indigenous people. Yet in Indigenous communities, additional sociospatial and structural determinants of health must be acknowledged. Notably, AI/AN people are disproportionately rural: approximately 29% of Indigenous people in the United States live in rural areas, as compared with 15% of the US population overall. Poverty rates are persistently higher in rural areas than in nonmetropolitan areas (19% and 15%, respectively), and there are increasingly few, if any, rural attorneys. These rural "legal deserts" are now formally recognized as a critical health determinant,[9] and their impacts on A2J are far-reaching in rural Tribal and state courts alike.[10]

Indigenous access to health and justice is also more broadly shaped by the pervasive effects of settler colonialism, or the ongoing exclusion, assimilation, and dehumanization of Indigenous people to legitimize non-Indigenous control over Native land and resources. Although we cannot sufficiently explore the extent of settler colonialism—including how it is differently navigated and resisted across diverse Sovereign nations—its impacts on health and legal outcomes are self-evident.

We know, for instance, that the persistent socioeconomic and political marginalization of Indigenous peoples has resulted in disproportionately high rates of racial and gendered violence, historical and transgenerational trauma, and postcolonial distress.[11] Indigenous people are overrepresented at every stage of the criminal legal system, from victimization to imprisonment.[12] And more broadly, federal Indian law actively undermines Indigenous political and cultural sovereignty by limiting access to land and water, cultural practices, and community safety. All of these factors, including heightened exposure to the criminal legal system and federal Indian law itself, are recognized as structural determinants of health.[13,14]

DOMINANT METHODOLOGIES AND WISE METHODOLOGIES

Even as scholars increasingly acknowledge the complex interplay of health and justice and how settler colonialism shapes Indigenous experiences within these systems, there remains a profound dearth of data around Indigenous A2J. Moreover, when data are collected, the methodologies employed typically prioritize Western institutions and research frameworks.

In the United States, for instance, prevailing legal needs assessments are largely designed with Anglo-adversarial justice systems in mind, thereby sustaining what Wanda D. McCaslin and Denise C. Breton describe as "'norms' that were never ours and do not fit us."[15] The positivist emphasis on "fair" or "objective" proves largely incompatible with Indigenous methodologies that prioritize context, relationality, and lived reality,[16] and we are left with data, measures, and A2J initiatives that fail to reflect the diverse values of Indigenous people and perpetuate alienating policies and funding priorities.

We ask the following in response: how might the health-harming legal needs of Indigenous people be meaningfully documented and addressed, acknowledging critical differences across Sovereign nations as well as shared experiences of colonization and marginalization? Critically, answers to this question exist, both within the robust body of literature on Indigenous research methods[17,18] and in A2J programs in the settler colonial nations of Canada, Australia, Aotearoa–New Zealand, and the United States. As we demonstrate subsequently, these models are upheld by Indigenous people and values and are actively informed by sound, community-relevant data collection and evaluation. Reflecting the turn from "best practices" to "wise practices,"[19] these models reassert and integrate locally situated belief systems, teachings, and healing practices into diverse legal settings.

These models include the Indigenous Legal Needs Project in Australia, in which research is conducted alongside community-based legal services to foster a more contextualized approach to Indigenous A2J. This approach has led to robust interprofessional partnerships between Aboriginal-controlled health services and legal service providers and to the training of First Nations community health workers to provide trusted legal advocacy.[20] Another example is Te Ao Mārama, an Aotearoa district court model that advances A2J and Māori self-determination via *Kaupapa Māori*, or the incorporation of Māori cultural protocols, knowledge, and participation.[21] Notably, the Te Ao Mārama model is expected to differ somewhat from place to place, ensuring that it accurately incorporates and reflects the different strengths of local communities.

AJPH November 2024, Vol. 114, No. 11

Other models include the Community Justice Worker program in Alaska, which trains individuals already embedded within Tribal agencies to provide targeted civil legal assistance and direct representation in court.[22] The development and advancement of this program have occurred in tandem with collaborative research that employs Indigenous methodologies and data sovereignty to identify the values, needs, and expectations of clients and other community members.

Finally, the Aboriginal Healing Foundation in Canada represented an Indigenous-led initiative to address intergenerational trauma through community-engaged research and resource development. Although no longer in existence, we include the Foundation because it directly involved Aboriginal people in the design, implementation, and assessment of programs that prevented or addressed health-harming legal needs, including culturally appropriate mental health services, 24-hour safe houses for survivors of abuse, and protocols for intervening in family violence situations.[23]

Taken together, these models demonstrate that expanding Indigenous A2J is fundamental in addressing health inequities among Indigenous peoples. They further evidence that this can be done, and evaluated, in a deeply relevant way. (Additional information about these models is provided in the Appendix, available as a supplement to the online version of this article at http://www.ajph.org.)

CONCRETE RECOMMENDATIONS FOR CHANGE

Health and justice are inextricably connected: unresolved civil issues compound medical problems, and vice versa. Yet even as there is increasing recognition of health-harming legal needs in the United States, we know considerably less about what issues are experienced in Indigenous communities, why, and how or whether these needs are resolved in a way that matters to Indigenous people themselves.

As we have shown here, Indigenous people in the United States experience complicated and distinct health determinants, many of which are rooted in the ongoing legacies of settler colonialism and uniquely implicate place, law, and justice. Although social science and medicine, and particularly Indigenous scholars within these fields, continue to rigorously demonstrate these complexities, Indigenous experiences are consistently neglected in A2J scholarship and policy.

This editorial serves as a modest starting point, challenging prevailing A2J metrics, outcomes, and conventional forms of assistance and acknowledging the multiple justice systems with which Indigenous people in the United States and other nations such as Canada, Australia, and Aotearoa–New Zealand regularly interact. We further recognize that there are approximately 400 Tribal courts in the United States, each a unique manifestation of Tribal sovereignty, addressing issues ranging from traditional dispute resolution to Anglo-adversarial models. The A2J programs and practices discussed here reflect these complex and locally situated realities. Drawing inspiration from these models, we offer several recommendations.

Address Marginalization in Data Collection

At best, dominant A2J data collection paradigms, policies, and funding priorities in the United States largely neglect the experiences and health contexts of Indigenous people within the civil justice system. At worst, they wholly undermine Indigenous A2J, perpetuating the marginalization and disenfranchisement of Indigenous communities. In response, we have highlighted Kaupapa Māori and the principles of ownership, control, access, and possession as examples of A2J data collection that are consistently informed by the diverse values, priorities, and expertise of Indigenous people and places. Adjusting research in this way will necessarily impact what—or whose—research questions are prioritized, what methods are chosen, whose experiences count, how data are managed and analyzed, and what policy and funding decisions are made.

Promote Community-Driven and Sovereign Initiatives

As evidenced in Australia and Aotearoa–New Zealand, community-driven and collaborative approaches must be central to A2J initiatives in Indigenous communities. Active participation from Tribal leaders, legal organizations, courts, community health centers, and other Tribal stakeholders ensures that Indigenous values and priorities inform nascent and long-term efforts. This approach is fundamental to decolonizing prevailing A2J norms and models.[24]

In addition, a tailored approach respecting the diverse backgrounds and circumstances of AI/AN communities is crucial. As in the mindful design of Te Ao Mārama, A2J initiatives should exhibit flexibility and acknowledge the distinct legal needs, cultural practices, challenges, and available resources within each Indigenous context. This increases the potential to address the unique health-harming legal needs of diverse Indigenous groups. Moreover, this attention facilitates trust and rapport with Indigenous communities, rendering legal and health services more accessible and effective by aligning them with the expectations of the individuals they serve.

Advance Interprofessional Approaches

A collaborative approach to Indigenous A2J must also involve diverse professionals, including community health workers, traditional healers, paralegals, social service providers, and so on. As demonstrated by the community justice worker model, the knowledge held by diverse individuals embedded in local institutions can provide salient advocacy, issue spotting, and practice insights. These individuals observe daily the urgent intersections of health and justice and are often most prepared, trusted, and willing to provide targeted assistance. By employing a comprehensive approach that encompasses both legal and nonlegal services, these initiatives recognize the complex nature of health-harming legal needs and address the underlying causes of health disparities faced by Indigenous individuals.

Move Beyond "Needs" and "Outcomes"

Although the models we have profiled offer compelling and replicable insights, many of these programs operate with inadequate resources or were shuttered owing to funding and policy changes. This significantly impacts the communities involved and poses a major obstacle to gathering comprehensive evaluative data, leaving our understanding of a program's potential incomplete. Therefore, we call for robust and sustained financial and policy backing from legal institutions, research entities, governmental bodies, and professional associations. Diverse stakeholder buy-in is essential.

We also recognize that prevailing A2J metrics are themselves limiting, often focusing narrowly on legal problems, costs, and case outcomes within Anglo-adversarial justice systems. Accordingly, we advocate for wise practices and evaluative measures of success that reflect the values and dimensions of access, health, and justice that matter to the community at hand. Indigenous methodologies remind us that these evaluative metrics must be expansive enough to honor an A2J initiative's ability to reveal knowledge, build relationships, rebalance power, honor sovereignty, and provide healing. This requires deep trust and concordance between everyone involved. And it is precisely why data collection, analysis, and evaluation must be driven by Indigenous experts in all contexts—local, scholarly, legal, and so on—and enacted in close, often interprofessional collaboration with Indigenous and non-Indigenous stakeholders. These steps are fundamental to self-determination.

Honor Indigenous Access to Justice as Health and Healing

As evidenced here, any A2J initiative undertaken in an Indigenous community must meaningfully recognize historical injustices and their continued impact on the health and legal needs of AI/AN people, particularly the intergenerational trauma resulting from forced assimilation policies, land dispossession, and systemic discrimination. This is precisely why Te Ao Mārama holistically acknowledges litigants' legal needs as well as their well-being within the court context. By actively working to address intergenerational trauma, Indigenous A2J models promote healing, prevent future health-harming legal needs, and empower Indigenous communities to advance their rights and well-being. We also recognize that providing training and resources to elevate Indigenous community members as community justice workers or legal advocates exemplifies a commitment to capacity building and self-determination.

As we have demonstrated here, understanding and addressing civil legal needs in Indigenous communities has profound impacts on community health. But it has to be done well. Drawing on the Anishinaabe concept of *Mino Bimaadiziwin*, we end this article by calling for Indigenous A2J research, analysis, and innovation done in a good way, one that reveals knowledge, decolonizes and rebalances power, creates relationships, and provides healing through culturally safe, relevant, and collaborative modalities as defined by Indigenous people themselves.[25] AJPH

CORRESPONDENCE

Correspondence should be sent to Michele Statz, PhD, University of Minnesota Medical School, 1035 University Dr, Duluth, MN 55812 (e-mail: mstatz@d.umn.edu). Reprints can be ordered at https://www.ajph.org by clicking the "Reprints" link.

PUBLICATION INFORMATION

Full Citation: Statz M, Watters B. An agenda for addressing health-harming legal needs in Indigenous communities. *Am J Public Health*. 2024; 114(11):1170–1174.

Acceptance Date: June 17, 2024.

DOI: https://doi.org/10.2105/AJPH.2024.307774

ORCID iD:
Michele Statz https://orcid.org/0000-0002-2497-5828

CONTRIBUTORS

Both authors conceptualized, drafted, and edited the article.

ACKNOWLEDGMENTS

We gratefully acknowledge the commitment and transformative work of the Tribal court personnel with whom we collaborate. We also recognize the institutional support of the Research for Indigenous Social Action and Equity Center at Northwestern University.

CONFLICTS OF INTEREST

The authors disclose no conflicts of interest.

REFERENCES

1. Cannon Y. Unmet legal needs as health injustice. Available at: https://scholarship.law.georgetown.edu/facpub/2394. Accessed November 6, 2023.
2. Genn H. When law is good for your health: mitigating the social determinants of health through access to justice. *Curr Leg Probl.* 2019;72(1):159–202. https://doi.org/10.1093/clp/cuz003
3. Cannon Y. Closing the health justice gap: access to justice in furtherance of health equity. Available at: https://scholarship.law.georgetown.edu/facpub/2394. Accessed November 6, 2023.
4. Legal Services Corporation. The justice gap: the unmet civil legal needs of low-income Americans. Available at: https://justicegap.lsc.gov. Accessed November 6, 2023.
5. SSRS. Pew Charitable Trusts Civil Legal Survey: topline report. Available at: https://www.pewtrusts.org/-/media/assets/2019/04/survey-topline-report.pdf. Accessed November 6, 2023.
6. Hague Institute for Innovation of Law. Justice needs and satisfaction in the United States of America. Available at: https://perma.cc/P6VU-VL82. Accessed November 6, 2023.
7. Simonds VW, Christopher S. Adapting Western research methods to Indigenous ways of knowing. *Am J Public Health.* 2013;103(12):2185–2192. https://doi.org/10.2105/AJPH.2012.301157
8. Walter M, Suina M. Indigenous data, Indigenous methodologies and Indigenous data sovereignty. *Int J Soc Res Methodol.* 2018;22(3):233–243. https://doi.org/10.1080/13645579.2018.1531228.
9. Statz M, Termuhlen P. Rural legal deserts are a critical health determinant. *Am J Public Health.* 2020;110(10):1519–1522. https://doi.org/10.2105/AJPH.2020.305807
10. Statz M. On shared suffering: judicial intimacy in the rural northland. *Law Soc Rev.* 2021;55(1):5–37. https://doi.org/10.1111/lasr.12537
11. Smallwood R, Woods C, Power T, Usher K. Understanding the impact of historical trauma due to colonization on the health and well-being of Indigenous young peoples: a systematic scoping review. *J Transcult Nurs.* 2021;32(1):59–68. https://doi.org/10.1177/1043659620935955
12. Cunneen C, Tauri JM. Indigenous peoples, criminology, and criminal justice. *Annu Rev Criminol.* 2019;2:359–381. https://doi.org/10.1146/annurev-criminol-011518-024630
13. LeMasters K, Renson A, Edwards JK, et al. Inequities in life course criminal legal system sanctions: measuring cumulative involvement. *Ann Epidemiol.* 2022;76:83–90. https://doi.org/10.1016/j.annepidem.2022.10.007
14. Hoss A. Federal Indian law as a structural determinant of health. *J Law Med Ethics.* 2019;47(4):34–42. https://doi.org/10.1177/1073110519898041
15. McCaslin WD, Breton DC. Justice as healing: going outside the colonizer's cage. In: Denzin NK, Lincoln YS, Smith LT, eds. *Handbook of Critical and Indigenous Methodologies.* Newbury Park, CA: Sage Publications; 2008:511–530. https://doi.org/10.4135/9781483385686.n26
16. Flicker S, O'Campo P, Monchalin R, et al. Research done in "a good way": the importance of indigenous elder involvement in HIV community-based research. *Am J Public Health.* 2015;105(6):1149–1154. https://doi.org/10.2105/AJPH.2014.302522
17. Denzin NK, Lincoln YS, Smith LT. *Handbook of Critical and Indigenous Methodologies.* Newbury Park, CA: Sage Publications; 2008. https://doi.org/10.4135/9781483385686
18. Chilisa B. *Indigenous Research Methodologies.* Vol 2. Newbury Park, CA: Sage Publications; 2020.
19. Nabigon H, Wenger-Nabigon A. Wise practices: integrating traditional teachings with mainstream treatment approaches. *Native Soc Work J.* 2012;8(1):43–55. Available at: https://www.collectionscanada.gc.ca/obj/thesescanada/vol2/OSUL/TC-OSUL-1981.pdf. Accessed December 1, 2024.
20. James Cook University. Indigenous Legal Needs Project. Available at: https://www.jcu.edu.au/indigenous-legal-needs-project/about. Accessed November 6, 2023.
21. Fa'amatuainu B. Self-represented litigation and meaningful access to justice in Aotearoa and Samoa. *AlterNative Int J Indig Peoples.* 2023;19(1):13–22. https://doi.org/10.1177/11771801221145843
22. Stremple C. Nonattorney advocates to represent Alaskans in court under new waiver. Available at: https://alaskabeacon.com/briefs/nonattorney-advocates-can-represent-alaskans-in-court-under-a-new-waiver. Accessed November 6, 2023.
23. Aboriginal Healing Foundation. Funded projects. Available at: https://www.ahf.ca/funded-projects. Accessed November 6, 2023.
24. Cochran PAL, Marshall CA, Garcia-Downing C, et al. Indigenous ways of knowing: implications for participatory research and community. *Am J Public Health.* 2008;98(1):22–27. https://doi.org/10.2105/AJPH.2006.093641
25. Denis JS, Duhaime G, Newhouse D. Indigenous conceptions of well-being: rejecting poverty, pursuing Mino-Bimaadiziwin. *J Aborig Econ Dev.* 2017;10(2):124–146. https://doi.org/10.29173/jaed387

Beyond Stigma: The Case Against the Criminalization of Sex Work for HIV Prevention and Health Equity

Tyler Cochran, JD, Leah Smith, MPA, Kara Ayers, PhD, and Maureen van Stone, MS, JD

ABOUT THE AUTHORS

Tyler Cochran is with the Maryland Center for Developmental Disabilities, Kennedy Krieger Institute, Baltimore. Leah Smith is with Cincinnati Children's Hospital Medical Center, Ohio. Kara Ayer is with Cincinnati Children's Hospital Medical Center, and University of Cincinnati, College of Medicine, Ohio. Maureen van Stone is with Maryland Center for Developmental Disabilities, Kennedy Krieger Institute, and The Department of Mental Health, Johns Hopkins Bloomberg School of Public Health, Baltimore.

The Joint United Nations Program on HIV/AIDS (UNAIDS) set a goal to record zero new HIV infections globally by 2030. Currently, more than one million new HIV infections are recorded annually.[1] As world governments and policymakers mobilize to pursue this goal, evidence suggests that among the most impactful policy changes in reducing HIV incidence is the decriminalization of sex work,[2] largely because of the disproportionate incidence of HIV infection among sex workers; for example, UNAIDS reports that female sex workers are 30 times more likely to become HIV-positive relative to the overall female population.[3]

However, a way forward remains: mathematical models from Imperial College London estimate that ending the criminalization of all aspects of sex work would prevent between 33% and 46% of global new HIV infections in sex workers and their clients—both of which are key populations particularly vulnerable to HIV infection.[4] Indeed, many experts argue that the total decriminalization of sex work would, "have a greater effect on the course of the HIV epidemic than any other structural intervention," by increasing key linkages to care and social support networks for sex workers living with HIV, as well as reducing the incidence of HIV infections for sex workers, their clients, and their clients' sexual networks.[5(p356)] Note that this essay will discuss evidence regarding both the decriminalization of sex work, meaning that consenting adults who are buying or selling sex are not committing a crime, and the legalization of sex work, which creates an affirmative regulatory scheme that creates rules governing the sale of sex between consenting adults.[6]

For the purposes of this article, sex work will be defined broadly, using the working definition put forward by Decriminalize Sex Work, a national organization that advocates the human rights of sex workers: "Sex work is the exchange of sexual services (sex, erotic dancing, pornography, etc.) for money or something of value."[7]

It is vital to note, however, that scholars and activists operationalize and define the broad category of sex work differently, and that works cited throughout will have slightly different operationalizations of the types of behavior included as sex work. Different forms of sex work present different levels of risk for HIV acquisition and violence. In-person forms of sex work most directly expose the worker to HIV and other sexually transmitted infections (STIs).

GLOBAL CONTEXT OF SEX WORK CRIMINALIZATION, VIOLENCE, AND HIV

Data demonstrate that punitive laws targeting sex workers and their clients are associated with increased rates of HIV infection among sex workers: sex workers who work in a jurisdiction that criminalizes sex work have a 7.7 times higher chance of acquiring HIV compared with sex workers who work in a jurisdiction that partially legalizes sex work.[3] Furthermore, evidence suggests that sex work–related stigma is higher in jurisdictions that criminalize sex work. Increased stigma leaves sex workers at a higher risk for contracting HIV, lowers their access to care and treatment, and leads to them being acutely vulnerable to violence and arrest.[8]

Violence as Key Driver of HIV Infection

One key driver of the disproportionate HIV infection rates of sex workers is the

AJPH November 2024, Vol. 114, No. 11

disproportionate levels of violence that sex workers experience.[8] A global systemic review of the relationship between legislation criminalizing sex work and HIV and other STIs outcomes points to the role of repressive policing in jurisdictions that criminalize sex work.[9] Sex workers who were exposed to repressive police activity, including extortion, blackmail, and physical and sexual violence perpetrated by police, had twice the likelihood of acquiring HIV and twice the likelihood of experiencing further physical and sexual violence at the hands of clients, police, and others, in comparison with sex workers who were not exposed to repressive policing.[9]

Across studies, up to 75% of adult female sex workers are assaulted or abused at least once in their lifetime.[3] Evidence suggests that criminalizing sex work contributes to sociocultural environments where sex workers are acutely vulnerable to HIV infection, as well as physical and sexual violence perpetrated not only by clients and partners but also at the hands of police, health workers, and other government officials who exploit the marginalization of sex workers in criminalized settings.[9]

Intersecting Marginalized Identities

When accounting for intersectional identities, the impacts of criminalization, marginalization, and stigma on violence and HIV transmission rates becomes even clearer. In a study conducted in Guatemala, men who have sex with men (MSM) sex workers and transgender sex workers were more than six times more likely to experience forced sex than MSMs and transgender people who are not sex workers.[8] Transgender sex workers in particular experienced higher levels of discrimination and physical violence than MSM, including MSM who participate in sex work.[8] This research indicates that identities and vulnerabilities do not exist in a vacuum: people with overlapping marginalized identities, including MSM and transgender sex workers, have a higher risk of both experiencing violence and acquiring HIV.

For disabled sex workers, this risk likely compounds upon existing vulnerabilities as well: people with disabilities are more than twice as likely to experience violence compared with people without disabilities,[10] and the HIV infection rate among people with disabilities is up to three times higher than among nondisabled people,[11] independent of any other factors such as engagement in sex work.

Researchers have concluded that the criminalization of sex work is a root cause of violence and marginalization experienced by sex workers, while also limiting sex workers' visibility, which limits research across settings.[8] Because of the limitations on robust research on the associations between sex work, violence, and HIV acquisition, further work needs to be done to develop better means to engage with sex worker communities for mutually beneficial research. It is clear, however, that the criminalization of sex work contributes to higher risks of death, HIV infection, physical and sexual violence, and abuse at the hands of police and health care workers, yet also pushes sex workers to the margins of society where they are less able to access safe and appropriate care.

UNAIDS's Evidence-Informed Recommendations

Responding to this ever-growing body of evidence, UNAIDS recommends that all member states take critical actions to protect sex workers. Their recommendations include, in part,

> Countries should implement evidence-informed responses to HIV and sex work that reduce inequalities and protect and promote human rights and public health. . . . Critical actions include ending the criminalization of all aspects of sex work, including the purchase, sale and management of sex work; extending labor protections; protecting sex workers from state and private actor violence; and ending stigma and discrimination.[1(p1)]

Despite this recommendation, many countries, including the United States, continue to criminalize sex work, increasing sex work–related stigma, risk of acquiring HIV, and vulnerability to violence and abuse.

CRIMINALIZATION OF SEX WORK IN THE UNITED STATES

Every jurisdiction in the United States criminalizes sex work.[12] Thirty states have laws that explicitly target people with HIV (such as laws that criminalize failure to disclose one's HIV status to one's sexual partners) or use sentence enhancements that add additional punishments for people with HIV committing certain crimes compared with people without HIV.[13] Many of these states punish sex workers with HIV more severely than sex workers without HIV, regardless of whether an individual has undetectable levels of HIV in their body, and is therefore unable to transmit HIV, or if they have taken steps to protect themself and their clients from exposure to HIV and other STIs.[12]

Florida's sentence enhancement statute is as an example: offering to exchange sex for any form of resources is punishable by up to 60 days of incarceration. However, if a person with HIV is alleged to have offered sex in exchange for resources, they can instead be charged with a felony punished by a five-year period of incarceration.[12] Notably, these types of charges do not require any actual exposure to HIV—merely the suggestion that a person might engage in sex work, often regardless of whether one's HIV status was disclosed, can lead to a person being arrested, lengthy imprisonment, and a felony criminal record.[12]

Instead of promoting condom use and adherence to antiretrovirals to promote public health, some jurisdictions use possession of condoms as evidence of intent to solicit or as evidence of a sex worker's knowledge of their HIV status.[12] Such penalties disincentivize sex workers to carry condoms, directly endangering the sexual health of both sex workers and their clients by reducing access to key means of risk reduction.

Mandatory Testing Upon Arrest

Another key intersection of HIV, sex work, and criminal law in the United States is the prevalence of mandatory HIV testing requirements upon arrest for solicitation or engaging in sex work. Multiple states mandate that a person arrested for alleged prostitution or solicitation offenses undergo HIV testing.[12] Unlike HIV testing voluntarily undertaken in a clinical setting— where informed consent is required, results are strictly confidential, and a person may elect to withdraw consent for testing at any time—states such as Connecticut, Michigan, Ohio, and Tennessee authorize law enforcement officials and judges to mandate that a detained person undergo a "venereal examination" upon arrest for an alleged sex work–related offense.[5] Such testing occurs before the person is convicted of any crime.

The results of such tests can often be used to support prosecution under the HIV criminalization laws discussed previously—either because the relevant statute authorizes such use, or because it fails to clearly identify such information as confidential and not to be used in prosecution. HIV testing of alleged sex workers upon arrest is, "not performed to protect their health but rather to establish a basis for prosecution and incarceration" serving to push sex workers further to the margins.[12(p3)]

CONCLUSION

Laws that criminalize sex work increase sex workers' vulnerability to violence and likelihood of developing an HIV infection, while directly contravening UNAIDS recommendations calling for the decriminalization of sex work. If the priority of public health policymakers is to enhance access to lifesaving care for people with HIV and to decrease the rate of new HIV infections to zero, the decriminalization of all aspects of sex work is likely the most effective place to start. AJPH

CORRESPONDENCE

Correspondence should be sent to Tyler Cochran, 716 N Broadway, Baltimore, MD 21205 (e-mail: tyler.cochran13@alumni.stanford.edu). Reprints can be ordered at https://www.ajph.org by clicking the "Reprints" link.

PUBLICATION INFORMATION

Full Citation: Cochran T, Smith L, Ayers K, van Stone M. Beyond stigma: the case against the criminalization of sex work for HIV prevention and health equity. *Am J Public Health*. 2024;114(11):1175–1178.

Acceptance Date: June 26, 2024.

https://doi.org/10.2105/AJPH.2024.307782

ORCID iD:

Tyler Cochran https://orcid.org/0009-0009-5611-4123

CONTRIBUTORS

T. Cochran and L. Smith created the first draft of this editorial. K. Ayers and M. van Stone helped rewrite it into what it is today.

ACKNOWLEDGMENTS

This article was completed in part through funding from the Administration for Community Living (90NCDE001) as a product of the National Center for Disability, Equity, and Intersectionality, a Project of National Significance.

The authors would like to acknowledge the work of Tracy Waller, JD, MPH, who provided both line and citation edits.

CONFLICTS OF INTEREST

The authors have no potential or actual conflicts of interest to report.

REFERENCES

1. UNAIDS. HIV and sex work. Human Rights Fact Sheets Series. 2021. Available at: https://www.unaids.org/sites/default/files/media_asset/05-hiv-human-rights-factsheet-sex-work_en.pdf. Accessed August 28, 2023.
2. Lyons CE, Schwartz SR, Murray SM, et al. The role of sex work laws and stigmas in increasing HIV risks among sex workers. *Nat Commun*. 2020; 11(1):773. https://doi.org/10.1038/s41467-020-14593-6
3. UNAIDS. Fact sheet: global HIV statistics. 2020. Available at: https://www.aidsdatahub.org/sites/default/files/resource/unaids-2020-global-aids-factsheets.pdf. Accessed August 28, 2023.
4. Wong S. Decriminalising sex work would cut HIV infections by a third. Imperial College London. July 24, 2014. Available at: https://www.imperial.ac.uk/news/154368/decriminalising-work-would-hiv-infections-third. Accessed August 28, 2023.
5. Baskin S, Ahmed A, Forbes A. Criminal laws on sex work and HIV transmission: mapping the laws, considering the consequences. *Denver Law Review*. 2016; 93(2):355–388. https://digitalcommons.du.edu/cgi/viewcontent.cgi?article=1071&context=dlr&_sm_nck=1
6. Decriminalize Sex Work. What about legalization of prostitution? 2020. Available at: https://decriminalizesex.work/why-decriminalization/briefing-papers/decriminalization-is-the-only-solution. Accessed May 17, 2024.
7. Decriminalize Sex Work. Why decriminalization of sex work. 2024. Available at: https://decriminalizesex.work/why-decriminalization. Accessed May 17, 2024.
8. Viswasam N, Schwartz S, Baral S. Characterizing the role of intersecting stigmas and sustained inequities in driving HIV syndemics across low- and middle-income settings. *Curr Opin HIV AIDS*.

2020;15(4):243–249. https://doi.org/10.1097/COH.0000000000000630

9. Platt L, Grenfell P, Meiksin R, et al. Associations between sex work laws and sex workers' health: a systematic review and meta-analysis of quantitative and qualitative studies. *PLoS Med.* 2018; 15(12):e1002680. https://doi.org/10.1371/journal.pmed.1002680
10. Office for Victims of Crime. Crimes against people with disabilities. 2018 National Crime Victims' Rights Week Resource Guide: Crime and Victimization Fact Sheets. Available at: https://ovc.ojp.gov/sites/g/files/xyckuh226/files/ncvrw2018/info_flyers/fact_sheets/2018NCVRW_VictimsWithDisabilities_508_QC.pdf. Accessed August 28, 2023.
11. Human Rights Watch. Fact sheet: HIV/AIDS and disability. June 8, 2011. Available at: https://www.hrw.org/news/2011/06/08/fact-sheet-hiv/aids-and-disability. Accessed August 28, 2023.
12. The National LGBTQ Taskforce and The Center for HIV Law and Policy. The intersection of sex work and criminalization: an advocate's toolkit. 2017. Available at: https://www.hivlawandpolicy.org/sites/default/files/Sex%20Work%20HIV%20Toolkit%20FINAL%20R2.pdf. Accessed August 28, 2023.
13. The Center for Law and HIV Policy. *HIV Criminalization in the United States.* 2022. Available at: https://www.hivlawandpolicy.org/sites/default/files/2024-01/HIV%20Criminalization%20in%20the%20U.S.%20A%20Sourcebook%20on%20State%20Fed%20HIV%20Criminal%20Law%20and%20Practice%20Jan24.pdf. Accessed May 17, 2024.

HIV Prevention in Foster Care Youths: Time for a Refocus

Casey W. Adrian, MSW, Stacey L. Shipe, PhD, MSc, MSW, and Kate Guastaferro, PhD, MPH

ABOUT THE AUTHORS

Casey W. Adrian is with the Bronfenbrenner Center for Translational Research, Cornell University, Ithaca, NY. Stacey L. Shipe is with the Department of Social Work, Binghamton University, Binghamton, NY. Kate Guastaferro is with the Department of Social and Behavioral Sciences, New York University, New York, NY.

Youths entering foster care have approximately the same rates of sexually transmitted infections as the general population of their peers.[1] Yet once in foster care and after emancipation, foster youths face a risk of sexually transmitted infection that is three to 14 times that of their nonfoster peers.[2] Indeed, during their time in the system, foster youths are disproportionately affected by HIV.[3] This indicates that foster youths could uniquely benefit from biomedical methods of HIV prevention (e.g., preexposure prophylaxis [PrEP]), which, over the past decade, have become a cornerstone of prevention strategies. The shift toward biomedical approaches to HIV prevention offers a way to supplement existing behavioral strategies with medically effective interventions. If taken as directed, PrEP can reduce the risk of contracting HIV through sex by 99%.[4] Yet as recently as 2021, data suggested that only 20% of people aged 16 to 24 years who could benefit from PrEP were prescribed the medication.[5] And despite their disproportionate risk of HIV infection, virtually nothing is known about how or if adolescents in the foster care system are accessing PrEP.

This gap in research stands in contrast to other sexual and reproductive health concerns facing foster youths. For instance, a small body of literature exists regarding family planning among foster adolescents, including information on how these particular young people access contraception and abortion services.[6] Lacking, however, is any mention of biomedical HIV prevention strategies within this population. In 2019, the Centers for Disease Control and Prevention (CDC) declared the goal of eliminating new HIV infections in the United States by 2030.[7] A key piece of this strategic plan involves expanding PrEP access to those with the highest need; specifically, of all people who could benefit from PrEP, 50% should be prescribed the medication by 2025.[7] If the goal of national HIV elimination is to be achieved, focus on PrEP access among this disproportionately affected population of adolescents is paramount.

DIMENSIONS OF PREEXPOSURE PROPHYLAXIS ACCESS

To create a taxonomical definition of access, Penchansky and Thomas[8] developed a framework to operationally measure the concept. The authors proposed that access is a measure of fitness between the characteristics of providers and health services and the characteristics and expectations of consumers. Penchansky and Thomas suggested five independent yet interconnected dimensions of access: accommodation (an organization's ability to adequately provide services); accessibility (proximity to consumer); availability (sufficient number and types of services); acceptability (consumer perceptions of services, including relevant social and cultural factors); and affordability (financial cost).[8] By this definition, nearly all adolescents face barriers to PrEP access. However, given their many unique lived and legal experiences, it is likely that adolescents in foster care face additional obstacles when attempting to access PrEP. These obstacles can be demonstrated through examining closely related and intersecting considerations.

Accommodation and Accessibility

For medications such as PrEP, parental consent laws vary widely between states. Although minors may consent to HIV testing and treatment in all 50 states and the District of Columbia, only 33 jurisdictions explicitly allow minors to consent independently to HIV prevention services; of these, only 18 specify confidentiality protections.[9] Whereas minors in other states may be able to consent to prevention services under the umbrella of testing and treatment, because of the ambiguous language within state policies, determining where or how youths can access PrEP, in addition to determining confidentiality protections, remains elusive.[9]

Several studies have highlighted that medical providers are more likely to prescribe PrEP if they are confident that the adolescent patient will receive and take the medication as intended.[10] However, for foster youths who experience frequent changes in foster placement, disruptions to routine preventative care are common[11]; this would require foster youths to reestablish PrEP care with several providers, and could lead to missing or incomplete medical documentation.[11] Indeed, medical providers are often unsure of their role in providing medical care to foster youths,[11] and there is a lack of studies examining how providers navigate ambiguous policies and changing foster placements to provide foster youths with consistent PrEP care. Given these factors, practitioners may feel unsure when providing PrEP to foster youths, and instead simply choose not to provide this population with such preventative care. This highlights how respective dimensions of accommodation and accessibility could uniquely intersect as a barrier for foster youths.

Availability

In states that do not allow minors to consent to prevention services, federally funded Title X clinics are able to override state policies and provide these services.[12] However, following federal regulations on Title X funding in 2020, many clinics began to publicly withdraw from Title X—including nearly all Planned Parenthood locations—to preserve their existing services, meaning that these could no longer meet the particular needs of adolescents without parental consent. Although evidence-based Title X guidelines were reenacted in late 2021 and many clinics reapplied for funding, this period of Title X withdrawal has had lasting impacts. States without minor consent laws saw a 29.7% decrease in Title X–funded clinics, leaving many minors with a prolonged lack of access to confidential sexual health services.[12] For a minor attempting to navigate fluctuating medicolegal landscapes without the help of a caregiver, understanding these complex policies could be daunting and exacerbate barriers to accessing care.

Acceptability

Youths in foster care face an additional obstacle related to acceptability. For foster youths who live in jurisdictions where parental consent is required, the identified parent is the state (i.e., their foster care caseworker), meaning that the young person must contact their state-appointed caseworker for permission.[13] For youths in an independent living or congregate care setting, in which they may only engage with their foster care worker once a month, the rapport needed for these sensitive discussions may not be established.

Affordability

In the event that a minor is able to access treatment and chooses to do so, they must also pay for the medication. All 50 states' Medicaid programs cover PrEP medication and care[14]; this is advantageous for foster youths, nearly all of whom are categorically eligible for Medicaid coverage.[15] However, any adolescent seeking PrEP treatment—either through Medicaid or using private insurance from a caregiver—would have an explanation of benefits (EOB) sent to their home address. This compromises confidentiality of services, a consequence that may jeopardize the safety and well-being of some minors. This could be particularly problematic for foster youths, who may be unaware of who will receive an EOB—or lack a relationship with the person receiving such information. Some states have passed legislation giving minors the ability to request private communication, such as having an EOB sent directly to the patient rather than the policyholder,[16] although this is not a universally available option. Regardless of ability to consent to PrEP-related care, issues of affordability and acceptability still serve as significant barriers for all young people, with nuances that are particularly troublesome for foster youths.

PRIORITIZING HIV PREVENTION STRATEGIES FOR FOSTER YOUTHS

When considering vulnerable populations and access to preventative care, a spotlight on foster youths showcases the unique barriers that these young people endure. Foster youths, compared with the general population of their peers, report higher rates of casual or transactional sex and are more likely to have sex without a condom.[2] Lesbian, gay, and bisexual (LGB) youths of color—including Black young men who have sex with men (YMSM), who account for 53% of all new HIV infections among those aged 13 to 24 years[17]—are overrepresented in the foster care system, and experience consistently higher rates of substance misuse or sexual health concerns than their non-LGB counterparts.[18] With each of these compounding factors, many adolescents in foster care stand at the intersection of several marginalized and particularly at-risk groups. Despite this, it can be inferred that barriers to PrEP access are exacerbated during their time in the foster care system.

To address the sexual health needs of adolescents in foster care, all five dimensions of Penchansky and Thomas'[8] concept of access must be examined in the context of PrEP-related care: availability, accessibility, accommodation, affordability, and acceptability. To understand how and if adolescents in foster care are accessing this important biomedical HIV prevention strategy, the perspectives and actions across researchers, public health professionals, medical providers, and policymakers are necessary.

Researchers

Given the protected status of foster youths, research on their sexual activity and sexual health includes several methodological and ethical roadblocks. In the 1990s, access to experimental HIV medication among foster children resulted in fear-mongering media coverage.[19] In one 2004 example, the British Broadcasting Corporation released *Guinea Pigs*, a documentary that presented foster children in HIV/AIDS clinical trials as helpless victims of biomedical research, erroneously framing these children as the latest case of unethical research practices facing low-income, African American communities.[19] Scholars posited that foster children in HIV/AIDS pediatric trials went through channels that were like those of pediatric cancer trials, in which patients receive treatment within a research protocol,[19] often incurring less risk and a higher degree of safety than if they received the same treatment in a clinical practice setting.

It is possible that contemporary adolescents in foster care are experiencing a period that is like that of the pediatric HIV/AIDS trials of the 1990s and early 2000s (2000–2010), in which the challenges of conducting research with a protected group—and accompanying public perceptions of providing sexual and reproductive care to members of this population—are hindering efforts to perform HIV research with foster youths. Given the ongoing impacts of HIV among young people—young Black men in particular, who are overrepresented in the foster care system—this barrier is no longer an excuse for a paucity of research involving this population. Because of the unique obstacles that foster care adolescents likely face when attempting to access PrEP, it is crucial for public health and child welfare researchers to develop rigorous, robust, and protective methods to accurately assess their HIV status, as well as determine PrEP access, usage, retention, and effectiveness.

Soliciting parental consent for foster youths in research trials may be particularly difficult, given that these minors may not (1) have an ongoing relationship with their legal parents, (2) may have fluctuating guardianship, or (3) may not wish for their guardian(s) to know about their PrEP use. However, there are avenues in which researchers can write grants and subsequent internal review board documentation. For example, to allow minors into research without parental consent, a researcher can state that the intervention offered (i.e., PrEP) is for purposes of treatment as well as prevention,[20] although we note that this differs based on individual state regulations. Another avenue is to create checks that determine whether the adolescent is mature enough to make informed decisions (e.g., mature minor doctrine). When this is available, a researcher can develop a line of questioning that helps illuminate whether youths can reasonably weigh the risks and benefits of the research in which they want to participate.

Public Health Professionals

Rates of HIV infections among White YMSM aged 13 to 24 years fell 45% between 2017 and 2021, whereas infections only fell 27% for Black YMSM in the same age demographic.[17] Given the disproportionate representation of sexual and racial/ethnic minorities within the foster care system,[18] it is imperative for public health professionals to center on this population.

In an amendment to Penchansky and Thomas' framework, Saurman[21] proposed awareness as a sixth dimension of access, defining awareness as effective communication and information-sharing with patients, clinicians, and the broader community—while being mindful of context and health literacy. Presently, it is unclear whether adolescents in foster care are either knowledgeable about or aware of how to access PrEP. The same can be said for the clinicians and community partners who serve them. Thus, public health practitioners should focus on awareness-raising campaigns that specifically target foster youths and members of their care network—providing education on PrEP, concise and age-appropriate information on how to begin the uptake process, and information that addresses the concerns of changing guardianship and place of residence. Given the unique experiences of foster youths, as well as the nuanced obstacles that they may face in attempting to access PrEP, it is important that awareness-raising materials be tailored to their needs.

Medical Providers

One may posit that medical providers can assist foster youths in their attempt to access PrEP; however, without their own thorough understanding of complicated child welfare policies and minor consent laws,[12] many adolescent health providers could be similarly baffled by this landscape. Likewise, previous studies involving child welfare social workers have noted that foster youths often have brief doctors' visits, indicating a potential lack of comprehensive, in-depth conversations with the patient.[22] With a lasting decrease in the number of Title X clinics after the 2020 funding regulations, it is especially important for medical providers to develop a standard of care and understand the circumstances in which they can provide young people with PrEP. Specific to adolescents in foster care, medical providers and child welfare practitioners must maintain an open dialogue about their respective and mutual responsibilities in providing preventative care to foster youths. By doing so, medical providers can confidently accommodate adolescents in foster care with services that fit their needs.

Policymakers

To date, there is a paucity of federal statutes on minors accessing health care outside of certain Title X programs. Instead, this responsibility remains at the state level, where the language for most professionals is unclear and inconsistent,[9] in addition to different states offering different levels of access. Particularly for foster youths, scholars have demonstrated how ambiguous health policies uniquely affect access to other forms of sexual and reproductive health care, such as unclear policies surrounding abortion and birth control.[6] This calls for a need to revisit foster care policies at both the federal and state levels to determine easier and more streamlined avenues for sexual and reproductive health care.[12] Because of its important role in HIV prevention, policymakers must critically examine PrEP access among this list of existing sexual and reproductive health care considerations.

CONCLUSION

Often standing at the intersection of several marginalized groups, adolescents in the foster care system are at a disproportionately high risk of contracting HIV. Concurrently, these young people likely face additional obstacles when attempting to access PrEP—a widely available and effective HIV prevention strategy. Yet virtually nothing is known about whether members of this population are accessing the medication, nor how they are navigating a complicated policy landscape to do so. Because of their high risk and unique characteristics, it is imperative that they be spotlighted separately from and in addition to the general population of their peers.

The intent of this editorial was to implore researchers, public health professionals, medical providers, and policymakers to address this population's access to PrEP from a number of appropriate dimensions. With the CDC's goal of markedly increased PrEP coverage among members of at-risk populations by 2025, the foster care system could be an opportunity for linking vulnerable young people with important care. AJPH

CORRESPONDENCE

Correspondence should be sent to Casey W. Adrian, 1201 Martha Van Rensselaer Hall, College of Human Ecology, Cornell University, Ithaca, NY 14853 (e-mail: cwa39@cornell.edu). Reprints can be ordered at https://www.ajph.org by clicking the "Reprints" link.

PUBLICATION INFORMATION

Full Citation: Adrian CW, Shipe SL, Guastaferro K. HIV prevention in foster care youths: time for a refocus. *Am J Public Health*. 2024;114(11): 1179–1183.

Acceptance Date: July 1, 2024.

DOI: https://doi.org/10.2105/AJPH.2024.307793

ORCID iDs:

Casey W. Adrian https://orcid.org/0009-0008-4470-6634

Stacey L. Shipe https://orcid.org/0000-0002-8145-4674

Kate Guastaferro https://orcid.org/0000-0002-5616-9708

CONTRIBUTORS

All authors made substantial contributions to this article. C. W. Adrian and S. L. Shipe conceptualized the essay. C. W. Adrian led the writing, revisions, and took point on the publication process. S. L. Shipe contributed to writing, a survey of existing literature, and provided invaluable mentorship. K. Guastaferro provided crucial feedback throughout each stage of the process.

ACKNOWLEDGMENTS

This editorial was conceptualized while C. W. Adrian studied and served as a graduate research assistant in the Department of Social Work at Binghamton University. C. W. Adrian thanks the department for their enduring support and generosity.

CONFLICTS OF INTEREST

The authors have no conflicts to disclose.

REFERENCES

1. Cheung KK, Montgomery D, Benjamins LJ. Prevalence of sexually transmitted infections among adolescents entering child protective services. *J Pediatr Adolesc Gynecol*. 2015;28(5):324–326. https://doi.org/10.1016/j.jpag.2014.09.011
2. Ahrens KR, McCarty C, Simoni J, Dworsky A, Courtney ME. Psychosocial pathways to sexually transmitted infection risk among youth transitioning out of foster care: evidence from a longitudinal cohort study. *J Adolesc Health*. 2013;53(4): 478–485. https://doi.org/10.1016/j.jadohealth.2013.05.010
3. Ramseyer Winter V, Brandon-Friedman RA, Ely GE. Sexual health behaviors and outcomes among current and former foster youth: a review of the literature. *Child Youth Serv Rev*. 2016;64:1–14. https://doi.org/10.1016/j.childyouth.2016.02.023
4. Centers for Disease Control and Prevention. Preexposure prophylaxis (PrEP). July 5, 2022. Available at: https://www.cdc.gov/hiv/risk/prep/index.html#:~:text=Pre%2Dexposure%20prophylaxis%20(or%20PrEP,use%20by%20at%20least%2074%25. Accessed July 19, 2024.
5. Centers for Disease Control and Prevention. HIV declines among young people and drives overall decrease in new HIV infections. May 23, 2023. Available at: https://www.cdc.gov/media/releases/2023/p0523-hiv-declines-among-young-people.html. Accessed February 21, 2024.

6. Svoboda DV, Shaw TV, Barth RP, Bright CL. Pregnancy and parenting among youth in foster care: a review. *Child Youth Serv Rev.* 2012;34(5):867–875. https://doi.org/10.1016/j.childyouth.2012.01.023
7. The White House. National HIV/AIDS Strategy 2023 Interim Action Report. 2023. Available at: https://files.hiv.gov/s3fs-public/2023-12/National-HIV-AIDS-Strategy-2023-Interim-Action-Report.pdf. Accessed February 21, 2024.
8. Penchansky R, Thomas JW. The concept of access. *Med Care.* 1981;19(2):127–140. https://doi.org/10.1097/00005650-198102000-00001
9. Nelson KM, Skinner A, Stout CD, et al. Minor consent laws for sexually transmitted infection and human immunodeficiency virus services in the United States: a comprehensive, longitudinal survey of US state laws. *Am J Public Health.* 2023;113(4):397–407. https://doi.org/10.2105/AJPH.2022.307199
10. Owens C, Currin JM, Hoffman M, Grant MJ, Hubach RD. Implementation factors associated with primary care providers' intention to prescribe HIV PrEP to adolescents in the United States. *J Adolesc Health.* 2023;73(1):181–189. https://doi.org/10.1016/j.jadohealth.2023.02.007
11. O'Donnell C. Accessing health care as a foster child. *J Health Care Law Policy.* 2021;24(2):157–177. https://digitalcommons.law.umaryland.edu/jhclp/vol24/iss2/2
12. Krass P, Tam V, Min J, et al. Adolescent access to federally funded clinics providing confidential family planning following changes to Title X funding regulations. *JAMA Netw Open.* 2022;5(6):e2217488. https://doi.org/10.1001/jamanetworkopen.2022.17488
13. Strassburger Z. Medical decision making for youth in the foster care system. *John Marshall Law Rev.* 2016;49(4):1103–1154. https://doi.org/10.31235/osf.io/ksauc
14. Seiler N, Heyison C, Dwyer G, et al. Navigating the Intersection of PrEP and Medicaid. *J Law Med Ethics.* 2022;50(S1):60–63. https://doi.org/10.1017/jme.2022.38
15. Child Welfare Information Gateway. Health-care coverage for children and youth in foster care—and after. US Dept of Health and Human Services, Administration for Children and Families, Children's Bureau. 2022. Available at: https://www.childwelfare.gov/resources/health-care-coverage-children-and-youth-foster-care-and-after. Accessed February 21, 2024.
16. Guttmacher Institute. Protecting confidentiality for individuals insured as dependents. August 31, 2023. Available at: https://www.guttmacher.org/state-policy/explore/protecting-confidentiality-individuals-insured-dependents. Accessed February 21, 2024.
17. *Diagnoses of HIV Infection in the United States and Dependent Areas, 2021: HIV Surveillance Report.* Atlanta, GA: Centers for Disease Control and Prevention; 2023.
18. Dettlaff AJ, Boyd R. Racial disproportionality and disparities in the child welfare system: why do they exist, and what can be done to address them? *Ann Am Acad Pol Soc Sci.* 2020;692(1):253–274. https://doi.org/10.1177/0002716220980329
19. Slomka J. Manufacturing mistrust: issues in the controversy regarding foster children in the pediatric HIV/AIDS clinical trials. *Sci Eng Ethics.* 2009;15(4):503–516. https://doi.org/10.1007/s11948-009-9179-5
20. Moore QL, Paul ME, McGuire AL, Majumder MA. Legal barriers to adolescent participation in research about HIV and other sexually transmitted infections. *Am J Public Health.* 2016;106(1):40–44. https://doi.org/10.2105/AJPH.2015.302940
21. Saurman E. Improving access: modifying Penchansky and Thomas's theory of access. *J Health Serv Res Policy.* 2016;21(1):36–39. https://doi.org/10.1177/1355819615600001
22. Aparicio EM, Kachingwe ON, Salerno JP, Geddings-Hayes M, Boekeloo BO. Addressing sexual health among youth in foster care group homes: a community-engaged grounded theory study. *Sex Res Soc Policy.* 2021;18(4):1136–1147. https://doi.org/10.1007/s13178-020-00519-w

The 2023 Maui Wildfires and the Mental Health Effects of Climate-Induced Relocation

Aditya Suresh, Lucy Tu, and Fatima Cody Stanford, MD, MPH, MPA, MBA

ABOUT THE AUTHORS

Aditya Suresh is with the Department of Molecular and Cellular Biology, University of California, Berkeley. Lucy Tu is with the Department of Sociology and Department of the History of Science, Harvard University, Cambridge, MA. Fatima Cody Stanford is with the Department of Medicine-Division of Endocrinology-Neuroendocrine, Department of Pediatrics-Division of Endocrinology, Weight Center, and Nutrition Obesity Research Center at Harvard, Massachusetts General Hospital, Boston, MA.

In August 2023, wildfires swept through the US state of Hawaii, predominantly on the island of Maui. The wind-driven fires prompted evacuations and caused widespread damage, killing at least 100 people and leaving more than 1100 others missing in Lāhainā.[1] Thousands of residents faced indefinite displacement as the wildfires decimated hundreds of residential buildings. These events occurred against a backdrop of worsening droughts and rising global temperatures, which have more than doubled the frequency and intensity of severe wildfires over the past two decades.[2]

Accordingly, the Lāhainā fires have become a significant case study for researchers worldwide as they examine the effects of climate change on human relocation. Beyond the immediate ecological and economic effects, a growing body of evidence emphasizes a less tangible but deeply significant aftermath of global environmental changes: the mental health implications of climate-related relocation. Indeed, the effects of climate-related relocation extend beyond the physical displacement of people, giving rise to a range of new psychological challenges that demand greater attention in current relocation initiatives.

OVERLOOKED TOLLS OF CLIMATE-RELATED RELOCATION

Climate-related relocation refers to the forced displacement of communities or individuals as a result of the adverse impacts of climate change. In 2020 alone, disasters induced by natural hazards drove more than 30 million displacements, and this number is projected to rise as a larger proportion of the global population settles in high-risk climate zones over the next decade.[3] Although precise epidemiological data on the prevalence of climate-related mental health issues are limited, individual case studies consistently show that displaced populations experience diverse and enduring mental health challenges that pervade many domains of life.[4] These effects differ from those associated with other forms of displacement owing to additional stressors stemming from ongoing environmental changes and uncertainty about future relocations, particularly as climate change–related disasters become more frequent.[5]

Thus, as climate change continues to reshape our world, the relationship between forced relocation and heightened mental health issues—including stress disorders, anxiety, suicidality, substance use, and symptoms akin to posttraumatic stress disorder—grows increasingly pronounced.[4,5] To that end, focusing solely on relocation's logistical and economic aspects while neglecting the correlated mental health repercussions leaves displaced populations vulnerable and underserved. Within this framework, we propose recommendations acknowledging the link between climate-related relocation and mental well-being, ensuring a holistic support system for affected communities.

Unfortunately, climate-related relocation initiatives have often neglected mental health.[6,7] As epidemiologists Torres and Casey note, discussions of climate migration's health impacts are limited and concentrate on infectious disease spread, increased violence, and reduced access to health care, overlooking a more integrated approach to psychosocial health and well-being.[5] Standard displacement interventions prioritize resources for shelter, food, and other necessities in the immediate aftermath of a disaster, but unaddressed mental health issues can hinder relocated communities' successful adaptation, diminishing the effectiveness of early physical aid.

For instance, a case study of communities in Nunatsiavut, Canada—whose residents experience significant climate change–induced challenges such as sporadic ice conditions and altered wildlife patterns—revealed heightened levels of family stress, drug and alcohol use, and suicidal ideation among those who had been displaced.[8] Notably, these mental health burdens persisted even when residents obtained physical or economic resources to manage environmental and geographic changes. Similarly, other studies have shown a strong association between climate-related relocation and an insidious constellation of mental health symptoms, sometimes termed "solastalgia," that are exacerbated by the damage to homes and possessions, feelings of alienation, and breakdowns in socioeconomic networks that typically accompany forced displacement.[4,5,9] These findings highlight the importance of mitigating climate-related relocation's short-, intermediate-, and long-term influence on mental and physical health.

INTEGRATING MENTAL HEALTH SUPPORT

To address these challenges, future disaster recovery and predisaster prevention initiatives must incorporate comprehensive mental health support, counseling, and community resilience programs to ensure that displaced individuals' mental and emotional needs are adequately addressed alongside their physical relocation needs. Mental health services should be embedded within resettlement programs to provide ongoing mental health and psychological support for relocated populations. For instance, community-based interventions such as peer support groups, supportive parenting programs, and assisted mourning and communal healing ceremonies have significantly improved the well-being of displaced populations.[10]

Proactive assessment and screening of at-risk communities within climate-related relocation programs is also crucial. Mental health professionals, including psychologists and social workers, may be deployed to relocation sites to conduct one-on-one assessments, which should account for several factors such as the nature of the displacement, the extent of trauma experienced, preexisting mental health conditions, and sociocultural factors. Tools such as the Impact of Event Scale–Revised can be used to gauge trauma severity. Also, the Patient Health Questionnaire-9 and the Generalized Anxiety Disorder-7 scale can be employed to screen for symptoms of depression and anxiety, respectively.[11,12] These tools enable health care providers to tailor their interventions and identify individuals in greatest need of specialized support amid relocation events.

In addition, as the effects of climate-related relocations become increasingly severe, digital mental health platforms offer a promising means to establish community support networks. Loss of social ties is one of the common deleterious stressors associated with climate-related relocation, a challenge that digital mental health platforms are uniquely equipped to address.[3,5] Some platforms provide accessible tools for communal stress reduction and virtual support groups, demonstrating particular effectiveness among younger and middle- to high-income groups.[13] In these community-based settings, displaced individuals can share their experiences, exchange coping mechanisms, and foster a sense of belonging, often eroded during climate-related relocation. Many digital mental health platforms combine these communal resources with individual-focused services such as providing access to crisis helplines and chat-based support, bridging the gap in immediate care.[9] Users can also track their moods and stress levels over time, facilitating self-awareness and helping them recognize patterns in their emotional well-being.

CULTURAL AND TRAUMA-INFORMED CARE FOR VULNERABLE GROUPS

Importantly, in accordance with international standards for delivering psychosocial services in emergency settings, interventions should aim not only to maximize support but also to minimize unintentional worsening of distress.[14] For example, prioritizing access to community and family support before introducing care, as well as involving primary care workers familiar with the displaced community when conducting mental health screenings, has proven beneficial in reducing potential harm and reinforcing long-term social support.[3,14] Effective interventions should also consider that the type of relocation affects the necessary services: short-term relocations may require immediate psychological first aid, whereas permanent relocations demand ongoing mental health care and integration support. Responsibility for delivering these services should be shared among government agencies, nongovernmental organizations, and international bodies, ensuring a cohesive response.

A successful example of such coordination is the Kiribati Climate Resilience Initiative of 2022.[15] Faced with severe relocation caused by rising sea levels, environmental degradation, and increased extreme weather events,

Kiribati collaborated with the International Organization for Migration, the Kiribati government, and various nongovernmental organizations to establish an efficient mental health support network. This initiative included community-based workshops to reduce stress, introduce constructive coping methods, and foster adaptation among affected populations. Support from the World Health Organization and the Korea International Cooperation Agency further strengthened Kiribati's health system, enhancing climate resilience in health care facilities and raising awareness of climate change's health effects.

Finally, a paramount consideration of climate-related relocation interventions must be cultural sensitivity, upholding displaced individuals' cultural, historical, and personal beliefs. Previous research has shown that the individuals most vulnerable to mental health complications from climate-related relocation are those who are generally most susceptible to climate change. These groups include children, elderly adults, members of racial and ethnic minority groups, and socioeconomically disadvantaged populations who often have fewer resources and less resilience when facing climate-related disasters and forced displacement.[4]

In addition, land-vulnerable communities and residents (e.g., those dependent on local natural resources for their livelihood), such as farmers, some indigenous communities, and individuals living in areas prone to droughts or natural disasters, are particularly susceptible to distress during climate-related relocation.[4,6] Importantly, these populations are among the most likely to face involuntary immobility, lacking the necessary economic and social resources to relocate during climate disasters. This nuance underscores the need for a proactive and culturally and trauma-informed approach to climate distress. By recognizing which groups are most vulnerable during ongoing or sudden climate events, health care providers will be better equipped to manage emerging psychosocial concerns or mitigate exacerbations of existing mental health issues triggered by climate-related disasters.

LOOKING FORWARD

As we navigate the complex landscape of climate-related relocation, this phenomenon's profound mental health implications emerge as a critical concern that demands our utmost attention. Therefore, it is not just a moral imperative but a health care necessity to prioritize mental health within climate-related relocation strategies. Such efforts will facilitate research into effective methods for mitigating climate-related health risks and expand our understanding of relocation's often-understudied mental health consequences. This, in turn, will enable health care providers to tailor future services to the unique needs resulting from various forms of climate-related relocation (e.g., international and intranational, short and long term). By implementing culturally and socially cognizant initiatives, we can offer holistic support, fortifying the well-being of affected communities in a changing world and securing a resilient future for generations to come. AJPH

CORRESPONDENCE

Correspondence should be sent to Fatima Cody Stanford, MD, MPH, MPA, MBA, 4th Floor, Weight Center, 50 Staniford St, Boston, MA 02114 (e-mail: fstanford@mgh.harvard.edu). Reprints can be ordered at https://www.ajph.org by clicking the "Reprints" link.

PUBLICATION INFORMATION

Full Citation: Suresh A, Tu L, Stanford FC. The 2023 Maui wildfires and the mental health effects of climate-induced relocation. *Am J Public Health*. 2024;114(11):1184–1187.

Acceptance Date: July 19, 2024.

DOI: https://doi.org/10.2105/AJPH.2024.307815

ORCID iDs:

Aditya Suresh https://orcid.org/0009-0002-5725-6384

Lucy Tu https://orcid.org/0000-0002-7649-6634

Fatima Cody Stanford https://orcid.org/0000-0003-4616-533X

CONTRIBUTORS

A. Suresh and L. Tu were co–first authors of the article. A. Suresh conceptualized the article. A. Suresh and L. Tu conducted literature reviews and authored initial drafts of the article. F. C. Stanford supervised all analyses and provided edits. All of the authors reviewed and revised the final article.

ACKNOWLEDGMENTS

This work was supported by the National Institute of Diabetes and Digestive and Kidney Diseases (grants U24 DK132733, P30 DK040561, and UE5 DK137285).

CONFLICTS OF INTEREST

The authors do not report any conflicts of interest.

REFERENCES

1. Holliday R, Krishnamurti LS, Jordan SE, Sia MA, Brenner LA, Monteith LL. The health and social impacts of the Maui wildfires: post-disaster care from a sociocultural lens. *Hawaii J Health Soc Welf*. 2024;83(3):85–87. https://doi.org/10.62547/KXYZ1785
2. Cunningham CX, Williamson GJ, Bowman DMJS. Increasing frequency and intensity of the most extreme wildfires on Earth. *Nat Ecol Evol*. 2024; 8:1420–1425. https://doi.org/10.1038/s41559-024-02452-2
3. International Federation of Red Cross and Red Crescent Societies. Displacement in changing climate. Available at: https://www.ifrc.org/sites/default/files/2021-11/2021-Climate-Displacement-Report-Final.pdf. Accessed June 20, 2024.
4. White BP, Breakey S, Brown MJ, et al. Mental health impacts of climate change among vulnerable populations globally: an integrative review. *Ann Glob Health*. 2023;89(1):66. https://doi.org/10.5334/aogh.4105
5. Torres JM, Casey JA. The centrality of social ties to climate migration and mental health. *BMC Public Health*. 2017;17(1):600. https://doi.org/10.1186/s12889-017-4508-0
6. Clayton S, Manning C, Speiser M, Hill AN. Mental health and our changing climate: impacts, inequities, and responses. Available at: https://www.apa.org/

news/press/releases/mental-health-climate-change.pdf. Accessed June 20, 2024.

7. Fry I. Addressing the human rights implications of climate change displacement including legal protection of people displaced across international borders. Available at: https://www.ohchr.org/en/press-releases/2023/06/un-expert-calls-full-legal-protection-people-displaced-climate-change. Accessed June 20, 2024.
8. Cunsolo Willox A, Harper SL, Ford JD, et al. Climate change and mental health: an exploratory case study from Rigolet, Nunatsiavut, Canada. *Clim Change.* 2013;121(2):255–270. https://doi.org/10.1007/s10584-013-0875-4
9. Schwerdtle P, Bowen K, McMichael C. The health impacts of climate-related migration. *BMC Med.* 2018;16(1):1. https://doi.org/10.1186/s12916-017-0981-7
10. Tol WA, Barbui C, Galappatti A, et al. Mental health and psychosocial support in humanitarian settings: linking practice and research. *Lancet.* 2011;378(9802):1581–1591. https://doi.org/10.1016/S0140-6736(11)61094-5
11. Weiss DS, Marmar CR. The impact of event scale–revised. In: Wilson JP, Keane TM, eds. *Assessing Psychological Trauma and PTSD.* New York, NY: Guilford Press; 1997:399–411.
12. Pranckeviciene A, Saudargiene A, Gecaite-Stoneciene J, et al. Validation of the Patient Health Questionnaire-9 and the Generalized Anxiety Disorder-7 in Lithuanian student sample. *PLoS One.* 2022;17(1):e0263027. https://doi.org/10.1371/journal.pone.0263027
13. Balcombe L, De Leo D. Evaluation of the use of digital mental health platforms and interventions: scoping review. *Int J Environ Res Public Health.* 2023;20(1):362. https://doi.org/10.3390/ijerph20010362
14. United Nations Office for the Coordination of Humanitarian Affairs. IASC guidelines on mental health and psychosocial support in emergency settings. Available at: https://interagencystandingcommittee.org/iasc-task-force-mental-health-and-psychosocial-support-emergency-settings/iasc-guidelines-mental-health-and-psychosocial-support-emergency-settings-2007. Accessed June 24, 2024.
15. World Health Organization. Kiribati's climate resilience set to get a boost with support from WHO and KOICA. Available at: https://www.who.int/westernpacific/about/how-we-work/pacific-support/news/detail/19-05-2023-kiribati-s-climate-resilience-set-to-get-a-boost-with-support-from-who-and-koica. Accessed June 19, 2024.

Kratom Products Are Widely Available Throughout the United States

Matthew E. Rossheim, PhD, MPH, Cassidy R. LoParco, PhD, Kayla K. Tillett, MPH, R. Andrew Yockey, PhD, Hsien-Chang Lin, PhD, and Carla J. Berg, PhD

ABOUT THE AUTHORS

Matthew E. Rossheim and Kayla K. Tillett are with the Department of Health Administration and Health Policy, School of Public Health, University of North Texas Health Science Center, Fort Worth, TX. Cassidy R. LoParco and Carla J. Berg are with the Department of Prevention and Community Health, Milken Institute School of Public Health, George Washington University, Washington, DC. R. Andrew Yockey is with the Department of Public Health, School of Applied Sciences, University of Mississippi, University, MS. Hsien-Chang Lin is with the Department of Applied Health Science, School of Public Health, Indiana University Bloomington, Bloomington, IN.

AJPH November 2024, Vol. 114, No. 11

According to nationally representative data from 2022, an estimated 1.9 million Americans (0.7%) used kratom in the past year.[1] Kratom use can have widely varied effects among users, including both stimulant and sedative effects, primarily attributed to mitragynine and 7-hydroxymitragynine.[2,3] 7-Hydroxymitragynine is present in low concentrations, but the concentration can increase during the drying process and after ingestion, contributing to kratom's effects.[2]

Kratom is often marketed as having pain-relieving and mood-enhancing properties, and for being a safer substitute for opioids and managing related withdrawal symptoms and cravings.[2–4] However, little clinical evidence exists on the effects of kratom, and according to the US Food and Drug Administration (FDA), kratom is not lawfully marketed as a drug, dietary supplement, or food additive because data supporting its safety are lacking.[4] Moreover, the FDA warns consumers not to use kratom products because of the risk of serious adverse effects, including liver toxicity, seizures, and the development of a substance use disorder.[4] The FDA also issued warnings when specific kratom products were found to be contaminated with salmonella or high levels of heavy metals.[4] Additional studies indicate serious health risks from using kratom that is highly concentrated, adulterated, or contaminated, or in combination with other substances.[5] These issues are compounded by a lack of standardized product labeling, leaving consumers potentially ill informed.[5] Given the many public health concerns regarding kratom use,[2,5] and that accessibility is a major determinant of substance use,[6] understanding kratom's accessibility has important policy implications. Previous studies have found that kratom products are available in tobacco specialty stores in many cities across the United States in various forms, including powder, pills, and liquid (e.g., shots).[7–9] However, little is known regarding its retail availability nationwide. Thus, we examined kratom product availability in tobacco specialty stores across the United States overall, as well as by state regulatory context.

From November 18 to December 19, 2023, we systematically identified, called, and completed brief surveys with 520 US tobacco specialty stores (n = 10 per state, Washington DC, and Puerto Rico). We established sampling frames by selecting the largest commercial airport and the capitol building in each state, Washington DC, and Puerto Rico, as landmarks because of their geographic prominence and accessibility. Using Google Maps, we identified 104 such landmarks and employed the "search nearby" feature to compile an initial list of tobacco specialty stores. These locations were screened to confirm that they were smoke–tobacco–vape shops and not licensed cannabis dispensaries. More information about the study methods is available elsewhere.[10]

To help optimize response rates, the survey was designed to be brief and focused on product availability. We asked, "Do you sell kratom?" Responses were recorded as yes or no. Overall, 661 stores were called to achieve our targeted sample of 520 tobacco specialty stores (response rate = 78.7%). Nonresponse (21.3%) occurred solely when a phone number was invalid or no one answered the phone. Information on state kratom laws, as of November 28, 2023, was obtained from a Congressional Research Service (CRS) report.[11] For each state or territory, we computed the percentage of tobacco specialty stores selling kratom.

Table 1 displays the percentage of stores selling kratom products in each of the 52 states and territories, along with information about their respective

TABLE 1— Kratom Availability in Tobacco Specialty Stores: United States, 2023

% of Stores With Kratom Products Available, by State or Jurisdiction[a]
Bans Mitragynine or 7-Hydroxymitragynine
0%
AL
AR
IN
VT
WI
40%
RI
Does Not Ban Mitragynine or 7-Hydroxymitragynine
50%
PA
WA
60%
AK
HI
ME
MN[b]
MS
MT
PR
70%
DC
DE
IA
KS
MO
NV[b]
NJ
OK[b]
OR[c]
SC
WY
80%
CT
ID
NM
NY
TX[b]
90%
AZ[b]
CA
CO[c]
MA
MD
NC
ND
NE
NH
OH
SD[c]
100%
FL[c]
GA[b]
IL[b]
KY
LA[c]
MI
TN[c]
UT[b]
VA[c]
WV[c]

Note. The sample size was n = 520. Additional details about state-level legislation regulating kratom products are provided in Appendix A, available as a supplement to the online version of this article at http://www.ajph.org.
[a]Percentage of stores with kratom products available is based on a sample of 520 stores, including 10 stores per state.
[b]Retailers in these states can only sell to customers aged 18 years or older.
[c]Retailers in these states can only sell to customers aged 21 years or older.

kratom laws. Overall, 72% of tobacco specialty stores sold kratom products (372/520). Across the 46 states and territories where kratom was legal, 80% of stores sold kratom (368/460), and at least 50% of stores in each of these states and territories reported selling kratom. Moreover, in 21 states, at least 90% of stores reported selling kratom. Among the six states with kratom bans, only Rhode Island had tobacco specialty stores reporting the sale of kratom (40%).

Although kratom products have been known to be available in US tobacco specialty stores, the extent to which they have been available across the United States was previously undocumented. This study marks an advancement addressing this gap and found that, across the 46 states and territories without bans, four out of five tobacco specialty stores reported selling kratom products. This finding underscores the substance's widespread market penetration, despite ongoing debates about its impacts on public health and safety.[2–4]

Interestingly, 40% of stores in Rhode Island sold kratom products despite statewide prohibitions. This finding is consistent with previous research, which identified high rates of noncompliance with local ordinances banning kratom in San Diego, California.[7] Overall, the availability of kratom was considerably lower in states with bans: 0% in five of six states with bans. However, four of these six states with bans (Indiana, Rhode Island, Vermont, and Wisconsin) have introduced bills to legalize and regulate its sale (more details in Appendix A, available as a supplement to the online version of this article at http://www.ajph.org). Thus, it is plausible that the retail availability of kratom will continue to rise.

We used a systematic and broad geographic sampling approach encompassing diverse regulatory environments across the United States. By conducting telephone surveys, we obtained direct responses from retailers, which provided current and specific information about kratom availability. However, the reliance on self-reported data from store representatives without further verification could introduce response bias, especially in the six states where it was illegal. There may also be nonresponse bias, related to the 21.3% of the stores that could not be contacted. Finally, the potential underrepresentation of rural areas could affect the generalizability of our findings. Future studies should include more representative samples and store types.

Growing national attention is being paid to kratom, as evidenced by the Federal Kratom Consumer Protection Act, which was introduced in the House and Senate in October 2023.[12] This bill is purportedly designed to "protect access to kratom" by requiring the FDA to form a committee to examine the health effects and safety of products with kratom. However, the only other major provision in this bill is that it would prohibit the FDA from applying regulations to kratom that are more stringent than those for food or dietary supplements or ingredients. Given kratom's unique properties, potential for abuse, and health risks not common to typical dietary supplements, it would likely be beneficial to have more tailored regulations addressing specific risks such as dependency and drug interactions.[2–5] Our findings underscore the scale of this issue nationally and therefore the critical need for effective consumer safety regulations.

A standardized federal approach is crucial given the widespread availability of kratom across the United States and the existing patchwork of state laws. Federal regulations should be evidence-based and crafted to protect consumer safety rather than industry profits. These regulations should mandate rigorous product testing, establish safety standards, and set marketing restrictions. They should also define upper limits for alkaloid content, set a minimum purchase age, and require clear labeling of product contents, ingredient lists, safety warnings, and directions for safe use, without implying therapeutic benefits or suggesting medical usage.

Policymakers, regulatory bodies, and public health professionals should collaborate to ensure that the marketing, accessibility, and attributes of kratom products are regulated in a manner that optimally protects public health and safety. Our study findings underscore the urgent need for additional studies examining the clinical effects of kratom use, and the impacts of regulatory changes on its marketing, use, and associated health effects. These studies will play a crucial role in informing and refining policies to effectively manage the risks—along with any potential harm reduction benefits—associated with kratom. AJPH

CORRESPONDENCE

Correspondence should be sent to Matthew Rossheim, Associate Professor, School of Public Health, University of North Texas Health Science Center, 3500 Camp Bowie Blvd, Fort Worth, TX 76107 (e-mail: Matthew.Rossheim@unthsc.edu). Reprints can be ordered at https://www.ajph.org by clicking the "Reprints" link.

PUBLICATION INFORMATION

Full Citation: Rossheim ME, LoParco CR, Tillett KK, Yockey RA, Lin HC, Berg CJ. Kratom products are widely available throughout the United States. *Am J Public Health*. 2024;114(11):1188–1190.

Acceptance Date: July 22, 2024.

DOI: https://doi.org/10.2105/AJPH.2024.307824

ORCID iDs:

Matthew E. Rossheim https://orcid.org/0000-0003-4388-5251

Kayla K. Tillett https://orcid.org/0000-0002-3681-3009

Hsien-Chang Lin https://orcid.org/0000-0001-9151-2172

Carla J. Berg https://orcid.org/0000-0001-8931-1961

CONTRIBUTORS

M. E. Rossheim conceptualized the study, collected data, conducted analyses, and drafted the initial version of the article. C. R. LoParco, K. K. Tillett, R. A. Yockey, H.-C. Lin, and C. J. Berg aided in conceptualizing the study and drafting and editing the article. All authors approved the final version of the article.

CONFLICTS OF INTEREST

The authors have no conflicts of interest to declare.

REFERENCES

1. Substance Abuse and Mental Health Services Administration. Key substance use and mental health indicators in the United States: results from the 2022 National Survey on Drug Use and Health. HHS Pub No. PEP23-07-01-006, NSDUH Series H-58. 2023. Available at: https://www.samhsa.gov/data/report/2022-nsduh-annual-national-report. Accessed May 26, 2024.
2. Kerrigan S, Basiliere S. Kratom: a systematic review of toxicological issues. *WIRES Forensic Sci.* 2022;4(1):e1420. https://doi.org/10.1002/wfs2.1420
3. National Institute on Drug Abuse. Kratom. March 2022. Available at: https://nida.nih.gov/research-topics/kratom. Accessed May 26, 2024.
4. US Food and Drug Administration. FDA and kratom. Updated February 22, 2024. Available at: https://www.fda.gov/news-events/public-health-focus/fda-and-kratom. Accessed May 26, 2024.
5. Veltri C, Grundmann O. Current perspectives on the impact of Kratom use. *Subst Abuse Rehabil.* 2019;10:23–31. https://doi.org/10.2147/SAR.S164261
6. Berg CJ, Henriksen L, Cavazos-Rehg PA, Haardoerfer R, Freisthler B. The emerging marijuana retail environment: key lessons learned from tobacco and alcohol retail research. *Addict Behav.* 2018;81:26–31. https://doi.org/10.1016/j.addbeh.2018.01.040
7. Bowdring MA, Leas EC, Vishwakarma M, et al. Kratom availability in California vape shops. *Prev Med Rep.* 2023;35:102380. https://doi.org/10.1016/j.pmedr.2023.102380
8. Berg CJ, Romm KF, Barker DC, et al. Changes in the point-of-sale among vape shops in six US metropolitan areas over time, 2018–2021. *Nicotine Tob Res.* 2023;25(7):1369–1377. https://doi.org/10.1093/ntr/ntad046
9. Berg CJ, Melena A, Wittman FD, et al. The reshaping of the e-cigarette retail environment: its evolution and public health concerns. *Int J Environ Res Public Health.* 2022;19(14):8518. https://doi.org/10.3390/ijerph19148518
10. Rossheim ME, LoParco CR, Tillett KK, et al. Intoxicating cannabis products in vape shops: United States, 2023. *Am J Prev Med.* 2024; S0749-3797(24)00229-0. https://doi.org/10.1016/j.amepre.2024.07.001
11. Heflin JO. Kratom regulation: federal status and state approaches. November 28, 2023. Available at: https://crsreports.congress.gov/product/pdf/LSB/LSB11082. Accessed May 26, 2024.
12. Federal Kratom Consumer Protection Act. H.R.5905, 118th Congress. Introduced in Senate October 4, 2023. Available at: https://www.congress.gov/bill/118th-congress/senate-bill/3039. Accessed May 26, 2024.

Kids No Longer Smoke Cigarettes. Why Aren't We Celebrating?

Kenneth E. Warner, PhD

ABOUT THE AUTHOR

Kenneth E. Warner is professor emeritus with the School of Public Health, University of Michigan, Ann Arbor.

The decrease in cigarette smoking among American youths is one of the great public health triumphs of the present century. Yet, few people are talking about it. Public health agencies and tobacco control organizations mention it, if at all, in passing. Media coverage is minimal. Should we not be shouting it from the mountaintops?

THE REMARKABLE DECLINE IN YOUTH SMOKING

In 2023, 1.9% of US high school students and 1.1% of middle school students reported smoking cigarettes at least once in the past 30 days.[1] Past-30-day smoking prevalence among 12th graders rose through the 1990s to 36.5% in 1997, a level from which it fell virtually annually thereafter. Smoking among 10th and 8th graders peaked in 1996 at 30.4% and 21%, respectively, before also decreasing nearly every year (Figure 1; https://bit.ly/4cM1hD2).

Past-30-day smoking includes everything from puffing on a cigarette once to smoking daily. Regarding the latter, in 1997, 24.6% of 12th graders—one of every four high school seniors—smoked every single day. Last year? It was 0.7%—one of every 143 seniors (https://bit.ly/4cM1hD2).

Youth cigar smoking has plummeted as well. Past 30-day use of cigars dropped from 11.3% of high school students in 2011 to 1.8% in 2023. Middle school cigar use was 1.1%, down from 3.7%.[1,3]

By any measure, youth smoking has nearly ceased to exist.

CAUSES OF THE DECREASE IN YOUTH SMOKING

How did we get here? The principal answer is a major change in social norms. Over time, smoking shifted from desirable, or at least acceptable, to a sizable subset of youths to universally undesirable and unacceptable. Policy changes[4] supported social norm change: clean indoor air laws, prohibition of ads attractive to young people, effective counteradvertising, and cigarette price increases.

The last of these reflects a combination of tax increases and industry-imposed wholesale price increases. The latter, exceeding general inflation in recent years, are of particular interest. With young people especially price sensitive,[4] industry's increasing prices indicate that they may be giving up their age-old pursuit of "replacement smokers," the newly smoking young people who replaced older customers who quit smoking or died. The increased prices likely mean that the industry is focusing on the near-term goal of extracting maximal revenue from their heavily addicted middle-aged and older customers.

The public health community has been fighting youth smoking for decades. Why, therefore, are we not celebrating what is essentially the demise of smoking by adolescents?

PUBLIC PERCEPTIONS OF TOBACCO AND NICOTINE

Several reasons come to mind. One is concern about youth tobacco use in all its forms. In 2023, 10% of middle and high school students had used any tobacco product in the past 30 days.[1] While less than half the rate in 2019 (23%),[5] this prevalence still represents a consequential proportion of students. Anyone concerned about youth tobacco product use may consider the demise of smoking per se only a step in the right direction. This is especially true for the many people, including public health professionals, who believe that smokeless products are as dangerous as smoking.

Survey data demonstrate the extent of this belief. In 2017, the Health Information National Trends Survey (HINTS) asked respondents, "Do you believe that some smokeless tobacco products, such as chewing tobacco and snuff, are less harmful than cigarettes?" Seventy-one percent answered "No." Only 13.4% answered "Yes" (https://bit.ly/4dGiZJv). Similarly, the 2020 HINTS asked respondents to compare electronic cigarettes with conventional cigarettes, and 62.2% perceived e-cigarettes to be as harmful as, or more harmful than, smoking. Only 11.2% considered e-cigarettes less harmful (https://bit.ly/3Z4N8hp). A recent survey of physicians

AJPH November 2024, Vol. 114, No. 11

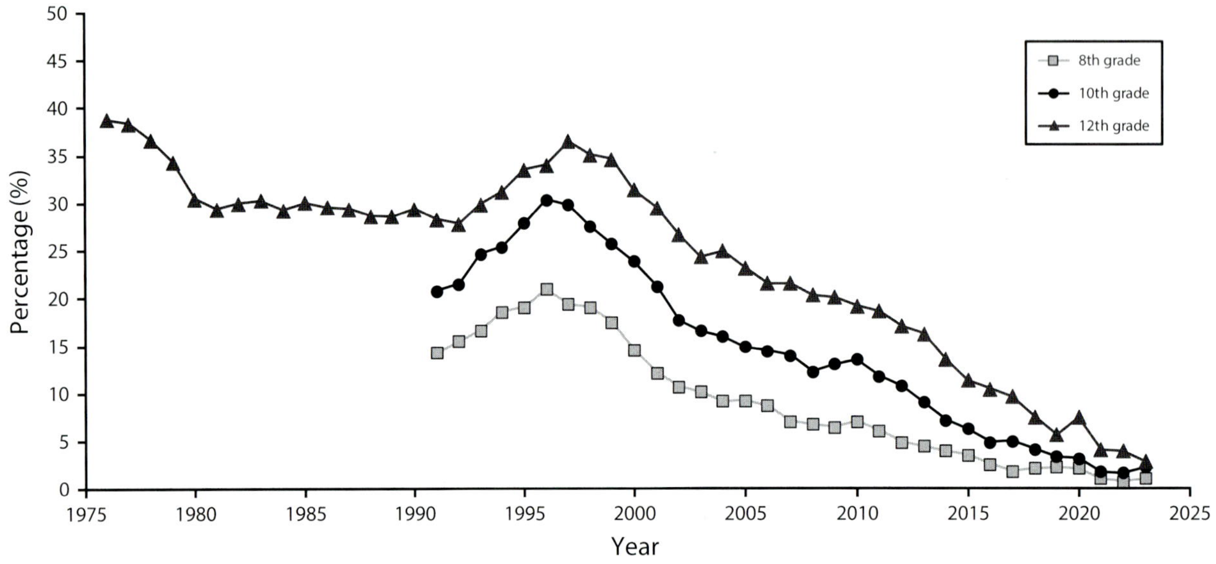

FIGURE 1— 30-Day Prevalence of Cigarette Smoking in 8th, 10th, and 12th Grade: United States, 1976–2023

Source. Miech et al.[2]

AJPH November 2024, Vol. 114, No. 11

found that "More than 60% . . . believed all tobacco products to be equally harmful."[6]

In fact, smokeless tobacco products sold in the United States create substantially less risk than does smoking.[7–9] And authoritative bodies have characterized e-cigarettes as significantly less dangerous than combusted tobacco products (https://bit.ly/4cRRdlJ; https://bit.ly/3Mxn9aB).[10] Smokeless tobacco products and e-cigarettes have many fewer toxins than does cigarette smoke (https://bit.ly/479xMKc).[10] Furthermore, for toxins the products have in common, yields tend to be much higher for cigarettes.[11,12] Smoking is responsible for nearly all tobacco-related disease and death. The Surgeon General urged us to keep our eyes on the prize: the elimination of the use of combusted tobacco products.[13] With kids, that elusive prize has been won.

A second reason we are not celebrating that victory is that all tobacco products contain nicotine, an addictive drug, and public health professionals and the general public understandably abhor adolescent nicotine use in any form. Adolescent exposure to nicotine per se is a genuine concern for several reasons, ranging from the psychological effects of dependence to the economic consequences (significant expenditures on tobacco products) to concerns that it may foster use of other drugs.[14,15] But conflating the issue of nicotine addiction with the presumed disease-producing equivalence of all tobacco products creates the expectation that addiction will lead to substantial risk of morbidity and mortality. Nicotine per se is not the direct cause of the diseases associated with tobacco. Rather, it causes persistent use of the products that expose users to the actual toxins.

Unfortunately, surveys find that the public views nicotine as a principal culprit in smoking-produced disease. In the 2019 HINTS, 56.5% of respondents agreed that "nicotine in cigarettes is the substance that causes most of the cancer caused by smoking." Only 21.4% disagreed (https://bit.ly/4e1zn7l). Large majorities of physicians incorrectly believe that "nicotine, on its own," is the direct cause of smoking-associated heart disease, respiratory disease, and cancer.[16]

THE SPECIAL CASE OF E-CIGARETTES

Nowhere have worries about adolescents using tobacco products and risking nicotine addiction played out more vividly than in the case of e-cigarettes. E-cigarettes gained popularity among adolescents a decade ago, leading to the JUUL-inspired leap in youth vaping in 2018 and 2019, widely labeled an epidemic. Especially because, unlike cigarette smoking, many adolescents from highly educated, affluent families tried vaping,[17] the state of alarm among parents reached Red Alert. Youth vaping has declined substantially since then, from 30-day prevalence of 27.5% in high school students in 2019[18] to 7.8% this year (https://bit.ly/4d9c5LJ). But the anxiety persists.

Worries about youth vaping focus on two issues. One is the contention that nicotine can damage developing adolescent brains or harm health in other ways. Most research regarding brain effects is based on animal models but with potential relevance for humans.[14,19] However, the lack of evidence of brain damage in previous generations of people who smoked mitigates this concern. Regarding other serious long-term adverse health consequences, use of e-cigarettes is too recent to know.

The second concern is that vaping can cause nicotine addiction. While warranted, evidence indicates that vaping-induced addiction may be less pervasive than commonly assumed.[20] Much adolescent e-cigarette use is experimental and transitory. Furthermore, frequent vaping, the behavior most consistent with addiction, is far more common among adolescents who either smoke or used to smoke and hence may have become nicotine dependent from their smoking. In 2022, 9% of never-smoking high school students had vaped in the past 30 days, 3% frequently (≥ 20 days). In contrast, 54% of ever-smoking students had vaped in the past 30 days, 34% frequently (https://bit.ly/3MqB4iY). Still, that 3% of never-smoking students vape frequently is a legitimate source of concern.

So, too, is the possibility that vaping has sustained, or even increased, the level of youth nicotine dependence compared with what it was when cigarettes were the principal source of addiction. Daily use of a nicotine product likely indicates addiction. In 2013, just before adolescent uptake of e-cigarettes, 8.5% of high school seniors smoked cigarettes daily. In 2019—the peak year of youth vaping—that rate was 2.4%, falling to 0.7% in 2023. The prevalence of daily vaping by 12th graders in 2019 was 11.6%, dropping to 5.8% in 2023.[2] The sum of daily smokers and daily vapers totaled 14% in 2019 and 6.5% in 2023. Thus, daily use of these products increased from the year before vaping to vaping's peak year. It then decreased by nearly 60% to the present. This measure of likely nicotine addiction dropped by a quarter over the decade from before vaping to 2023, and today's source of likely addiction, e-cigarettes, is substantially less dangerous than was the product in 2013, combustible cigarettes.

Even so, to many observers, worries regarding e-cigarettes have supplanted concerns about youth cigarette smoking. For anyone with this view, vaping's perceived perils may make celebrating the demise of youth smoking seem unwarranted.

THE LEGACY OF THE DISAPPEARANCE OF YOUTH SMOKING

But is it really? Just over 100 years ago, a medical professor told his students, observing the autopsy of a lung cancer victim, that they were unlikely to ever see this then extraordinarily rare disease again.[21] Today, lung cancer is the leading cause of cancer death in both men and women, with smoking responsible for 80% to 90% of cases. The near disappearance of smoking among today's young people means that a few decades hence, lung cancer is likely to be a relatively minor cause of cancer. Deaths from chronic obstructive pulmonary disease—80% attributable to smoking—will likely fall as well, as may age-adjusted heart disease mortality.

THE LOGICAL—AND CRUCIAL—NEXT STEP

The rapid and nearly complete disappearance of adolescent smoking is arguably the single most dramatic, and ultimately important, tobacco control achievement to date. Next on the docket is the elimination of adult smoking. Like youth smoking, adult smoking has declined substantially, albeit more slowly, to 11.5%. The benefits of the decrease are uneven, however. Reductions in smoking by younger adults have driven the decline. Smoking has not decreased among older adults, the group most at risk for near-term illness and death.[22] Twenty-eight million Americans smoke, and cigarettes continue to claim 480 000 lives every year.[23] Furthermore, the overall 11.5% prevalence masks significant disparities in prevalence and mortality. Increasingly, smoking's victims are society's marginalized groups—people with lower income and education, those suffering from mental health problems, Indigenous people, and sexual and gender minoritized groups.[24] Having essentially eliminated youth smoking, it is time to focus attention on reducing adult smoking[25]—the prize in tobacco control, according to the Surgeon General.

In the process, and perhaps as a model of success, let us celebrate the near elimination of cigarette smoking among our young people. They will live longer, healthier lives than their parents and grandparents. AJPH

CORRESPONDENCE

Correspondence should be sent to Kenneth E. Warner, Department of Health Management and Policy, School of Public Health, University of Michigan, 1415 Washington Heights, Ann Arbor, MI 48109-2029 (e-mail: kwarner@umich.edu).
Reprints can be ordered at https://www.ajph.org by clicking the "Reprints" link.

PUBLICATION INFORMATION

Full Citation: Warner KE. Kids no longer smoke cigarettes. Why aren't we celebrating? *Am J Public Health*. 2024;114(11):1191–1194.

Acceptance Date: August 7, 2024.

DOI: https://doi.org/10.2105/AJPH.2024.307841

ORCID iD:
Kenneth E. Warner https://orcid.org/0000-0002-8214-1776

CONFLICTS OF INTEREST

The author has no conflicts of interest.

REFERENCES

1. Birdsey J, Cornelius M, Jamal A, et al. Tobacco product use among US middle and high school students—National Youth Tobacco Survey, 2023. *MMWR Morb Mortal Wkly Rep.* 2023;72(44):1173–1182. https://doi.org/10.15585/mmwr.mm7244a1
2. Miech RA, Johnston LD, Patrick ME, O'Malley PM. Monitoring the Future national survey results on drug use, 1975–2023: overview and detailed results for secondary school students. Monitoring the Future Monograph Series. Institute for Social Research, University of Michigan. Available at: https://monitoringthefuture.org/results/annual-reports. Accessed June 16, 2024.
3. Wang TW, Gentzke A, Sharapova S, Cullen KA, Ambrose BK, Jamal A. Tobacco product use among middle and high school students—United States, 2011–2017. *MMWR Morb Mortal Wkly Rep.* 2018;67(22):629–633. https://doi.org/10.15585/mmwr.mm6722a3
4. Warner KE. Tobacco policy research: insights and contributions to public health policy. In: Warner KE, ed. *Tobacco Control Policy.* San Francisco: Jossey-Bass; 2006:3–86.
5. Wang TW, Gentzke AS, Creamer MR, et al. Tobacco product use and associated factors among middle and high school students—United States, 2019. *MMWR Surveill Summ.* 2019;68(12):1–22. https://doi.org/10.15585/mmwr.ss6812a1
6. Delnevo CD, Jeong M, Teotia A, et al. Communication between US physicians and patients regarding electronic cigarette use. *JAMA Netw Open.* 2022;5(4):e226692. https://doi.org/10.1001/jamanetworkopen.2022.6692
7. Fisher MT, Tan-Torres SM, Gaworski CL, et al. Smokeless tobacco mortality risks: an analysis of two contemporary nationally representative longitudinal mortality studies. *Harm Reduct J.* 2019;16(1):27. https://doi.org/10.1186/s12954-019-0294-6
8. Accortt NA, Waterbor JW, Beall C, Howard G. Chronic disease mortality in a cohort of smokeless tobacco users. *Am J Epidemiol.* 2002;156(8):730–737. https://doi.org/10.1093/aje/kwf106
9. Levy DT, Mumford EA, Cummings KM, et al. The relative risks of a low-nitrosamine smokeless tobacco product compared with smoking cigarettes: estimates of a panel of experts. *Cancer Epidemiol Biomarkers Prev.* 2004;13(12):2035–2042. https://doi.org/10.1158/1055-9965.2035.13.12
10. National Academies of Sciences, Engineering, and Medicine. *Public Health Consequences of E-Cigarettes.* Washington, DC: The National Academies Press; 2018. https://doi.org/10.17226/24952
11. Majeed B, Linder D, Eissenberg T, Tarasenko Y, Smith D, Ashley D. Cluster analysis of urinary tobacco biomarkers among US adults: Population Assessment of Tobacco and Health (PATH) biomarker study (2013–2014). *Prev Med.* 2020;140:106218. https://doi.org/10.1016/j.ypmed.2020.106218
12. Goniewicz ML, Smith DM, Edwards KC, et al. Comparison of nicotine and toxicant exposure in users of electronic cigarettes and combustible cigarettes. *JAMA Netw Open.* 2018;1(8):e185937. https://doi.org/10.1001/jamanetworkopen.2018.5937
13. National Center for Chronic Disease Prevention and Health Promotion, Office on Smoking and Health. *The Health Consequences of Smoking—50 Years of Progress: A Report of the Surgeon General.* Atlanta, GA: Centers for Disease Control and Prevention; 2014. Available at: https://www.ncbi.nlm.nih.gov/books/NBK179276. Accessed September 16, 2024.
14. Kandel ER, Kandel DB. A molecular basis for nicotine as a gateway drug. *N Engl J Med.* 2014;371(10):932–943. https://doi.org/10.1056/NEJMsa1405092
15. Lau L, Conti AA, Hemmati Z, Baldacchino A. The prospective association between the use of e-cigarettes and other psychoactive substances in young people: a systematic review and meta-analysis. *Neurosci Biobehav Rev.* 2023;153:105392. https://doi.org/10.1016/j.neubiorev.2023.105392
16. Bover Manderski MT, Steinberg MB, Wackowski OA, Singh B, Young WJ, Delnevo CD. Persistent misperceptions about nicotine among US physicians: results from a randomized survey experiment. *Int J Environ Res Public Health.* 2021;18(14):7713. https://doi.org/10.3390/ijerph18147713
17. Simon P, Camenga DR, Morean ME, et al. Socioeconomic status and adolescent e-cigarette use: the mediating role of e-cigarette advertisement exposure. *Prev Med.* 2018;112:193–198. https://doi.org/10.1016/j.ypmed.2018.04.019
18. Cullen KA, Gentzke AS, Sawdey MD, et al. e-Cigarette use among youth in the United States, 2019. *JAMA.* 2019;322(21):2095–2103. https://doi.org/10.1001/jama.2019.18387
19. Leslie FM. Unique, long-term effects of nicotine on adolescent brain. *Pharmacol Biochem Behav.* 2020;197:173010. https://doi.org/10.1016/j.pbb.2020.173010
20. Jackson SE, Brown J, Jarvis MJ. Dependence on nicotine in US high school students in the context of changing patterns of tobacco product use. *Addiction.* 2021;116(7):1859–1870. https://doi.org/10.1111/add.15403
21. Blum A. Alton Ochsner, MD, 1896–1981, anti-smoking pioneer. *Ochsner J.* 1999;1(3):102–105.
22. Meza R, Cao P, Jeon J, Warner KE, Levy DT. Trends in US adult smoking prevalence, 2011 to 2022. *JAMA Health Forum.* 2023;4(12):e234213. https://doi.org/10.1001/jamahealthforum.2023.4213
23. Le TTT, Mendez D, Warner KE. New estimates of smoking-attributable mortality in the US from 2020 through 2035. *Am J Prev Med.* 2024;66(5):877–882. https://doi.org/10.1016/j.amepre.2023.12.017
24. Balfour DJK, Benowitz NL, Colby SM, et al. Balancing consideration of the risks and benefits of e-cigarettes. *Am J Public Health.* 2021;111(9):1661–1672. https://doi.org/10.2105/AJPH.2021.306416
25. Califf RM, King BA. The need for a smoking cessation "care package." *JAMA.* 2023;329(3):203–204. https://doi.org/10.1001/jama.2022.24398

Rethinking Rankings in Public Health Graduate Education—Who Are They For?

Jonathon P. Leider, PhD

ABOUT THE AUTHOR

Jonathon P. Leider is the founding director of the Center for Public Health Systems, Division of Health Policy and Management, University of Minnesota School of Public Health, Minneapolis.

US News and World Report (*USNWR*) rankings are a force in education. They drive strategy and investments, and influence campaigns.[1] Forty years after their inception, they still provoke significant controversy. Yearly ranking is now the norm. The "why" seems obvious from *USNWR*'s perspective. The "market" rationale for student benefit rings less true; publishing more rankings, of more schools, more frequently, does not seem to in fact enhance student choice or fit, if it is not done well.[1,2]

Institutions contend that the methodology used for *USNWR* rankings further disadvantages the already disadvantaged populations they serve, and is misleading to applicants.[1] Administrators have been charged with crimes for trying to fraudulently enhance their rankings, or called out on supplying bad data.[3,4] In all the cases in question, those rankings are based, ostensibly, on several points of data. Unfortunately, for many programs, both in public health and in graduate programs in the health sciences more broadly, the assessment is based on an even more tenuous foundation. In the case of public health, the entirety of the *USNWR* rankings comes down to a single question. Staff are asked to assess the quality of each peer academic program on a scale of 1 (marginal) to 5 (outstanding).[5] And fewer than half of eligible public health schools responded to that question in 2024.

So much rides on a ranking, and the question is regularly asked: Why, still, must prospective students (and schools and programs) settle for this?

Rankings as a concept are easily digestible and are supposed to be a proxy for the quality of an institution or program. It seems reasonable to ask whether that is, or was ever, true in the case of the health sciences rankings in general, or public health specifically. Can a single measure based solely on peer assessment help guide a student to finding a good fit, much less good value? As more and more schools are added to the contest, and response rates decrease, the quality of the single measure may be further called into question.

Consider Figure 1, which shows rankings by group and peer score over time. The horizontal bar represents the minimum peer score for the group ranked 11 to 50 in a given year. It is notable that peer scores vary, sometimes substantially, year to year. A single metric drives the ranking. However, the combination of (1) far more schools participating and, perhaps, (2) greater frequency of publication was associated with dramatic change from the mid-2010s through 2021 in the category of public health. The vaunted "top 10" (and up through top 20) has been relatively stable, but the addition of more schools has proved more variable for much of the rest who are ranked. Between 2019 and 2021, a number of schools saw their peer scores improve when more peers were added. This effect was even more pronounced in 2022; in addition, rankings overall shuffled quite a bit. The rankings appear somewhat stable now, but that is only detectable several years after the fact, as is the period of stability. Did the quality of institutions in fact change between 2019 and 2022, or is the fluctuation in rankings a function of who was added to the pool? Whether a given school happens to fall into or out of the top 10, the top 50, or the top 100 may partially be a function of the number of programs (and new programs) in that year and who happens to respond (the response rate) that year, even if the overall objective quality of the school is relatively similar, year to year.

One might expect the plurality or majority of academic programs to remain relatively stable in structure, size, employment outcomes of graduates, and approach year to year. Therefore, an annually varying "quality" measure, as observed in these peer scores, is methodologically problematic. Moreover, even when the peer scores are relatively close (changing by 0.1 to 0.2 points, on average), dramatic movement is observed in rankings, even as far as moving into new top groups

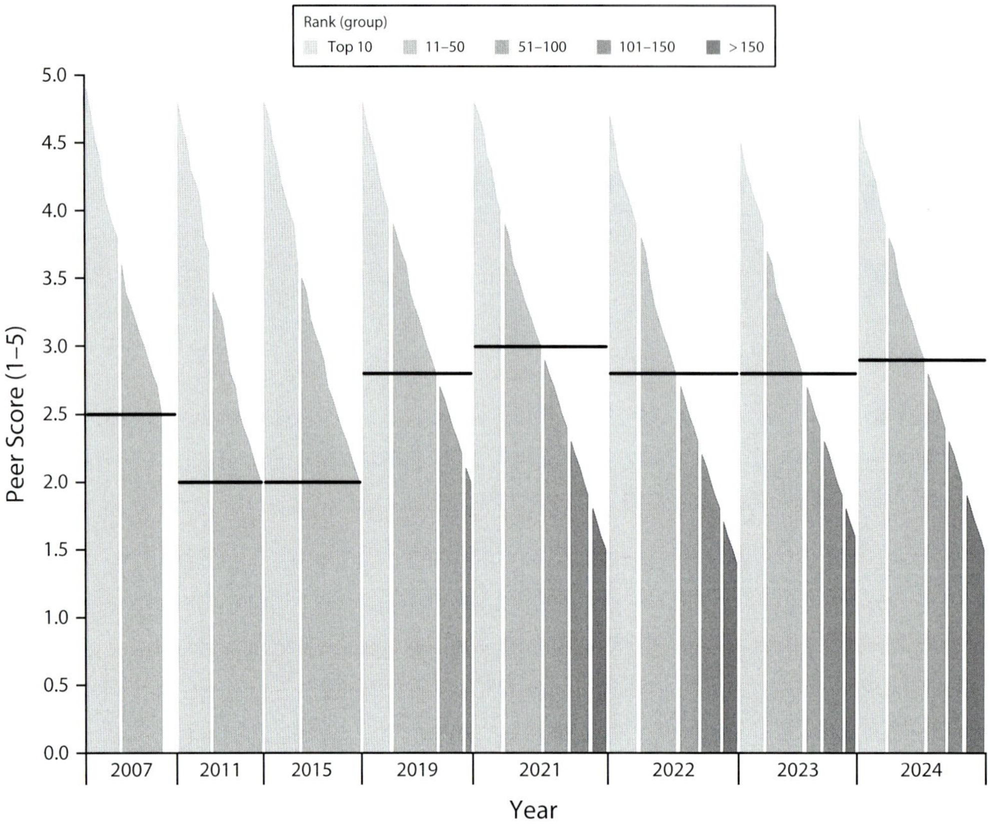

FIGURE 1— ***US News and World Report* Rankings of Public Health Schools, 2007–2024**

Note. Bar represents minimum peer score of the group ranked 11 to 50 in a given year. The x-axis is the *US News and World Report* rankings of each institution by year, grouped as indicated in the legend. Peer scores are the average of the single-item survey each institution is asked of others. Per *US News and World Report* methodology,[6] "Respondents rated the academic quality of programs on a scale of 1 (marginal) to 5 (outstanding). They were instructed to select 'don't know' if they did not have enough knowledge about a program to rate it. Only fully accredited programs in good standing during the survey period are ranked."
Source. Author analysis of *US News and World Report* rankings and National Center for Education Statistics graduation data.

(Appendix Figure A, available as a supplement to the online version of this article at http://www.ajph.org).

The top 10 sees relatively little change. Since 2007, two entrants reached that vaunted list after increasing (improving) their peer scores by only 0.2 and 0.1; of those that were bumped out, one fell from grace even though their peer score improved by 0.3, and the other after receiving a decreased 0.2 average peer score compared with the previous cycle.

Despite great interest in the top 10, substantially more movement occurs outside it, though by similarly small margins. Eight entrances to the 11 to 50 rank occurred (generally by improving peer scores 0.1 to 0.3 points), and 18 exits occurred (generally by decreasing peer scores 0.1 to 0.4 points). Among the top 50, a cycle-to-cycle change of 0.3 to 0.5 points regularly moved institutions up dozens of rankings, often into higher groups. However, even nominal or no change may result in (substantially) lower rankings. In 2024, there were 16 transitions from the 101 to 150 rank to the 151 and over rank. Five had no change in peer score, nine were 0.1 points worse, one was 0.2 points worse, and one was 0.3 points worse. For such a high-stakes enterprise, that a nominal peer score change could result in such a drastic swing in rankings—and opaquely to the public—is severely problematic.

Public health and the health sciences are not trivial fields. Any ranking or rating-based system should merit more substantive metrics than "How much do you like me?" or "Have you heard of me?" Public health now confers over 20 000 graduate degrees and as many undergraduate degrees annually from more than 600 schools and programs, of which more than 250 are accredited.[6–9] Applicants deserve more than a reflection of how well programs are marketed cross-institutionally. Our institutions report data to all sorts of entities, data that prospective students could use: application counts, acceptance rates, yield, degree-associated and cumulative student loan debt, first-destination graduate outcomes, faculty–student ratios, on-time graduation rates, faculty productivity in paper publishing, and grant and contract awards, to name a few. There are more. Some of these *USNWR* deigns to use to rank the programs it considers worthwhile—but not public health.

Interest in public health as a profession, like other health sciences, grew during the COVID-19 pandemic; between challenging macroeconomic conditions and growing awareness of the field as a viable career, public health applications skyrocketed. But a correction is likely on the horizon, and has already arrived for some. In a field where schools and programs are colleagues, but also competitors, the rankings are often a differentiator.[10] Especially for those up top. Breaking those incentives is a problem.

But here is the counter. Those who are recognized by their peers at the top have good reason to feel secure in that status.[10] It is almost certainly true that in any multifactorial ranking, no set of institutions would hold the crown for all subcategories. Those who perform well in individual items that peer institutions recognize as promoting student fit will necessarily perform well overall. If there is any validity at all to the *USNWR* rankings, then different data points would bear out the relative rankings that exist at a high level, and prospective students would have more information and be better off. But if there is not internal validity here, it is unconscionable to use these rankings, however much one may benefit.

Rankings are a cottage industry built on a sinkhole, but one postsecondary institutions continue to try and fill in, instead of digging it out and rebuilding around the foundation. Some are trying.[2,10–12] Institutions and programs in other fields, recognizing the problems associated with *USNWR*'s methodologies, have chosen to pull out of rankings altogether. This action is laudable, and although it is a hopeful sign that the same could be done in public health, it is not a reasonable ask of any one institution to make that change on their own. It is challenging to contemplate a path forward that would benefit the field as a whole. *USNWR* has not moved on the health sciences ranking methods, public health included, despite public requests. As a field, frankly, public health's import to *USNWR* is too low to motivate change. If the pandemic did not change that, no momentum from the base will.

What, then, is the alternative? Withdrawing from the rankings, as participants in other fields have done, is one path. The membership of the Association of Schools and Programs of Public Health could create an alternative ratings or rankings system—a practical approach, perhaps, but fraught with political ramifications. An independent third party could emerge to create new rankings or ratings, although that would entail more data reporting for participants. Institutions could collectively agree to "best fit" measures—employment, debt, earnings, net tuition, student and faculty diversity, faculty productivity, and so forth—and transparently post these data points on their own. Although that approach would not be centralized, nor as consumer-friendly as the rankings, it would be a substantial improvement.

Many options would provide better data for promoting student fit for public health programs than rankings, which have, reasonably or unreasonably, become associated with an overall measure of perceived quality. After all, even cursory analysis of the data suggests that the relationship between ranking, debt, and first-destination earnings is complex.[13] Although the rankings methodology acknowledges the importance of other items in determining fit,[5] these are not assessed by *USNWR*.

USNWR explicitly states that their rankings should not be the sole factor in any student decision-making. That does not obviate their responsibility to be a rigorous and trustworthy source. And so it is, somewhat unreasonably, incumbent on the applicant to beware the ranking—something not so easily done.

It is time for a true alternative. The first step is to move beyond the dependence on the current rankings and offer our applicants something better, something meaningful, something grounded in what our field cares about: data. Not just whether enough people think you are outstanding . . . or merely marginal. AJPH

CORRESPONDENCE

Correspondence should be sent to Jonathon Leider, D312 Mayo Building, MMC 729, 420 Delaware St SE, Minneapolis, MN 55455 (e-mail: lleider@umn.edu). Reprints can be ordered at https://www.ajph.org by clicking the "Reprints" link.

PUBLICATION INFORMATION

Full Citation: Leider JP. Rethinking rankings in public health graduate education—who are they for? *Am J Public Health*. 2024;114(11):1195–1198.

Acceptance Date: August 11, 2024.

DOI: https://doi.org/10.2105/AJPH.2024.307848

ORCID iD:
Jonathon P. Leider https://orcid.org/0000-0001-9905-476X

ACKNOWLEDGMENTS

I thank peer reviewers Jennifer McGuire and Michelle Niemann for their feedback on an earlier version of this commentary.

CONFLICTS OF INTEREST

The author has no conflicts of interest to disclose.

REFERENCES

1. Meredith M. Why do universities compete in the ratings game? An empirical analysis of the effects of the *US News and World Report* college rankings. *Res High Educ.* 2004;45(5):443–461. https://doi.org/10.1023/B:RIHE.0000032324.46716.f4
2. Humphrey HJ, Levinson D, Carter K. Medical school rankings—bad for the health of the profession and the public. *JAMA.* 2023;329(16):1343–1344. https://doi.org/10.1001/jama.2023.2815
3. Moshtaghian A. Columbia University acknowledges submitting inaccurate data for consideration in college rankings. *CNN.* September 11, 2022. Available at https://www.cnn.com/2022/09/11/media/columbia-university-us-news-world-report-college-rankings/index.html. Accessed April 25, 2024.
4. Levenson E, Westhoff K. Former dean of Temple University convicted of fraud for using fake data to boost its national ranking. *Philadelphia Inquirer.* November 30, 2021. Available at: https://www.cnn.com/2021/11/30/us/temple-university-dean-guilty/index.html. Accessed April 25, 2024.
5. Morse R, Brooks EF. Methodology: best health school rankings. *US News and World Report.* 2024. Available at: https://www.usnews.com/education/best-graduate-schools/articles/health-schools-methodology. Accessed April 25, 2024.
6. *Technical Documentation: College Scorecard Data by Field of Study.* Washington, DC: National Center for Education Statistics; 2022.
7. Leider JP, Burke E, Nguyen RHN, et al. Trends in degree conferrals, degree-associated debt, and employment outcomes among undergraduate public health degree graduates, 2001–2020. *Am J Public Health.* 2023;113(1):115–123. https://doi.org/10.2105/AJPH.2022.307113
8. National Center for Education Statistics. IPEDS Data Center [data set]. 2020. Available at: https://nces.ed.gov/ipeds/datacenter/DataFiles.aspx?gotoReportId=7&fromIpeds=true&sid=f5e09d18-62c7-4305-b8ff-25d2cfb84f53&rtid=7. Accessed April 25, 2024.
9. Council on Education for Public Health. List of accredited schools and programs. 2024. Available at: https://ceph.org/about/org-info/who-we-accredit/accredited. Accessed June 28, 2024.
10. Dugerdil A, Babington-Ashaye A, Bochud M, et al. A new model for ranking schools of public health: The Public Health Academic Ranking. *Int J Public Health.* 2024;69:1606684. https://doi.org/10.3389/ijph.2024.1606684
11. Hartocollis A. Yale and Harvard law schools withdraw from the US News rankings. *New York Times.* November 16, 2022. Available at: https://www.nytimes.com/2022/11/16/us/yale-law-school-us-news-rankings.html. Accessed December 2022.
12. Tuttle WA, O'Connor SJ, Borkowski N, Hernandez SR, Szychowski J. The influence of *US News and World Report* rankings of graduate programs in healthcare management on applicant pool quality and student job placement of graduates. *J Health Adm Educ.* 2020;37(3):193–212.
13. Center for Public Health Systems. Debt and earnings of public health graduates. 2022. Available at: https://www.sph.umn.edu/research/centers/cphs/dashboards/debt-and-earnings-of-public-health-graduates. Accessed June 28, 2024.

Public Health Monitoring: An Active Phrase for Vigilance, Warning, Guidance, and Accountability

Nancy Krieger, PhD

ABOUT THE AUTHOR

Nancy Krieger, PhD is with the Department of Social and Behavioral Sciences, Harvard T. H. Chan School of Public Health, Boston, MA.

Kudos to *AJPH* for calling the long overdue question: Should the field of public health use "public health monitoring" instead of "public health surveillance" or even "public health data"?"[1(p662)] Tellingly, "public health monitoring" leads the list, as it should—a term to be preferred, because it uniquely encompasses people, technology, and systems and actively connotes vigilance, warning, guidance, and accountability.

In 2023, Kassler and Bowman cogently argued in their essay "Overcoming Public Health 'Surveillance': When Words Matter" that the field of public health needs to drop the phrase "surveillance," given its deep links to state and corporate efforts to collect data to control people as political subjects and as consumers.[2] Reminding readers of the etymology of "surveillance"—as "derived from the French roots *sur* (over) and *veiller* (to watch)"[2(p1102)]—they called for a reframing of "public health surveillance" so that it prioritizes "protecting data privacy and restoring public trust as foremost objectives."[2(p1104)] They did not, however, offer alternative terminology to describe their alternative: "epidemiological regime."[2(p1104)]

"Public health monitoring" fits the bill. To support this claim, I offer three lines of argument: etymology, scope of work, and recognition that social justice has been the foundation of public health since the mid–19th-century emergence of public health agencies.[3]

"Monitoring" and the word "monitor"—which can be either a verb or a noun—are, according to the *Oxford English Dictionary* (*OED*), terms that are "a borrowing from Latin," whereby "monit-" is the "past participial stem of *monēre* to advise, warn, or remind."[4] As the dictionary explains, "monitor" simultaneously can refer to instruments, systems, and people, with the *OED* definitions including both "something that advises or monitors" and "a person who advises or monitors."[4]

Examples accompanying these definitions include, for instruments, "an instrument or device for continuously measuring some quantity or property" (e.g., radiation monitor, fetal heart monitor, apnea monitor), "a computer program which monitors and controls the running of other programs; an operating system," and "a visual display unit connected to a computer to display text and images; a computer screen."[4] For people, examples of those who are monitors include "a person who oversees or observes; one who observes or comments on a process or activity, esp. in an official capacity to ensure that correct procedure is followed" (e.g., human rights monitor) and "a person who uses monitoring equipment to check levels, standards, etc."[4] All of these examples involve familiar public health roles and technology.

From the standpoint of both etymology and scope of work, "monitoring" is thus vastly preferable to both "surveillance" and "data." To begin with, it is an active word and makes clear that someone or something is doing the monitoring—and this monitoring can be implemented by individuals and by communities for themselves to advance their health and thus is not reducible to surveillance conducted by government agencies or corporations to control populations and behaviors. It also avoids the problem of "data" being a passive word[5]—effectively meaning "that which is given," since it is derived from the "neuter past participle of *dare* to give."[4] Stated bluntly, data are never simply a "given" but instead are a social product whose content and cost reflect societal priorities and intellectual frameworks—with the work and resources required to obtain the data necessarily involving human labor, technology, and concepts regarding the phenomena to be measured.[3,5]

Additionally, "monitoring," unlike "surveillance," provides a sense of purpose that is in accord with a public health focus on prevention: monitors warn to guide action to prevent harm.

AJPH November 2024, Vol. 114, No. 11

It is also connotes "vigilance," a term notably used in the name of the Brazilian public health agency Agência Nacional de Vigilância Sanitária (Brazilian Health Regulatory Agency)[6,7] that is becoming more common in the English-language public health literature.[8,9] Thus, as observed by Alvarez da Silva et al., "Brazil has its own specific expression for health surveillance—'health vigilance'—but their actions are of a universal practice."[7] Similarly, Wier and Mykhalovskiy argued in their 2010 book *Global Public Health Vigilance: Creating a World on Alert*:

> Vigilance directs analytic attention to apparatuses that continuously monitor phenomena that may give rise to catastrophic events. In the public health sense, vigilance refers to an attitude of being attentive, alert, and watchful; vigilance is an ethical standard to be used by public health officials in the course of their work.[8(p9)]

No such ethical standard is implied by "public health surveillance" or "public health data."

"Monitoring," additionally, is compatible not only with public health activities to promote population health and health equity and individual and community efforts to monitor their own health but also with civil society engagement to monitor how actions by governments and corporations affect people's health and planetary health.[3,5] Monitoring involves both accountability and agency[3,5]: one monitors to give warning and to hold accountable those who cause harm. Such monitoring is central to advancing health justice and stands in opposition to older frameworks emphasizing surveillance, whose roots extend back to 18th- and 19th-century conceptions of "medical police."[3,10]

Changing long-used terms is not easy, but it is feasible. "Surveillance" has long been interwoven with public health discourse, practice, and systems.[2,10–12] It is central to the US Centers for Disease Control and Prevention's Office of Public Health Data, Surveillance, and Technology, including its new "data modernization" initiative.[13] Yet concepts and standards can and do change if people decide to and are able to implement these changes.

One instructive example is the name change, in the mid-1990s, of the venerable publication *Control of Communicable Diseases in Man* to *Control of Communicable Diseases Manual*.[14] This change occurred because I initiated and circulated with colleagues a petition at the American Public Health Association's annual meeting in 1992[14] titled "APHA Publications Should Not Use 'Man' to Mean 'Women and Men.'" The text stated:

> We, the undersigned members of APHA, petition APHA to change the title of its publication *Control of Communicable Diseases in Man*. The use of the term "man" to refer to women and men is irritating and outdated. We suggest that APHA update the title so that it is inclusive of women; a more accurate title would be: *Control of Communicable Diseases in Human Populations*.[14(p20)]

Agreeing with the need to shift to a "gender neutral"[14(p20)] title, the APHA Executive Board devised a pithy solution, whereby it replaced "in man" with "manual." This new title was conceptually valid and more accurate (describing the book as a "manual"), was typographically feasible (both "in man" and "manual" had the same character count of six characters), and allowed the book to retain its "well-known acronym, *CCDM*."[14(p20)]

Similarly, the 2024 decision of the journal *Substance Abuse* to take the major step of revising its name, after 15 years, to *Substance Use* exemplifies shifts in public health terminology paralleling shifts in understandings and values.[15] In an editorial tellingly titled "What's in a Name? Destigmatizing Language Regarding People Who Use Alcohol or Drugs in Publications and Journal Title[s]," the journal editors Stuart and Ramsey offered two reasons for the name change:

> 1. Scholars have compellingly argued that use of certain terminology, such as "substance abuse," carries a variety of negative connotations. Renaming the journal is motivated largely by our desire to move away from stigmatizing language and the harms it causes. . . . Referring to people as substance abusers defines them by their problem and increases stigma, increases blame and culpability, and decreases help-seeking behavior.
> 2. [We] had another important reason to change the journal title. We are interested in research with a focus that is broader than problematic substance use. Specifically, we are interested in research on substance use, not solely disordered use.[15]

The name change thus simultaneously offered greater conceptual clarity, expanded the journal's scope, removed stigmatizing language, and institutionalized the new language in a way that will affect what it publishes and the public health discourse going forward.

In closing, changes in terminology are evidence of people's thoughtful engagement with changes in ideas, values, and knowledge.[3,10] It is time, past time, to replace "public health surveillance" with "public health monitoring." AJPH

CORRESPONDENCE

Correspondence should be sent to Nancy Krieger, PhD, Professor of Social Epidemiology, Department of Social and Behavioral Sciences, Harvard T. H. Chan School of Public Health (Kresge 717), 677 Huntington Ave, Boston, MA 02115 (e-mail: nkrieger@hsph.harvard.edu). Reprints can be ordered at https://www.ajph.org by clicking the "Reprints" link.

PUBLICATION INFORMATION

Full Citation: Krieger N. Public health monitoring: an active phrase for vigilance, warning, guidance, and accountability. *Am J Public Health*. 2024; 114(11):1199–1201.

Acceptance Date: August 9, 2024.

DOI: https://doi.org/10.2105/AJPH.2024.307850

ORCID iD:

Nancy Krieger https://orcid.org/0000-0002-4815-5947

ACKNOWLEDGMENTS

This work was supported in part by the American Cancer Society Clinical Research Professor Award to N. Krieger.

CONFLICTS OF INTEREST

The author has no conflicts of interest to declare.

REFERENCES

1. Morabia A, Dasgupta N, Thorpe L. Public health surveillance, monitoring, or data? Time to decide. *Am J Public Health.* 2024;114(7):661–662. https://doi.org/10.2105/AJPH.2024.307709
2. Kassler WJ, Bowman CL. Overcoming public health "surveillance": when words matter. *Am J Public Health.* 2023;113(10):1102–1105. https://doi.org/10.2105/AJPH.2023.307348
3. Krieger N. *Epidemiology and the People's Health: Theory and Context.* 2nd ed. New York, NY: Oxford University Press; 2024. https://doi.org/10.1093/oso/9780197695555.001.0001
4. Oxford University Press. *Oxford English Dictionary.* Available at: https://www.oed.com. Accessed July 9, 2024.
5. Krieger N. The making of public health data: paradigms, politics, and policy. *J Public Health Policy.* 1992;13(4):412–427. https://doi.org/10.2307/3342531
6. Brazilian Health Regulatory Agency [Agência Nacional de Vigilância Sanitária (ANVISA)]. Available at: https://www.gov.br/anvisa/en. Accessed July 8, 2024.
7. Alvarez da Silva JA, Alvas Costa E, Lucchese G. Unified health system 30th birthday: health surveillance. *Ciênc saúde colet.* 2018;23(6). https://doi.org/10.1590/1413-81232018236.04972018
8. Weir L, Mykhalovskiy E. *Global Public Health Vigilance: Creating a World on Alert.* New York, NY: Routledge; 2010. https://doi.org/10.4324/9780203857724
9. Williams J, Mayes C, Flint-Peterson E, Degeling C. Vigilance in infectious disease emergencies: expanding the concept. *Soc Sci Med.* 2024;344: 116648. https://doi.org/10.1016/j.socscimed.2024.116648
10. Rosen G. *From Medical Police to Social Medicine: Essays on the History of Health Care.* New York, NY: Science History Publications; 1974.
11. Centers for Disease Control and Prevention. Public health surveillance in the United States: evolution and challenges. *MMWR Suppl.* 2012;61(3): 3–9. Available at: https://www.cdc.gov/mmwr/preview/mmwrhtml/su6103a2.htm?s_cid%3Dsu6103a2_x. Accessed July 8, 2024.
12. Groseclose SL, Buckeridge DL. Public health surveillance systems: recent advances in their use and evaluation. *Annu Rev Public Health.* 2017;38:57–79. https://doi.org/10.1146/annurev-publhealth-031816-044348
13. Centers for Disease Control and Prevention. Office of Public Health Data, Surveillance, and Technology (OPHDST). Available at: https://www.cdc.gov/ophdst/index.html. Accessed July 8, 2024.
14. American Public Health Association. CCDM undergoes slight name change. *The Nation's Health.* 1993;20.
15. Stuart GL, Ramsey SE. What's in a name? Destigmatizing language regarding people who use alcohol or drugs in publications and journal title[s]. *Subst Use.* 2024;18:11782218231222908. https://doi.org/10.1177/11782218231222908

Community Organizations, Local Health Equity Action Teams, and a Learning Collaborative to Address COVID-19 Disparities in Urban and Rural Communities

Edward F. Ellerbeck, MD, MPH, Vicki L. Collie-Akers, PhD, MPH, Elizabeth Ablah, PhD, MPH, Sarah Landry, LMSW, Allison Honn, MBA, Sara Obermeier, MA, Mariana Ramirez, LCSW, Yvonnes Chen, PhD, Ian R. Knight, MA, Crystal Y. Lumpkins, PhD, Mary Ricketts, Tony Carter, BA, Ullyses Wright, BASc, Christal Watson, MA, Daniel L. Kurz, MPH, Stacy McCrea-Robertson, MS, Sarah Finocchario-Kessler, PhD, MPH, Joseph LeMaster, MD, MPH, Erin Corriveau, MD, MPH, Broderick Crawford, BS, Jianghua He, PhD, and K. Allen Greiner, MD, MPH

See also Notes From the Field, pp. 1207–1231.

Rapid Acceleration of Diagnostics–Underserved Populations (RADx-UP) Kansas worked with 10 Kansas counties from November 2020 through June 2022 to form local health equity action teams (LHEATs), develop COVID-19 testing strategies, foster communication about COVID-19, and share best practices through a learning collaborative. Participating counties documented 693 distinct COVID-19 testing and 178 communication activities. Although the intervention was not associated with changes in the proportion of positive COVID-19 tests, LHEATs in the learning collaborative implemented new testing strategies and responded to emerging COVID-19 challenges. (*Am J Public Health*. 2024;114(11): 1202–1206. https://doi.org/10.2105/AJPH.2024.307771)

AJPH November 2024, Vol. 114, No. 11

The success of public health emergency responses often depends upon the ability of communities and institutions to work together.[1] Community engagement in public health initiatives can have an impact on health behaviors and health outcomes, but there are limited data to guide how to organize community groups and help them respond to rapidly changing circumstances in the midst of a public health crisis.[2] Learning collaboratives have the potential to empower community members who seek to work with institutions to improve public health responses in an emergency.[3–6] Learning collaboratives can provide members with details on what to do (i.e., what works and what does not) and how to get the work done—the critical knowledge needed to support implementation.[6,7]

INTERVENTION AND IMPLEMENTATION

RADx-UP Kansas was funded through the federal Rapid Acceleration of Diagnostics-Underserved Populations (RADx-UP) initiative designed to improve COVID-19 testing in high-risk communities and reduce the impact of COVID-19. In the intervention, health departments and community organizations in 10 Kansas counties received funding to recruit staff, form local health equity action teams (LHEATs), launch COVID-19 testing and communication activities, and participate in a learning collaborative. We conducted monthly and often biweekly check-in meetings with county partners to discuss their progress and troubleshoot problems.

The lead organization in each county developed an LHEAT to engage historically excluded and marginalized groups and elicit an authentic community voice to inform COVID-19 testing and mitigation efforts. In forming their LHEATs, counties were encouraged to take advantage of existing community organizations that already had grassroots connections and identify community members who could help them leverage existing communication channels. Many of the LHEAT members had connections with community-based organizations that were already working in high-risk areas in their county, including faith-based organizations, social service agencies, and health care providers.

Representatives from each county participated in learning collaborative meetings held 1 or 2 times each month. These meetings brought county representatives together with local and state public health representatives leading the COVID-19 response. The meetings provided a platform for peer support and helped foster the sharing of community-driven interventions and best practices in COVID-19 control. To support the collaborative, our research team compiled a virtual repository of tools, support materials, and resources.[8]

PLACE, TIME, AND PERSONS

RADx-UP Kansas was conducted in 10 Kansas counties (6 rural, 4 urban) disproportionately impacted by the COVID-19 epidemic.[9] Interventions and follow-up occurred between November 2020 and June 2022. The project was co-led by community members and faculty at the Kansas University Medical Center and engaged the support of staff from local health departments and community organizations in each of the 10 participating counties. A team of community consultants was engaged to guide plans for community engagement and the design of interventions. The 10 LHEATs were composed of 117 community members who helped drive local COVID-19 testing and communication activities.

PURPOSE

RADx-UP Kansas was designed to help local community organizations form LHEATs and bring them together in a learning collaborative designed to rapidly adapt, test, and implement community-driven solutions to improve COVID-19–related communication and address disparities in COVID-19 testing.

EVALUATION AND ADVERSE EFFECTS

RADx-UP Kansas used a 3-fold evaluation strategy: a process evaluation to capture local community activities, a quantitative evaluation of COVID-19 test positivity rates, and an assessment of barriers and facilitators of program implementation.

Process Evaluation

The process evaluation captured community-level testing and communication activities reported by county representatives through the Community Check Box.[10] This reporting platform allowed the central research team to measure progress, display data, and highlight major accomplishments. Results of this process evaluation demonstrated a variety of activities to promote COVID-19 testing (Box 1), including pop-up testing events affiliated with churches, businesses, and community organizations. Testing was offered at multiple group events including sporting events, back-to-school events, youth summer camps, and job fairs. In total, the counties reported conducting 604 one-time testing events and 89 recurring testing activities in addition to testing already being conducted within local health departments and clinical sites. Testing activities were primarily focused on reaching low-income populations (n = 472 out of 693; 68.1%), Latinx (n = 402; 58.0%), immigrants or refugees (n = 268; 38.7%), and Blacks/African Americans (n = 267; 38.5%). As they became available, COVID-19 home test kits were also distributed in high-risk communities. Through these efforts, a total of 104 006 COVID-19 tests were made available.

Each county also launched communication activities, including efforts to advertise testing opportunities through newsletters, social media (particularly Facebook), newspaper, radio, and television (Box 1). LHEAT members helped to design and distribute messages through their own organizational channels (e.g., church newsletters, e-mail lists). Several learning collaborative meetings focused specifically on best practices for businesses; this led to worksite seminars and town hall meetings focused on recommendations for employers. Counties reported 178 different COVID-19–related communication activities that were estimated to directly reach 217 774 individuals. A coordinated multimedia campaign entitled Community Workers Beat the Virus was also launched across the participating counties; the results of this campaign have been reported elsewhere and are not included in these numbers.[11]

Quantitative Evaluation

The quantitative evaluation focused on the rate of positive tests as a proxy measure for test availability and demand. We compared test positivity rates[12] from April 2020 through November 2021 in intervention versus control counties matched on population size, rurality, race/ethnicity, or

BOX 1— Testing and Communication Innovations Developed and Shared in the RADx-UP Kansas Collaborative

Innovations
Testing • Pop-up testing sites (irregular schedules, sites changing but typically community settings) • Regularly scheduled testing at community (non–health care) settings (primarily churches, also community centers, libraries, laundromats) • Worksite testing • School-based testing for staff and students • Testing and vaccination drive-up events • Testing with food packages and food trucks • Testing with raffles, gift cards, other tangible incentives • Mobile testing units deployed to community settings • Distribution of home test kits through community events (e.g., back-to-school fairs, Pride festivals) • Distribution of home test kits through holiday events (e.g., Juneteenth, Thanksgiving, Easter, Eid al-Fitr) • Distribution of home test kits through nonprofit organizations • Summer camp testing programs
Communication • Social and traditional media promoting testing activities occurring locally • Social and traditional media promoting testing generally • Locally, regionally, and RADx-UP Kansas–produced communications featuring local and regional community members promoting testing and other mitigation activities • Canvassing and door-to-door communications (e.g., flyers, brochures) to promote testing events or availability • Townhall meetings or educational presentations (e.g., Spanish-speaking panel discussion COVID-19 mitigation efforts) • Sponsorships aimed at promoting testing and vaccination (e.g., college football game communications) • RADx-UP Kansas–produced webinars focused on specific sectors or audiences disseminated to communities (worksites, Divine Nine: African American Sororities and Fraternities) • Distribution of materials produced by RADx-UP Kansas team (e.g., one-pager describing why testing was necessary) through social and traditional media

Note. RADx-UP = Rapid Acceleration of Diagnostics–Underserved Populations.

geographic proximity (Figure 1). Pre- and postintervention testing rates in intervention and matched control counties are shown in Table A (available as a supplement to the online version of this article at https://ajph.org). Using a mixed logistic regression model, we estimated the impact of the intervention by modeling the monthly rate of positive tests at the county level controlling for time (post- vs preintervention) and group (intervention vs control). The change in

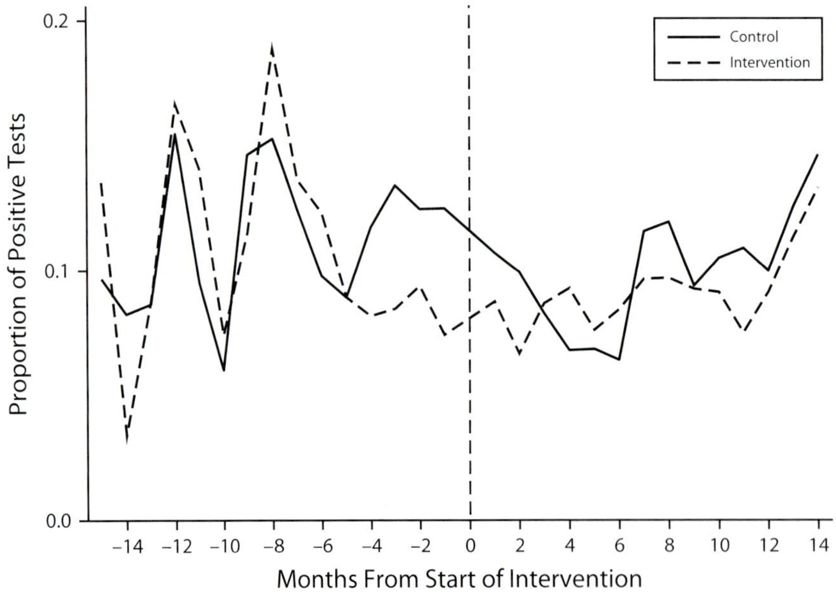

FIGURE 1— Proportion of Positive COVID-19 Tests in 9 Intervention and 21 Control Counties in Kansas Before and After the Start of the Intervention: April 2020–November 2021

COVID-19 test positivity before and after the interventions was not significantly different in intervention versus control counties ($P = .75$; Table B, available as a supplement to the online version of this article at https://ajph.org).

Barriers and Facilitators to Program Implementation

Using the Consolidated Framework for Implementation Research as a guide,[13] we reached out to key informants from each of our 10 partners and completed 19 semistructured interviews. We probed on 3 Consolidated Framework for Implementation Research domains that were determined a priori to be most critical to the success of this intervention: intervention characteristics, outer setting, and inner setting.

A summary of the barriers and facilitators to implementing COVID-19 testing activities in their communities is presented in Table C (available as a supplement to the online version of this article at https://ajph.org). In describing intervention characteristics, respondents described the value of forming an LHEAT and engaging collaborators with meaningful lived experiences noting that "they're the heart of it all . . . they are trusted members of our community for those underserved populations." They noted how the learning collaborative allowed them to connect with public health leaders who could help with "understanding and just interpreting what [the guidelines] mean." The collaborative allowed them to "borrow things from other counties" and see how testing interventions done in another county might be adapted for use in their own community.

In terms of the outer setting, respondents noted the importance of testing resources available from the state, but also noted that "whenever there was a spike [in COVID-19], there was a shortage of testing, and whenever there was a lull, we had to incentivize testing." COVID-19 responses became political, and there were many local groups that were opposed to testing and to wearing a mask, but despite this political turmoil, many historically disadvantaged communities "were not 'being political' and were more friendly to us than other populations."

In discussing the inner setting domain, respondents noted problems with space (e.g., "The office that we have is not ideal for testing"), but they took advantage of other local resources, such as a church available for rent. Staffing could be an issue, but some organizations were able to adapt—"Once we hired Spanish-speaking [community health workers], it got so much easier." Many respondents reported a competing need to prioritize vaccinations over testing, noting that vaccination, as soon as it became available, was "where everyone's attention, energy, everything went."

SUSTAINABILITY

Based on our preliminary findings, the Kansas Department of Health and the Environment authorized the formation of Communities Organizing to Promote Equity in 20 counties across Kansas. Like RADx-UP Kansas, Communities Organizing to Promote Equity has supported existing LHEATs or formed new ones and supported an ongoing learning collaborative. It has also provided support for local community health workers to directly work with high-risk members of their local community.[14] Efforts are being coordinated with local health departments and federally qualified health centers to integrate LHEATs and provide long-term support of community health workers.

PUBLIC HEALTH SIGNIFICANCE

The LHEATs in each of the communities provided a critical avenue for expanding access to COVID-19 testing and communication messages at the local level and supporting community engagement. This engagement may be particularly important for communities that have previously been excluded from power.[2,15] The LHEATs were not only able to leverage local resources to respond to the epidemic but also created a bidirectional communication channel with public health leaders. RADx-UP Kansas showed how a learning collaborative could support communities in their response to a crisis, providing a vehicle for sharing best practices and helping community partners adapt to new challenges that arose during the course of the COVID-19 pandemic. AJPH

ABOUT THE AUTHORS

Edward F. Ellerbeck, Vicki L. Collie-Akers, Sarah Landry, Sara Obermeier, Mariana Ramirez, Daniel L. Kurz, and Stacy McCrea-Robertson are with the Department of Population Health, University of Kansas Medical Center, Kansas City. Elizabeth Ablah and Allison Honn are with the Department of Population Health, University of Kansas Medical Center, Wichita. Yvonnes Chen is with the School of Journalism and Mass Communication, University of Kansas, Lawrence. Ian R. Knight is a community member, Phoenix, AZ. Crystal Y. Lumpkins is with the Department of Communication, Huntsman Cancer Institute, University of Utah, Salt Lake City. Mary Ricketts is with Turning Point Training and Consultation, Overland Park, KS. Tony Carter is with Salem Missionary Baptist Church, Kansas City, KS. Ullyses Wright is a community member, Overland Park, KS. Christal Watson is with Kansas City Kansas Schools Foundation, Kansas City, KS. Sarah Finocchario-Kessler, Joseph LeMaster, Erin Corriveau, and K. Allen Greiner are with the Department of Family Medicine, University of Kansas Medical Center, Kansas City. Broderick Crawford was with the NBC Community Development Corporation, Kansas City, KS. Jianghua He is with the Department of Biostatistics and Data Science, University of Kansas Medical Center, Kansas City.

CORRESPONDENCE

Correspondence should be sent to Edward F. Ellerbeck, MD, MPH, 3901 Rainbow Blvd, MS 3044, Kansas City, KS 66160 (e-mail: eellerbe@kumc.edu). Reprints can be ordered at https://www.ajph.org by clicking the "Reprints" link.

PUBLICATION INFORMATION

Full Citation: Ellerbeck EF, Collie-Akers VL, Ablah E, et al. Community organizations, local health equity action teams, and a learning collaborative to address COVID-19 disparities in urban and rural communities. *Am J Public Health*. 2024;114(11): 1202–1206.

Acceptance Date: June 17, 2024.

DOI: https://doi.org/10.2105/AJPH.2024.307771

ORCID iDs:

Edward F. Ellerbeck https://orcid.org/0000-0002-7774-2729

Elizabeth Ablah https://orcid.org/0000-0003-4550-2162

Allison Honn https://orcid.org/0000-0002-6764-9133

CONTRIBUTORS

B. Crawford contributed to the study design, co-led the application for funding, trained community staff, and led many community interventions described in this study. All other authors reviewed and contributed to the final content of the article. E. F. Ellerbeck, S. Finocchario-Kessler, and K. A. Greiner co-designed the study, procured study funding, and oversaw study implementation, data collection, and analysis. V. L. Collie-Akers, E. Ablah, S. Landry, A. Honn, S. Obermeier, D. L. Kurz, and S. McCrea-Robertson were engaged in implementation of the interventions, data collection, analysis, and reporting. J. He oversaw collection and analysis of quantitative data. M. Ramirez, Y. Chen, I. R. Knight, C. Y. Lumpkins, M. Ricketts, T. Carter, U. Wright, C. Watson, J. LeMaster, and E. Corriveau guided the design of intervention tools, community engagement, and communication plans.

ACKNOWLEDGMENTS

This research was supported by the National Institutes of Health under award UL1 Tr002366-04S3.

This article is dedicated to the memory of Broderick Crawford, a community-based, co-principal investigator, who has inspired his co-authors to continue to advocate for higher levels of community engagement and co-leadership in research. He tragically died November 27, 2022, prior to completion of the final analysis of the study findings.

The authors would like to thank the numerous staff and volunteers at both the state and county level in Kansas that spent so much time and effort in responding to the needs of their communities during the COVID-19 epidemic and were ultimately responsible for the work described in this article.

Note. The content is solely the responsibility of the authors and does not necessarily represent the official views of the National Institutes of Health.

CONFLICTS OF INTEREST

The authors declare that they have no relevant or material financial interests that relate to the research described in this article.

HUMAN PARTICIPANT PROTECTION

This study was reviewed and approved by the University of Kansas Medical Center institutional review board (study 00146321).

REFERENCES

1. Ramsbottom A, O'Brien E, Ciotti L, Takacs J. Enablers and barriers to community engagement in public health emergency preparedness: a literature review. *J Community Health*. 2018;43(2):412–420. https://doi.org/10.1007/s10900-017-0415-7
2. O'Mara-Eves A, Brunton G, Oliver S, Kavanagh J, Jamal F, Thomas J. The effectiveness of community engagement in public health interventions for disadvantaged groups: a meta-analysis. *BMC Public Health*. 2015;15(1):129. https://doi.org/10.1186/s12889-015-1352-y
3. Varda DM, Chandra A, Stern SA, Lurie N. Core dimensions of connectivity in public health collaboratives. *J Public Health Manag Pract*. 2008;14(5): E1–E7. https://doi.org/10.1097/01.PHH.0000333889.60517.46
4. Ayers LR, Beyea SC, Godfrey MM, Harper DC, Nelson EC, Batalden PB. Quality improvement learning collaboratives. *Qual Manag Health Care*. 2005;14(4):234–247. https://doi.org/10.1097/00019514-200510000-00010
5. Joly BM, Booth M, Shaler G, Conway A. Quality improvement learning collaboratives in public health: findings from a multisite case study. *J Public Health Manag Pract*. 2012;18(1):87–94. https://doi.org/10.1097/PHH.0b013e3182367db1
6. Nix M, McNamara P, Genevro J, et al. Learning collaboratives. Insights and a new taxonomy from AHRQ's two decades of experience. *Health Aff (Millwood)*. 2018;37(2):205–212. https://doi.org/10.1377/hlthaff.2017.1144
7. Rohweder C, Wangen M, Black M, et al. Understanding quality improvement collaboratives through an implementation science lens. *Prev Med*. 2019;129S:105859. https://doi.org/10.1016/j.ypmed.2019.105859
8. Kansas University Medical Center. RADx-UP Kansas. Available at: https://www.kumc.edu/school-of-medicine/academics/departments/population-health/research/radxup.html. Accessed November 1, 2023.
9. Kansas Department of Health and the Environment. COVID-19 cases in Kansas. Available at: https://www.coronavirus.kdheks.gov/160/COVID-19-in-Kansas. Accessed August 2, 2020.
10. Center for Community Health and Development. Community Check Box Evaluation System. Available at: https://checkbox.ctb.ku.edu. Accessed November 1, 2023.
11. Chen Y, Ramirez M, Lumpkins CY, Crawford B, Allen Greiner K, Ellerbeck E. Lessons learned from Community Workers Beat the Virus, a multimedia campaign cocreated with trusted community leaders. *Am J Public Health*. 2022;112(suppl 9):S909–S912. https://doi.org/10.2105/AJPH.2022.307071
12. Centers for Disease Control and Prevention. COVID Data Tracker. Available at: https://covid.cdc.gov/covid-data-tracker/#datatracker-home. Accessed July 20, 2023,
13. Damschroder LJ, Aron DC, Keith RE, Kirsh SR, Alexander JA, Lowery JC. Fostering implementation of health services research findings into practice: a consolidated framework for advancing implementation science. *Implement Sci*. 2009;4:50. https://doi.org/10.1186/1748-5908-4-50
14. Kansas University Medical Center. Communities Organizing to Promote Equity. Available at: https://www.kumc.edu/school-of-medicine/academics/departments/family-medicine-and-community-health/research/communities-organizing-to-promote-equity.html. Accessed August 5, 2023.
15. Brunton G, Thomas J, O'Mara-Eves A, Jamal F, Oliver S, Kavanagh J. Narratives of community engagement: a systematic review-derived conceptual framework for public health interventions. *BMC Public Health*. 2017;17(1):944. https://doi.org/10.1186/s12889-017-4958-4

Reach and Engagement With Population Health Management Interventions to Address COVID-19 Among Safety-Net Health Care Systems

Chelsey R. Schlechter, PhD, MPH, Tatyana V. Kuzmenko, PhD, Brian Orleans, MS, Jennifer Wirth, MS, Kimberly A. Kaphingst, ScD, Bryan Gibson, DPT, PhD, Kensaku Kawamoto, MD, PhD, MHS, Tracey Siaperas, Alan Pruhs, Courtney Pariera Dinkins, MS, Tom Greene, PhD, Yue Zhang, PhD, Jonathan J. Chipman, PhD, Michael Friedrichs, MS, Cho Y. Lam, PhD, Joni H. Pierce, MBA, MS, Emerson P. Borsato, PhD, Ryan C. Cornia, Leticia Stevens, Anna Martinez, MEd, Richard L. Bradshaw, PhD, MS, Rachel Hess, MD, MS, Guilherme Del Fiol, MD, PhD, and David W. Wetter, PhD

See also Notes From the Field, pp. 1202–1231.

Interventions designed to address COVID-19 needed to be rapidly scaled up to the population level, and to address health equity by reaching historically marginalized populations most affected by the pandemic (e.g., racial/ethnic minorities and rural and low socioeconomic status populations). From February 2021 to June 2022, SCALE-UP Utah used text messaging interventions to reach 107 846 patients from 28 clinics within seven safety-net health care systems. Interventions provided informational and motivational messaging regarding COVID-19 testing and vaccination, and were developed using extensive community partner input. (*Am J Public Health*. 2024;114(11):1207–1211. https://doi.org/10.2105/AJPH.2024.307770)

AJPH November 2024, Vol. 114, No. 11

The SCALE-UP Utah trial used population health management strategies to increase COVID-19 testing and vaccination among Community Health Center patients.

INTERVENTION AND IMPLEMENTATION

SCALE-UP Utah used proactive, bidirectional text messages regarding risk, motivation for COVID-19 testing and vaccination, and provision of scheduling information to increase COVID-19 testing and vaccination among patients in federally qualified and community health centers (CHCs) across Utah. Text messages (Figure 1) were sent on behalf of the patient's CHC in English or Spanish based on the patient's preferred language in the electronic health record (EHR). Reports containing demographics and phone numbers for patients seen at participating CHCs for three years before the intervention start date were obtained from CHCs and were uploaded into a population health management (PHM) platform. Phone numbers were validated using a telecommunications application programming interface that checked that numbers were active and could receive SMS.

SCALE-UP Utah was conducted in partnership with the Association for Utah Community Health (AUCH, Utah's federally designated primary care association), the Utah Department of Health and Human Services (UDHHS), and CHCs throughout Utah.[1] The project used a multimethod engagement approach to develop and adapt PHM interventions[2] in real-time rapid cycles according to changing recommendations for testing and vaccination, CHC preferences, and individually tailored information (e.g., local case rates). The approach included consultation meetings with AUCH and UDHHS, meetings with leadership at each CHC, quarterly meetings with a Patient Advisory Committee (consisting of CHC patients) and Study Advisory Committee (consisting of CHC patients, CHC staff, AUCH, and UDHHS), and a weekly stakeholder

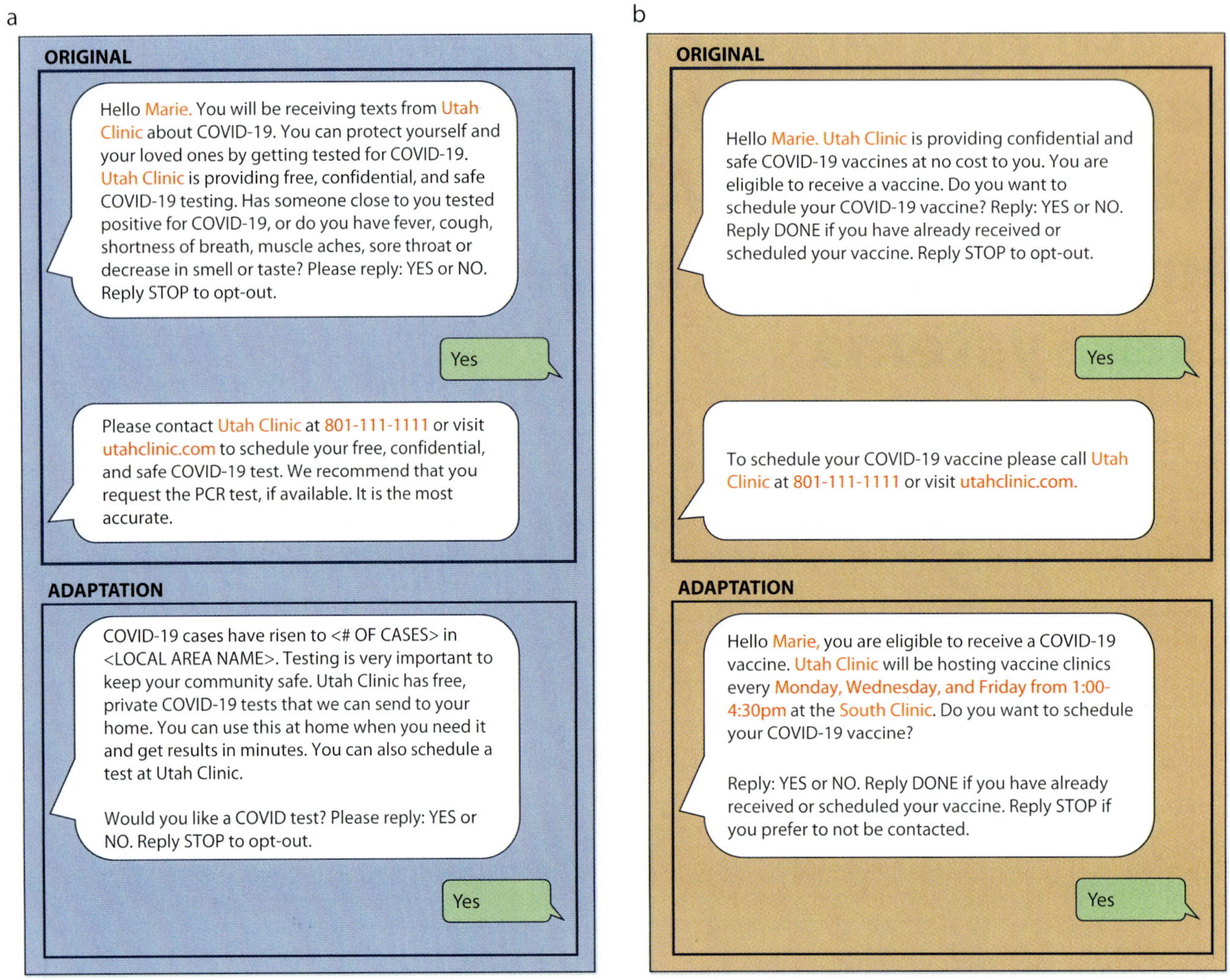

FIGURE 1— Examples of Original and Adapted Text Messages Sent Regarding COVID-19 (a) Testing and (b) Vaccination: Utah, 2021–2022

meeting with AUCH, UDHHS, and the research team. The project relied on shared data and resources across project partners to identify priority groups for PHM interventions.

PLACE, TIME, AND PERSONS

Seven of 13 CHCs in Utah participated in SCALE-UP Utah; 114 485 of their patients met inclusion criteria (≥ 18 years, encounter at CHC in last three years, English or Spanish primary language in EHR). Six percent of patients (n = 6639) did not have a validated, text-enabled phone number listed in the EHR. Ninety-four percent (n = 107 846) had a validated, text-enabled phone number listed in the EHR and were sent at least one text message. Of these 107 846 patients, 54.8% were female, 44.9% Hispanic/Latino, 17.0% rural (rural–urban commuting area ≥ 4), 58.7% uninsured, and 34.6% had Spanish as primary language in the EHR. Patients' mean age was 42.1 years (SD = 16.1). The Patient Advisory Committee consisted of four patients (50% spoke Spanish, 75% were from rural areas), and the seven clinic representatives on the committee included two clinic managers, three providers, one operations director, and one pharmacist. The project was conducted from February 2021 to June 2022.

PURPOSE

Populations from racial/ethnic minority, rural, and low socioeconomic status (SES) groups were disproportionately affected by COVID-19.[3] CHCs provide comprehensive primary care regardless of insurance status and faced substantial challenges throughout the pandemic, including restrictions to in-person visits and shifts to telehealth. These challenges underscored the need to proactively identify groups disproportionately at risk for COVID-19 and to address COVID-19 outside of clinical encounters.[4]

PHM[5] strategies such as proactive text messaging have been promoted for improving chronic disease prevention and control, are beneficial for multiple racial/ethnic groups, have the potential to improve COVID-19 testing and vaccination, and have substantial reach.[2,6,7] Even in households with annual incomes less than $30 000, 97% own a cellphone and 76% own a smartphone.[8] Incorporating community partner priorities for rapid, real-time adaptation of messaging has the potential to improve relevance, timeliness, and acceptability of text messaging. Furthermore, ensuring equitable reach of interventions such as text messaging is necessary to ensure that interventions do not inadvertently exacerbate health inequities.

EVALUATION AND ADVERSE EFFECTS

The goal of this evaluation was to evaluate reach (i.e., patients had a valid, text-enabled phone number in the EHR and were sent a text), engagement, (i.e., patients responded with a text other than opt out), and opt out (i.e., responded with only an opt out) of text messaging. Data presented herein include only results from the first text campaign for which each individual patient was included. From February 2021 to June 2022, SCALE-UP Utah reached 107 846 CHC patients via text messaging to promote COVID-19 testing and vaccination. Of those patients, 7% (n = 7862) opted out of receiving additional texts as their only response, 15% (n = 16 191) responded to at least one text that was not an opt out, and 77% (n = 83 793) did not respond.

To understand potential impacts on health equity, we examined differences in outcomes by demographic characteristics using logistic regression models (Table 1). Although most CHC patients had a valid, text-enabled phone number in the EHR, the odds of being a patient without a text-enabled phone number were higher among patients who were older (vs younger), rural (vs urban), non-Hispanic/Latino or missing ethnicity (vs Hispanic/Latino), male or other/unknown (vs female), or had public insurance (vs private insurance). Among Hispanic/Latino patients, the odds of being a patient without a text-enabled phone number were higher among patients whose primary language was English (vs Spanish).

Among those with valid phone numbers, the odds of being a patient who opted out of messaging were higher among patients who were older (vs younger), non-Hispanic/Latino or missing ethnicity (vs Hispanic/Latino), and had private insurance (vs public insurance or no insurance). Among Hispanic/Latino patients, the odds of being a patient who opted out of messaging were higher among patients whose primary language was English (vs Spanish).

Among those with valid phone numbers, the odds of being a patient who engaged with text messaging (i.e., responded with a message other than opt out) were higher among patients who were older (vs younger), urban (vs rural), non-Hispanic/Latino or missing ethnicity (vs Hispanic/Latino), female (vs male or other/unknown), and had private insurance (vs public or no insurance).

SUSTAINABILITY

SCALE-UP Utah interventions were designed to use existing infrastructure at CHCs and AUCH; all CHCs throughout Utah currently employ texting to send patients appointment reminders and prompts to complete routine health screenings. Furthermore, the research–practice partnership was leveraged to obtain additional funding to continue addressing COVID-19 in Utah CHCs through 2024.

PUBLIC HEALTH SIGNIFICANCE

To make a public and population health impact, interventions need to be effective and also reach populations in need.[9,10] COVID-19 highlighted long-standing health inequities among racial/ethnic minority, rural, and low SES populations, and underscored the need to reach these communities to affect health inequities. SCALE-UP Utah was conducted using a community-engaged approach that leveraged a research–practice partnership between AUCH, CHCs throughout Utah, UDHHS, and the University of Utah.[1,2] Intervention procedures and content were developed and adapted in conjunction with community partners, including patient and staff representatives from CHCs.[2] The community-engagement approach ensured that interventions met the needs of CHCs and were appropriate for patients; as a result, SCALE-UP Utah reached virtually entire populations of patients seen at CHCs to motivate and facilitate COVID-19 testing and vaccination. Future researchers and practitioners should continue to engage community partners to ensure high reach among historically marginalized populations.

TABLE 1— Logistic Regression Models Assessing the Adjusted Association Between Demographics and Outcomes of Reach and Engagement: Utah, 2021–2022

	Total No.	No Valid Mobile Number (Model 1)[a]		Total No. Messaged	Opt Out Only (Model 2)[a]		Engaged With Text Message (Model 3)[a]	
		% (No.)	AOR (95% CI)		% (No.)	AOR (97.5%[a] CI)	% (No.)	AOR (97.5%[a] CI)
Age,[b] y								
<30	30 964	5.4 (1 661)	1 (Ref)	29 303	7.5 (2 205)	1 (Ref)	10.1 (2 970)	1 (Ref)
30–64	71 732	5.7 (4 105)	1.08 (1.02, 1.15)	67 627	7.1 (4 822)	0.99 (0.93, 1.05)	15.7 (10 642)	1.68 (1.59, 1.76)
≥65	11 789	7.4 (873)	1.01 (0.91, 1.12)	10 916	7.6 (835)	1.11 (1.00, 1.23)	23.6 (2 574)	2.51 (2.34, 2.70)
Rurality[c]								
Rural (Ref)	21 243	13.9 (2 960)	1 (Ref)	18 283	11.3 (2 057)	1 (Ref)	19.4 (3 539)	1 (Ref)
Urban	93 292	3.9 (3 679)	0.69 (0.63, 0.75)	89 563	6.5 (5 805)	1.06 (0.96, 1.16)	14.1 (12 652)	1.19 (1.11, 1.28)
Ethnicity[b]								
Hispanic or Latino	49 675	2.6 (1 275)	1 (Ref)	48 400	4.5 (2 200)	1 (Ref)	12.4 (6 009)	1 (Ref)
Non-Hispanic	53 549	8.9 (4 790)	2.19 (2.04, 2.35)	48 759	9.7 (4 749)	2.12 (1.99, 2.27)	17.8 (8 661)	1.27 (1.21, 1.33)
Missing	11 261	5.1 (574)	1.64 (1.47, 1.82)	10 687	8.5 (913)	2.13 (1.93, 2.34)	14.2 (1 521)	1.14 (1.06, 1.23)
Gender[b]								
Female	62 151	4.9 (3 039)	1 (Ref)	59 112	7.3 (4 325)	1 (Ref)	15.7 (9 304)	1 (Ref)
Male	47 614	6.7 (3 195)	1.30 (1.24, 1.38)	44 419	7.2 (3 212)	0.97 (0.91, 1.02)	14.1 (6 272)	0.85 (082, 0.89)
Other/unknown	4 720	8.6 (405)	1.23 (1.09, 1.38)	4 315	7.5 (325)	1.06 (0.91, 1.22)	14.3 (615)	0.86 (0.77, 0.95)
Insurance[b]								
Private	26 279	6.9 (1 804)	1 (Ref)	24 475	8.6 (2 263)	1 (Ref)	18.5 (4 533)	1 (Ref)
Public	22 100	9.4 (2 081)	1.46 (1.35, 1.57)	20 019	7.6 (1 514)	0.72 (0.67, 0.78)	18.0 (3 598)	0.77 (0.73, 0.82)
Uninsured	66 106	4.2 (2 754)	1.01 (0.95, 1.09)	63 352	6.4 (4 085)	0.87 (0.81, 0.93)	12.7 (8 060)	0.74 (0.70, 0.78)
Primary language[d] (Hispanic/Latino patients only)								
English	14 667	3.9 (577)	1 (Ref)	14 090	5.6 (786)	1 (Ref)	11.4 (1 608)	1 (Ref)
Spanish	35 008	2.0 (698)	0.62 (0.55, 0.71)	34 310	4.1 (1 414)	0.71 (0.64, 0.78)	12.8 (4 401)	0.97 (0.90, 1.03)

Note. AOR = adjusted odds ratio; CI = confidence interval.

[a]Model 1 included all patients in our sample and utilized α at 0.05. Models 2 and 3 included only those found to have a valid mobile phone number. The outcome for models 2 and 3 utilized a three-level outcome of no response, engaged, or opted out and derived two categorical variables defined as opted out (versus no response or engaged) for model 2, and engaged (versus no response or opted out) for model. Because of our hypothesized interrelation between model 2 and 3 outcomes, α was set to 0.025.

[b]Models included the following covariates: ethnicity, gender, urban/rural, insurance, age, community health center (CHC), category of text message content (i.e., test only, vaccine only, combination), days since start of study, intervention group (e.g., whether patient was offered patient navigation in addition to text messaging).

[c]Model included ethnicity, gender, insurance, age, text message content, days since start of study, and intervention group as covariates.

[d]Model included gender, urban/rural, insurance, age, CHC, text message content, days since start of study, and intervention group as covariates; model restricted to Hispanic/Latino patients.

Although the majority of patients in participating CHCs (94%) had valid, text-enabled phone numbers listed in the EHR, the odds of having a text-enabled phone number differed between populations. For example, 14% of rural patients did not have a text-enabled phone number in the EHR compared with 4% of urban patients. Similarly, there were differences in odds of engaging with text messaging between population groups: 17% of patients who were privately insured versus 12% of patients who were uninsured engaged with text messaging. These results suggest that researchers and practitioners need to closely monitor PHM interventions to ensure they do not exacerbate health inequities among historically marginalized populations. AJPH

ABOUT THE AUTHORS

Chelsey R. Schlechter, Cho Y. Lam, and David W. Wetter are with the Department of Population Health Sciences, Center for Health Outcomes and Population Equity, Huntsman Cancer Institute, University of Utah, Salt Lake City. Tatyana V. Kuzmenko, Kensaku Kawamoto, Joni H. Pierce, Emerson P. Borsato, Ryan C. Cornia, Leticia Stevens, Richard L. Bradshaw, and Guilherme Del Fiol are with the Department of Biomedical Informatics, University of Utah School of Medicine, Salt Lake City. Brian Orleans, Jennifer Wirth, and Anna Martinez are with the Center for Health Outcomes and Population Equity, Huntsman Cancer Institute, University of Utah, Salt Lake City. Kimberly A. Kaphingst is with the Department of Communication, Huntsman Cancer Institute, University of Utah, Salt Lake City. Bryan Gibson is with the School of Medicine, University of Utah, Salt Lake City. Tracey Siaperas, Alan Pruhs, and Courtney Pariera Dinkins are with the Association for Utah Community Health, Salt Lake City. Tom Greene, Yue Zhang, and Jonathan J. Chipman are with the Department of Population Health Sciences, University of Utah, Salt Lake City. Michael Friedrichs is with the Utah Department of Health and Human Services, Salt Lake City. Rachel Hess is with the Departments of Population Health Sciences and Internal Medicine, Spencer Fox Eccles School of Medicine, University of Utah, Salt Lake City.

CORRESPONDENCE

Correspondence should be sent to Chelsey R. Schlechter, 2000 Circle of Hope Dr, Salt Lake City, UT 84112 (e-mail: chelsey.schlechter@hci.utah.edu). Reprints can be ordered at http://www.ajph.org by clicking the "Reprints" link.

PUBLICATION INFORMATION

Full Citation: Schlechter CR, Kuzmenko TV, Orleans B, et al. Reach and engagement with population health management interventions to address COVID-19 among safety-net health care systems. *Am J Public Health*. 2024;114(11):1207–1211.

Acceptance Date: June 17, 2024.

DOI: https://doi.org/10.2105/AJPH.2024.307770

ORCID iDs:

Kimberly A. Kaphingst https://orcid.org/0000-0003-2668-9080

David W. Wetter https://orcid.org/0000-0002-4013-1932

CONTRIBUTORS

C. R. Schlechter, J. Wirth, K. A. Kaphingst, B. Gibson, K. Kawamoto, A. Pruhs, C. P. Dinkins, T. Greene, Y. Zhang, M. Friedrichs, C. Y. Lam, J. H. Pierce, A. Martinez, R. Hess, G. Del Fiol, and D. W. Wetter contributed to the concept and design. T. V. Kuzmenko, B. Orleans, C. R. Schlechter, J. Wirth, K. A. Kaphingst, B. Gibson, K. Kawamoto, E. P. Borsato, R. C. Cornia, L. Stevens, R. L. Bradshaw, G. Del Fiol, and D. W. Wetter contributed to the analysis and interpretation of the data. C. R. Schlechter drafted the manuscript. All authors contributed to the revision of the manuscript and approved the final manuscript.

ACKNOWLEDGMENTS

Research reported in this Rapid Acceleration of Diagnostics–Underserved Populations (RADx-UP) publication was supported by the National Institutes of Health under Award Numbers UL1TR002538, 3UL1TR002538-03S4, P30CA042014; and by the Huntsman Cancer Foundation.

We are extremely grateful to the Community Health Center staff and patients who have contributed their time and insight to the conduct of this project. We acknowledge and thank the Association for Utah Community Health staff, including our patient navigators. We also acknowledge the Utah Department of Health and Human Services for their support in this project and willingness to share their expertise and data.

Note. The contents of this article are solely the responsibility of the authors and do not necessarily represent the official views of the National Institutes of Health.

CONFLICTS OF INTEREST

The authors report no conflicts of interest.

HUMAN PARTICIPANT PROTECTION

This research was reviewed and approved by the University of Utah institutional review board (#IRB_00136001).

REFERENCES

1. Schlechter CR, Del Fiol G, Lam CY, et al. Application of community-engaged dissemination and implementation science to improve health equity. *Prev Med Rep*. 2021;24:101620. https://doi.org/10.1016/j.pmedr.2021.101620
2. Schlechter CR, Reese TJ, Wirth J, et al. Rapid-cycle designs to adapt interventions for COVID-19 in safety-net healthcare systems. *Transl Behav Med*. 2023;13(6):389–399. https://doi.org/10.1093/tbm/ibac101
3. McGowan VJ, Bambra C. COVID-19 mortality and deprivation: pandemic, syndemic, and endemic health inequalities. *Lancet Public Health*. 2022;7(11):e966–e975. https://doi.org/10.1016/S2468-2667(22)00223-7
4. Mann DM, Chen J, Chunara R, Testa PA, Nov O. COVID-19 transforms health care through telemedicine: evidence from the field. *J Am Med Inform Assoc*. 2020;27(7):1132–1135. https://doi.org/10.1093/jamia/ocaa072
5. Steenkamer BM, Drewes HW, Heijink R, Baan CA, Struijs JN. Defining population health management: a scoping review of the literature. *Popul Health Manag*. 2017;20(1):74–85. https://doi.org/10.1089/pop.2015.0149
6. Vodopivec-Jamsek V, de Jongh T, Gurol-Urganci I, Atun R, Car J. Mobile phone messaging for preventive health care. *Cochrane Database Syst Rev*. 2012;12(12):CD007457. https://doi.org/10.1002/14651858.CD007457.pub2
7. Nelson LA, Greevy RA, Spieker A, et al. Effects of a tailored text messaging intervention among diverse adults with type 2 diabetes: evidence from the 15-month REACH Randomized Controlled Trial. *Diabetes Care*. 2021;44(1):26–34. https://doi.org/10.2337/dc20-0961
8. Pew Research Center. Mobile fact sheet. Available at: https://www.pewresearch.org/internet/fact-sheet/mobile. Accessed March 15, 2021.
9. Glasgow RE, Vogt TM, Boles SM. Evaluating the public health impact of health promotion interventions: the RE-AIM framework. *Am J Public Health*. 1999;89(9):1322–1327. https://doi.org/10.2105/AJPH.89.9.1322
10. Glasgow RE, Harden SM, Gaglio B, et al. RE-AIM planning and evaluation framework: adapting to new science and practice with a 20-year review. *Front Public Health*. 2019;7:64. https://doi.org/10.3389/fpubh.2019.00064

Reach, Adoption, Implementation, and Sustainability of the Mobile Health for Migrant Health (mHealth-4-Mhealth) Program: Nebraska, 2022–2023

Russell J. McCulloh, MD, Ellen Kerns, PhD, MPH, Chad Abresch, PhD, Michelle Warren, PhD, Fernando Sanchez, Gisela Marfileno, Lisvey Rivera, and M. Jana Broadhurst, MD, PhD

See also Notes From the Field, pp. 1202–1231.

Migrant families face challenges to health and well-being from COVID-19. We deployed Mobile Health for Migrant Health (mHealth-4-Mhealth) to migrant families, a household-based program with mHealth-assisted at-home testing and linkages to community resources. We assessed the reach, adoption, and implementation of the program among rural migrant families enrolled in the Title IC Nebraska Migrant Education Program from February 2022 to July 2023. We describe successful adoption and longitudinal use of mHealth screening tools for severe acute respiratory syndrome coronavirus 2 infection risk and social determinants of health. (*Am J Public Health*. 2024;114(11):1212–1216. https://doi.org/10.2105/AJPH.2024.307746)

AJPH November 2024, Vol. 114, No. 11

Families living in rural areas face significant barriers to accessing health care resources,[1–5] including information on severe acute respiratory syndrome coronavirus 2 (SARS-CoV-2) and access to high-quality diagnostic testing.[6] More than 95% of Nebraska counties are designated health care shortage areas. Migrant agricultural workers face additional barriers to accessing care and community resources as they are newly arrived to the area and are isolated from existing social infrastructure and capital. Mobile health (mHealth) technologies can overcome geographic barriers to accessing high-quality health care information and can be adapted for use in multiple languages. This technology, when combined with at-home SARS-CoV-2 testing and linkages to community resources and aid, may empower families to make optimal health and well-being decisions, thus enhancing families' resiliency in the face of disruptions such as the COVID-19 pandemic.

INTERVENTION AND IMPLEMENTATION

Families enrolled in the Title IC Nebraska Migrant Education Program (MEP) are eligible to participate in mHealth-4-Mhealth. Nebraska MEP eligibility is based on a family's work in agriculture and movement between school districts; most enrolled families identify as Hispanic, Latino, or Spanish origin. Our study team includes bilingual, bicultural community coordinators based in central Nebraska, facilitating engagement with families at community events and Spanish-language informed consent. All study materials, including the mHealth app, are available in Spanish or English.

mHealth-4-Mhealth study interventions are home-based and occur at the household level. The designated head of household is guided to download the mHealth tool[7] and receives at-home SARS-CoV-2 testing kits (Quidel QuickVue, QuidelOrtho, San Diego, CA). Families use the mHealth tool for daily symptom screening to assess household risk of SARS-CoV-2 infection and to access up-to-date public health guidance. A positive screen prompts at-home antigen testing by all household members, with recording of test results prompted by the app. The app also facilitates weekly screening for household challenges related to social determinants of health (SDOH) and provides links to community aid and resources. When requested, a family navigator engages with households to assist with identifying and accessing community resources. Participants are interviewed regarding engagement with program elements and reasons for testing or declining to test.

PLACE, TIME, AND PERSONS

MEP-enrolled families were referred to the study from MEP community events hosted in rural Nebraska. Here we report data from the first enrollments from February 2022 to July 2023.

PURPOSE

The aim of the mHealth-4-Mhealth program is to improve migrant families' resiliency through mHealth-facilitated SARS-CoV-2 risk screening and SDOH challenges screening.[8] Risk screening provides decision support for use and interpretation of at-home antigen testing, and SDOH challenges screening provides linkages to community resources and aid. The objective of the present study is to summarize reach and engagement of the mHealth-4-Mhealth program among migrant families in Nebraska.

EVALUATION AND ADVERSE EFFECTS

We evaluated interim program performance using measures organized under the Reach, Efficacy, Adoption, Implementation, Maintenance (RE-AIM) framework.[9] We characterized program reach by the number and demographics of study participants and representativeness of Nebraska MEP enrollees. We describe program adoption using the proportion of households with the mHealth tool downloaded and antigen test kits delivered. We measured program implementation based on household use of the mHealth screening tools, performance of at-home testing when prompted, and requests for household assistance.

Reach

As of July 2023, a total of 82 households comprising 318 participants (range = 2–8 participants per household) have been enrolled across 19 Nebraska counties and 20 school districts. Nearly all participants (n = 306; 96%) resided in a nonmetropolitan zip code (Rural-Urban Commuting Area code of 4 or greater[10]; Figure 1). More than half of participants (n = 165; 52%) were children; 82 (26%) were heads of household, and 71 (22%) were other adults in the household. All primary and secondary school grades (K–12) were represented (16 children in kindergarten; 27 children in grades 1 through 3; 31 children in grades 4 through 6; 29 children in grades 7 through 9; 11 children in grades 10 through 12). A total of 241 out of 248 (97%) participants indicated an ethnicity self-identified as Hispanic, Latino, or Spanish origin as compared with 70% among Nebraska MEP households; 132 out of 245 respondents (54%) identified as female. A total of 92% of heads of household spoke Spanish as their preferred language as compared with 46% of Nebraska MEP students with limited English proficiency.

Adoption

One hundred percent of participating households have downloaded the mHealth tool and received antigen testing kits.

Implementation

mHealth symptom screening. Households have performed a total of 5062 symptom screens to date, averaging two screens per household per week (Figure 2). A total of 130 (2.6%) of screens resulted in a prompt to test. Among households, 35 out of 82 (43%) have been prompted to test at least once since enrollment; 32 out of 35 (91%) households reported agreeing to test when prompted to do so (Figure 2). However, 56 out of 82 (68%) households reported using their test kits at least once since enrollment.

At-home SARS-CoV-2 antigen testing. A total of 24 household testing events (i.e., times when at-home antigen tests were both used by the family and had results sent to the study team) have been reported with 52 individual test results recorded. Current Food and Drug Administration guidelines require up to three valid negative tests, each performed 24 to 48 hours apart, to determine a negative result. Of the 52 individual test results recorded, seven (14%) participants recorded positive antigen tests, 34 (65%) recorded valid negative antigen tests, and 11 (21%) recorded antigen tests were indeterminate because of invalid or incomplete testing (Figure 2).

mHealth household challenges screening. Households have performed a total of 2954 household challenges screens

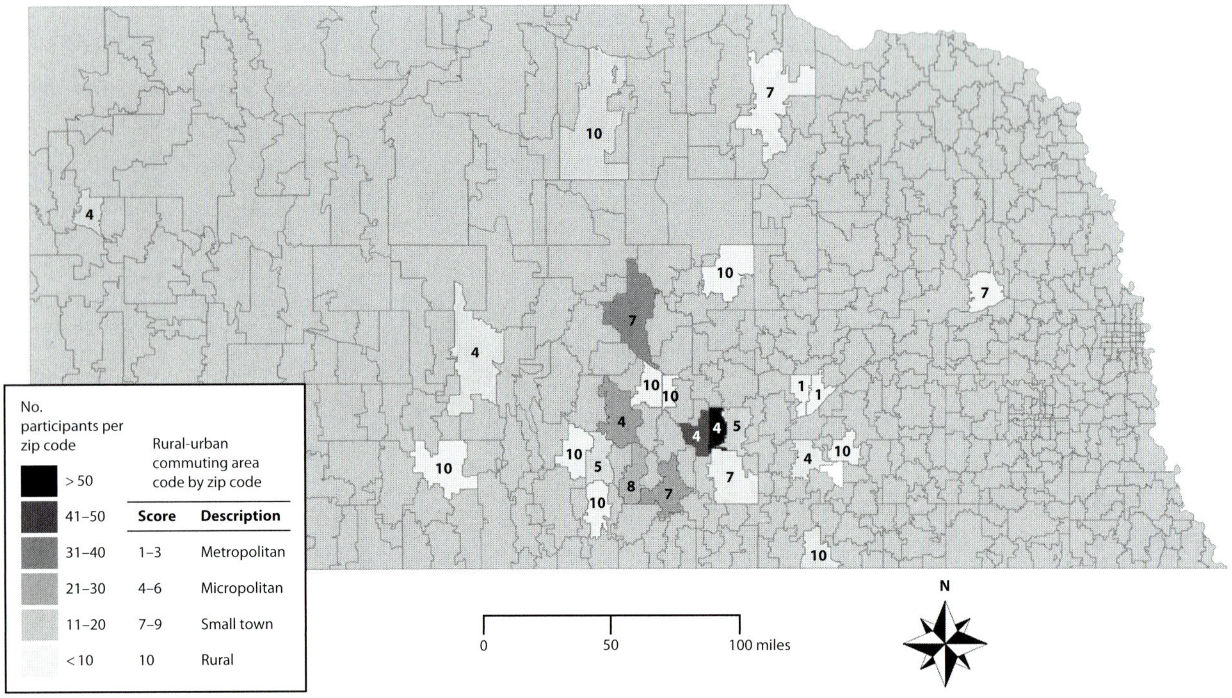

FIGURE 1— mHealth-4-Mhealth Program Reach and Participant Characteristics: Nebraska, 2022–2023

Note. Map of Nebraska zip codes indicating distribution of study participants. Inset numbers indicate Rural-Urban Commuting Area codes; codes 4 and greater denote nonmetropolitan zip codes.

to date, averaging one screen per household per week (Figure A, available as a supplement to the online version of this article at https://ajph.org). Frequently reported challenges included lost income, inability to afford expenses, inability to cope, delays in medical care, inability to afford healthy food, and childcare access (Figure A).

Community navigation assistance. A total of 197 (6.7%) household challenges screens reported one or more challenges. A total of 30 out of 82 (37%) households reported challenges (Figure A), all of

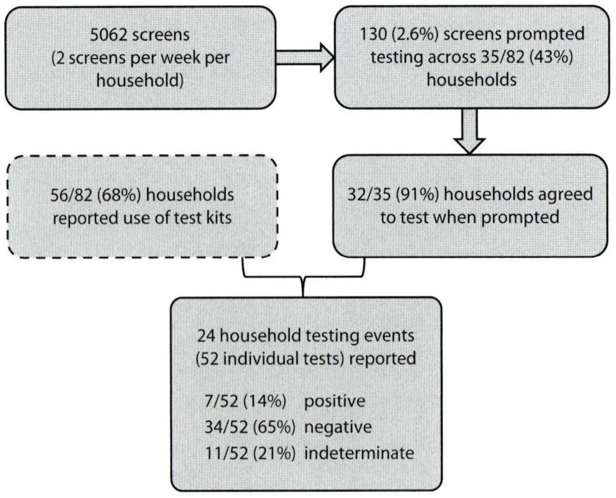

FIGURE 2— mHealth-4-Mhealth Program Implementation Metrics: Nebraska, 2022–2023

Note. Utilization and outcomes of mHealth-assisted screening for household risk of severe acute respiratory syndrome coronavirus 2 (SARS-CoV-2) infection and at-home SARS-CoV-2 rapid antigen test kits (Quidel QuickVue, QuidelOrtho, San Diego, CA).

whom requested family navigator assistance. Household contact and responses have been narratively recorded by the family navigator and are being analyzed to identify themes.

SUSTAINABILITY

Our results demonstrate the feasibility and scalability of mHealth-targeted at-home SARS-CoV-2 testing and of mHealth-targeted surveillance for SDOH challenges and facilitated referrals to community assistance among migrant households. Given our partnership with Nebraska MEP, our findings can inform future, larger-scale implementation of such programs in partnership with other MEPs across the country. Our program could also be adapted for use in other public health programs and community settings.

PUBLIC HEALTH SIGNIFICANCE

The mHealth-4-Mhealth program successfully engaged migrant families in rural Nebraska through partnership with the Nebraska MEP. An interim program performance evaluation using the RE-AIM framework demonstrates the following:

1. Program interventions were successfully delivered to rural, predominantly Spanish-speaking migrant families across a broad geographic range, including adults and children across all school grades.
2. All enrolled households successfully downloaded the mHealth app, received testing kits, and used the screening functions of the program's interventions.
3. Families sustained weekly screening activities across the study period, and nearly all families were willing to use at-home antigen test kits when prompted by the app.
4. mHealth-facilitated SDOH challenges screening is feasible and acceptable to rural, primarily Spanish-speaking migrant families. Families who reported challenges universally requested assistance, demonstrating the importance of linking mHealth screening to personnel with expertise in navigating community resources.

Results will provide evidentiary support to scale the intervention to migrant-serving programs nationally, inform health policy development, and drive future programs aimed at improving community resilience in public health emergencies. AJPH

ABOUT THE AUTHORS

Russell J. McCulloh and Ellen Kerns are with the Department of Pediatrics, College of Medicine, University of Nebraska Medical Center, Omaha. Chad Abresch is with the Department of Health Promotion, College of Public Health, University of Nebraska Medical Center. Michelle Warren is with the Department of Modern Languages, College of Arts and Sciences, University of Nebraska Kearney. Fernando Sanchez and Gisela Marfileno are with the Child Health Research Institute, University of Nebraska Medical Center. Lisvey Rivera is with the Nebraska Migrant Education Program, Hastings. M. Jana Broadhurst is with the Department of Pathology and Microbiology, College of Medicine, University of Nebraska Medical Center.

CORRESPONDENCE

Correspondence should be sent to Russell McCulloh, Department of Pediatrics, University of Nebraska Medical Center, 987878 Nebraska Medicine, Omaha, NE 68198-7878 (e-mail: russell.mcculloh@unmc.edu). Reprints can be ordered at https://ajph.org by clicking the "Reprints" link.

PUBLICATION INFORMATION

Full Citation: McCulloh RJ, Kerns E, Abresch C, et al. Reach, adoption, implementation, and sustainability of the Mobile Health for Migrant Health (mHealth-4-Mhealth) program: Nebraska, 2022–2023. *Am J Public Health*. 2024;114(11): 1212–1216.

Acceptance Date: May 24, 2024.

DOI: https://doi.org/10.2105/AJPH.2024.307746

ORCID iD:

Russell J. McCulloh https://orcid.org/0000-0002-0403-6639

CONTRIBUTORS

R. J. McCulloh and M. J. Broadhurst conceptualized the overall study design; supervised data acquisition, analysis, and interpretation; drafted the work; and approved the final version to be published. E. Kerns, C. Abresch, and M. Warren conceptualized the study design; contributed to data acquisition, analysis, and interpretation; critically revised the article; and approved the final version to be published. F. Sanchez, G. Marfileno, and L. Rivera contributed to data acquisition, analysis, and interpretation; critically revised the article; and approved the final version to be published.

ACKNOWLEDGMENTS

This research was supported by the National Institutes of Health under award 3OT2HD108106-01S1.

We are grateful for the contributions of Jera Hinkle, Laura Gamboa, Jonathan Figliomeni, Ricky Flores, Nicholas Reynolds, Julie Carstens, Alice Sato, and David Brett-Major, and leadership of the Nebraska Migrant Education Program including Sue Henry, Benjamin Zink, Cesar Duran, Dulce Valdez, and Veronica Estevez.

Note. The content is solely the responsibility of the authors and does not necessarily represent the official views of the National Institutes of Health.

CONFLICTS OF INTEREST

E. Kerns and R. J. McCulloh receive research grant support from the Merck Investigator Studies Program for vaccine communication research. M. J. Broadhurst received a speaker honorarium from Shoreland Inc.

HUMAN PARTICIPANT PROTECTION

This research project was approved by the University of Nebraska Medical Center institutional review board.

REFERENCES

1. Ferdows NB, Aranda MP, Baldwin JA, Baghban Ferdows S, Ahluwalia JS, Kumar A. Assessment of racial disparities in mortality rates among older adults living in US rural vs urban counties from 1968 to 2016. *JAMA Netw Open*. 2020;3(8): e2012241. https://doi.org/10.1001/jamanetworkopen.2020.12241
2. Leider JP, Meit M, McCullough JM, et al. The state of rural public health: enduring needs in a new decade. *Am J Public Health*. 2020;110(9): 1283–1290. https://doi.org/10.2105/AJPH.2020.305728

3. Herstein JJ, Degarege A, Stover D, et al. Characteristics of SARS-CoV-2 transmission among meat processing workers in Nebraska, USA, and effectiveness of risk mitigation measures. *Emerg Infect Dis*. 2021;27(4):1032–1038. https://doi.org/10.3201/eid2704.204800
4. Reyes S, Acosta LM, Domínguez V, Ramos AK, Andrews AR. Immigrant and US-born migrant farmworkers: dual paths to discrimination-related health outcomes. *Am J Orthopsychiatry*. 2022;92(4):452–462. https://doi.org/10.1037/ort0000625
5. Soto S, Yoder AM, Aceves B, Nuño T, Sepulveda R, Rosales CB. Determining regional differences in barriers to accessing health care among farmworkers using the national agricultural workers survey. *J Immigr Minor Health*. 2023;25(2):324–330. https://doi.org/10.1007/s10903-022-01406-9
6. Souch JM, Cossman JS. A commentary on rural-urban disparities in COVID-19 testing rates per 100,000 and risk factors. *J Rural Health*. 2021;37(1):188–190. https://doi.org/10.1111/jrh.12450
7. Honcoop AC, Kerns EK, McCulloh RJ, Lowndes BR, Clarke MA. Improving the usability of visual displays for a COVID-19 household screener. In: Ahram TZ, Falcão CS, eds. *Advances in Usability, User Experience, Wearable and Assistive Technology. AHFE 2021. Lecture Notes in Networks and Systems*. Vol 275. Cham, Switzerland: Springer; 2021. https://doi.org/10.1007/978-3-030-80091-8_102
8. Goldman JL, Kalu IC, Schuster JE, et al. Building school–academic partnerships to implement COVID-19 testing in underserved populations. *Pediatrics*. 2023;152(suppl 1):e2022060352C. https://doi.org/10.1542/peds.2022-060352C
9. Sweet SN, Ginis KA, Estabrooks PA, Latimer-Cheung AE. Operationalizing the RE-AIM framework to evaluate the impact of multi-sector partnerships. *Implement Sci*. 2014;9(1):74. https://doi.org/10.1186/1748-5908-9-74
10. US Department of Agriculture. Rural-Urban Commuting Area Codes. Economic Research Service. March 22, 2023. Available at: https://www.ers.usda.gov/data-products/rural-urban-commuting-area-codes. Accessed August 7, 2023.

Implementation of Neighborhood-Level Wastewater-Based Epidemiology to Measure and Mitigate Inequities in SARS-CoV-2 Infection in Boston, Massachusetts

Tori L. Cowger, PhD, MPH, Madeline T. Sharp, ScB, Justin D. Hart, MS, Bisola O. Ojikutu, MD, MPH, Shoba Nair, PhD, and Kathryn T. Hall, PhD, MPH

See also Notes From the Field, pp. 1202–1231.

Starting October 2022, the Boston Public Health Commission implemented a neighborhood-level wastewater-based epidemiology program to inform strategies to reduce COVID-19 inequities. We collected samples twice weekly at 11 neighborhood sites, covering approximately 18% of Boston, Massachusetts's population. Results from the program's first year revealed inequities unobservable in regional wastewater data both between the City of Boston and the greater Boston area and between Boston neighborhoods. We report program results and neighborhood-specific recommendations and resources to help residents interpret and use our findings. (*Am J Public Health*. 2024;114(11):1217–1221. https://doi.org/10.2105/AJPH.2024.307749)

AJPH November 2024, Vol. 114, No. 11

In Boston, Massachusetts, communities made vulnerable by systems of oppression have disproportionately borne COVID-19's impact, with inequities in SARS-CoV-2 (severe acute respiratory syndrome coronavirus 2) testing, COVID-19 vaccine uptake, and treatment.[1,2] Wastewater-based epidemiology is an important tool for measuring community-level infection independent of disease severity or access to testing and clinical care and can inform public health efforts to address structural inequities.[3–5] Wastewater SARS-CoV-2 testing has been ongoing in the greater Boston area since March 2020 through the Massachusetts Water Resources Authority. However, this regional program samples north and south influent covering 43 municipalities at Deer Island Treatment Plant and thus cannot identify inequities between the greater Boston area's cities and towns and between the City of Boston neighborhoods.[6]

INTERVENTION AND IMPLEMENTATION

The Boston Public Health Commission (BPHC) developed a neighborhood-level, wastewater-based epidemiology program to elucidate inequities in the SARS-CoV-2 burden between the City of Boston and the greater Boston region and between Boston's neighborhoods. These data inform the implementation of community-based strategies to reduce racialized and socioeconomic inequities in COVID-19 outcomes. We outline a concept to practice model for planning, implementing, and validating a neighborhood-level wastewater-based epidemiology program at a local health department.

BPHC launched a wastewater-based epidemiology program in October 2022 in collaboration with City of Boston partners and Biobot Analytics, a local wastewater-based epidemiology company.

Sampling Site Identification

Neighborhoods structure the health and well-being of residents through multiple intersecting pathways.[7] Boston and the surrounding metro area are economically and racially segregated, with persistent inequities across neighborhoods (Figure A; Table A, available as a supplement to the online version of this article at http://www.ajph.org).[1]

To evaluate potential sampling sites, we compared the size and sociodemographics of sewershed populations to those of surrounding neighborhoods (Table B; Figure B, available as a supplement to the online version of this article at http://www.ajph.org). We selected 11 sites covering 13 neighborhoods to maximize population coverage and representativeness citywide and by neighborhood, prioritizing neighborhoods most affected by persistent health inequities (Figure C; Supplementary Methods [available as a supplement to the online version of this article at http://www.ajph.org]). We excluded sampling along major roadways, which would have required hiring police officers to direct traffic.[8] This enabled us to maintain a consistent sampling schedule and reduce program costs while avoiding traffic disruptions, occupational hazards for sample collectors, and additional police presence.

Wastewater Sampling and Processing

We collected time-weighted, 24-hour composite samples at each site twice weekly using autosamplers mounted in sewer holes. We processed samples according to previously described Biobot Analytics methods, including using a concentration of pepper mild mottle virus to normalize the concentration of the SARS-CoV-2 N1 gene (Supplementary Methods).[9]

PLACE, TIME, AND PERSONS

The 11 selected neighborhood sampling sites cover an estimated 119 179 people (~18% of Boston's population; Figure C). Sites ranged in estimated population from 1869 to 34 412 (Figure C), with 60% identifying as Black, Indigenous, Latinx, or other People of Color (Table C, available as a supplement to the online version of this article at http://www.ajph.org). In addition, this population was representative of the wider City of Boston on a range of sociodemographic characteristics that may shape the risk of SARS-CoV-2 exposure and severe COVID-19 outcomes, including educational attainment, poverty, household crowding, health insurance, and transportation to work (Table C). We collected samples twice weekly from each site and used data collected over the program's first year in our analyses (October 2022–September 2023).

PURPOSE

To describe and validate program data as a measure of community-level SARS-CoV-2 infection, we compared wastewater SARS-CoV-2 concentrations to greater Boston area regional wastewater data and other COVID-19 clinical indicators (Table D, available as a supplement to the online version of this article at http://www.ajph.org), focusing on both Boston citywide average comparisons and neighborhood-level comparisons.

We compared the citywide, population-weighted average SARS-CoV-2 concentration across all sites to regional wastewater concentrations to elucidate any inequities between the City of Boston and the greater Boston region. Next, we assessed the strength of correlation and timeliness of citywide average SARS-CoV-2 concentrations compared with regional wastewater trends and other citywide COVID-19 indicators with various lead or lag times (Table D).

We examined neighborhood-level inequities by comparing average SARS-CoV-2 concentrations across neighborhood sites. Finally, we compared spatial patterns observed in neighborhood-level wastewater data to those observed in clinical indicators (Table D).

EVALUATION AND ADVERSE EFFECTS

In the program's first year, Boston's citywide population-weighted average SARS-CoV-2 concentrations were consistently higher than regional wastewater concentrations (Figure D, available as a supplement to the online version of this article at http://www.ajph.org): approximately 67% and 56% higher than Massachusetts Water Resources Authority North and South, respectively (Table E, available as a supplement to the online version of this article at http://www.ajph.org). Temporal trends in citywide average SARS-CoV-2 concentrations were consistent with those observed in Massachusetts Water Resources Authority North regional wastewater (Figure 1). Citywide SARS-CoV-2 wastewater concentrations were also strongly correlated with subsequent clinical indicators: COVID-19 case rates (two-day lead; $r = 0.89$), emergency department visits (three-day lead; $r = 0.94$), new hospital admissions (10-day lead; $r = 0.89$), total inpatient hospitalizations (15-day lead; $r = 0.94$), total adult intensive care unit hospitalizations (17-day lead; $r = 0.90$), and COVID-19 deaths (21-day lead; $r = 0.77$; Figure 1; Figure E, available as a supplement to the online version of this article at http://www.ajph.org).

We observed substantial inequities in average SARS-CoV-2 concentrations across neighborhoods (Figure 2). In Roxbury, the neighborhood with the highest average values, wastewater concentrations were 2.5 times those

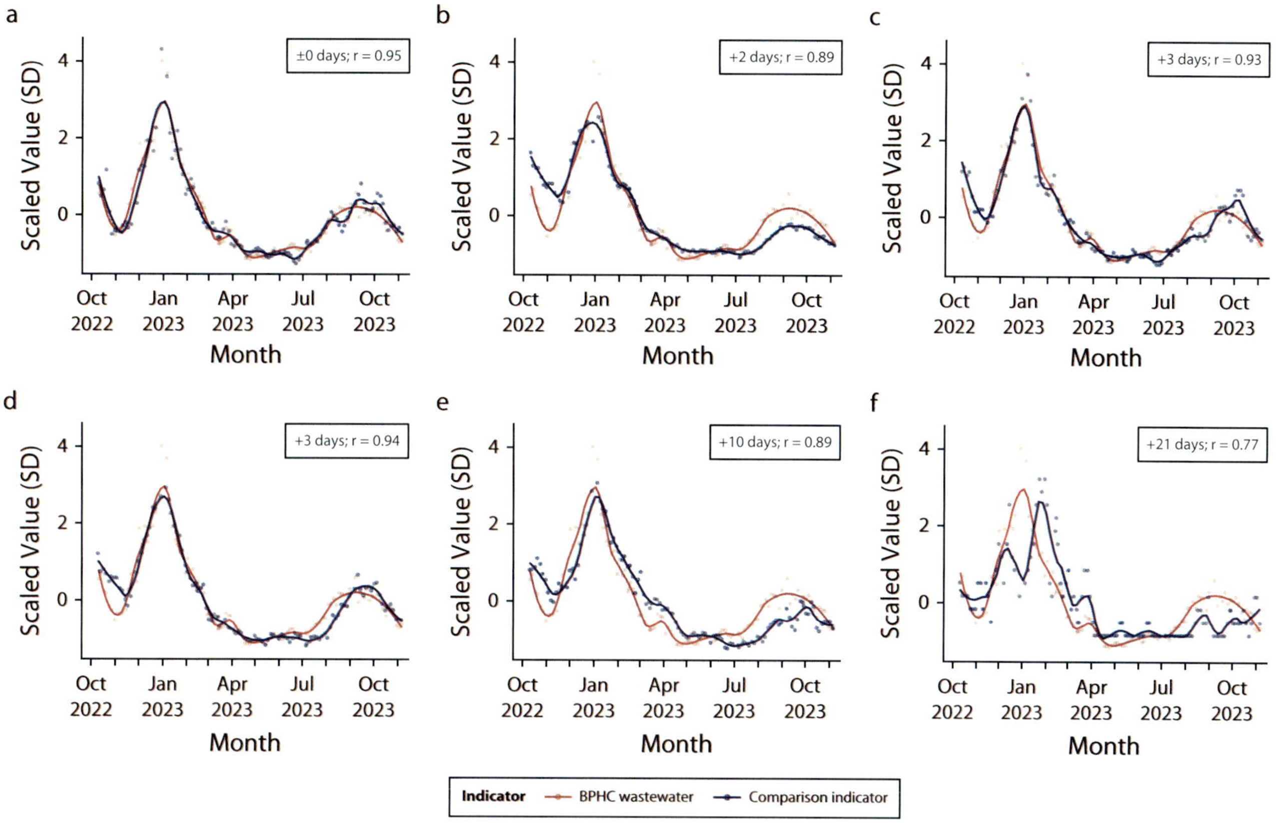

FIGURE 1— Trends, Lead Time, and Correlation in Citywide Population-Weighted Average SARS-CoV-2 Concentration Observed Across BPHC Sampling Sites Compared With (a) MWRA North Location Wastewater Concentration, (b) Reported COVID-19 Case Rates, (c) MWRA South Location Wastewater Concentration, (d) COVID-19 Emergency Department Visits, (e) New COVID-19 Hospital Admissions, and (f) COVID-19 Deaths: Boston, MA, October 2022–September 2023

Note. BPHC = Boston Public Health Commission; MWRA = Massachusetts Water Resources Authority; MWRA North = northern location; MWRA South = southern location. Red lines show SARS-CoV-2 concentration. Blue lines show COVID-19 indicators. COVID-19 clinical indicators included Boston-area regional wastewater concentrations from MWRA. All indicators were scaled and centered, with mean zero and units in SDs from the mean and shown with a LOESS (locally estimated scatterplot smoothing) line with a span of 0.15. Indicators were ordered by shortest lead time (MWRA North, 0 d) to longest lead time (COVID-19 deaths, +21 d). Details for each individual data source can be found in Table D (available as a supplement to the online version of this article at http://www.ajph.org), and corresponding data for total inpatient hospitalizations and total adult intensive care unit hospitalizations can be found in Figure E (available as a supplement to the online version of this article at http://www.ajph.org).

observed in Charlestown, the neighborhood with the lowest average values (1179 copies/mL vs 463 copies/mL, respectively; Table F, available as a supplement to the online version of this article at http://www.ajph.org). Overall, neighborhood-level inequities in wastewater concentrations corresponded with inequities in COVID-19 case rates and COVID-19 emergency department visits over the same period (Figure 2; Table F; Figure F, available as a supplement to the online version of this article at http://www.ajph.org) and also corresponded with neighborhood-level social vulnerability indices (Figure G, available as a supplement to the online version of this article at http://www.ajph.org). In some neighborhoods, wastewater concentrations may supplement clinical data. For example, in Allston–Brighton, the neighborhood with the highest test positivity, wastewater concentrations were relatively high compared with reported COVID-19 case rates and emergency department visits (Table F; Figure F).

We are unaware of any adverse effects of our intervention.

SUSTAINABILITY

Wastewater data are a robust, leading indicator of COVID-19 hospitalizations and reveal inequities across Boston neighborhoods unobservable in regional wastewater data, demonstrating the value of sustaining this program.[10] Additionally, reported COVID-19 case rates rely on polymerase chain reaction testing and have become increasingly unreliable as at-home testing has increased and accessibility of clinical testing has decreased, highlighting the importance of wastewater data.

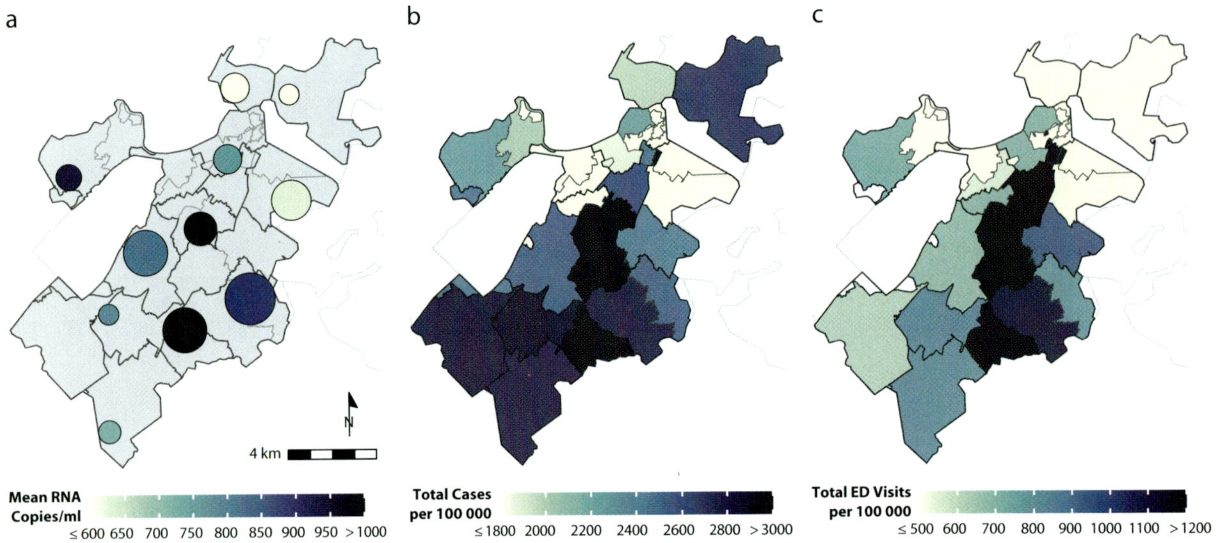

FIGURE 2— Representation of (a) Wastewater SARS-CoV-2 Concentration at BPHC Wastewater Neighborhood Sampling Sites, (b) Cumulative Reported COVID-19 Case Rates per 100 000 Population Across Boston ZCTAs, and (c) Cumulative COVID-19 Emergency Department (ED) Visits per 100 000 Population Across Boston ZCTAs: Boston, MA, October 2022–September 2023

Note. Sample size was n = 11. BPHC = Boston Public Health Commission; RNA = ribonucleic acid; ZCTA = zip code tabulation area. In panel a, the size of the circle corresponds to the population covered by the neighborhood sampling site. Table D (available as a supplement to the online version of this article at http://www.ajph.org) provides indicator definitions and sampling site description and details. Figure C (available as a supplement to the online version of this article at http://www.ajph.org) provides a list of neighborhood sampling sites.

PUBLIC HEALTH SIGNIFICANCE

Results from the first year of BPHC's program underscore the importance of city-specific and neighborhood-level wastewater epidemiology as a supplement to measuring trends at larger spatial scales. Despite widespread population immunity during the study period, citywide wastewater levels were strongly correlated with and provided critical lead time to increases in hospitalizations and deaths, consistent with previous work.[11] As an early indicator of severe disease, wastewater data signal the onset of emerging COVID-19 surges and are shared to inform local interventions, including policies on masking and preparedness for health care capacity in local hospitals. However, although citywide and regional temporal trends were similar, citywide wastewater levels in Boston were consistently higher, which may indicate higher burden in Boston compared with surrounding cities and towns. Reliance on regional wastewater data alone, therefore, may not be an accurate measure of community SARS-CoV-2 infection, masking inequities if City of Boston rates are higher than those in surrounding areas.

Neighborhood-level wastewater results revealed stark inequities in community burden of SARS-CoV-2 infection. These neighborhood-level wastewater patterns were largely consistent with reported COVID-19 case rates and emergency department visits. However, in several instances, wastewater data added key information not observed in clinical data, specifically in neighborhoods where community-level SARS-CoV-2 infection is less likely to be reported or to result in severe COVID-19 (owing to, e.g., low testing rates, younger ages).

Nevertheless, the persistence of social and environmental inequities, exacerbated by the COVID-19 pandemic, underscores the need for equitable implementation of wastewater epidemiology programs.[4,12] Structural barriers to health equity continue, including discriminatory housing policies and practices resulting in racialized socioeconomic segregation in the Boston area.[7] BPHC's program uniquely addresses these issues via neighborhood-level sampling so that inequities in SARS-CoV-2 infection across neighborhoods can be identified and addressed. Primarily, this community-based wastewater epidemiology program will inform mitigation strategies and reduce health inequities through neighborhood-level interventions (e.g., vaccine clinics), prioritizing neighborhoods for increased provision of personal protective equipment (e.g., high-quality masks and antigen tests) and enhancing outreach to community organizations serving residents at high risk (e.g., congregate care settings) in these neighborhoods.

We routinely report program results alongside recommendations and neighborhood-specific resources to help residents interpret and act on our findings. Given the findings that wastewater signals precede upcoming increases in clinical care requirements, BPHC uses wastewater data to inform area hospitals, government officials, and community-based organizations of impending COVID-19 surges.

This work had several limitations. We were unable to directly account for variation introduced by differences in sewer network engineering, climate, and SARS-CoV-2 evolution. Although this is likely somewhat addressed via normalizing with pepper mild mottle virus, these factors may also partially explain observed differences in SARS-CoV-2 concentrations. Additionally, because of sewerage infrastructure and resource constraints, two neighborhoods did not have sampling sites, and several covered small shares of the neighborhood populations. Future work will further examine spatiotemporal trends in wastewater and clinical indicators to assess whether wastewater data serve as a sentinel at the neighborhood level.

Our concept to practice model for a neighborhood-level wastewater-based epidemiology program measures and informs actions to mitigate inequities in community SARS-CoV-2 infection. The program's first-year results revealed inequities between the City of Boston and the greater Boston area and between neighborhoods in the City of Boston unobservable in regional wastewater data. This program's results will continue to inform community-based mitigation strategies to reduce health inequities. AJPH

ABOUT THE AUTHORS

All authors are with the Boston Public Health Commission, Boston, MA. Tori L. Cowger is also with the François-Xavier Bagnoud Center for Health and Human Rights, Harvard T. H. Chan School of Public Health, Boston, MA. Bisola O. Ojikutu and Kathryn T. Hall are also with Brigham and Women's Hospital, Harvard Medical School, Boston, MA.

CORRESPONDENCE

Correspondence should be sent to Tori L. Cowger, François-Xavier Bagnoud Center for Health and Human Rights, Harvard T.H. Chan School of Public Health, 651 Huntington Ave, 7th Floor, Boston, MA 02115 (e-mail: vcowger@hsph.harvard.edu). Reprints can be ordered at https://www.ajph.org by clicking the "Reprints" link.

PUBLICATION INFORMATION

Full Citation: Cowger TL, Sharp MT, Hart JD, Ojikutu BO, Nair S, Hall KT. Implementation of neighborhood-level wastewater-based epidemiology to measure and mitigate inequities in SARS-CoV-2 infection in Boston, Massachusetts. *Am J Public Health*. 2024;114(11):1217–1221.

Acceptance Date: May 30, 2024.

DOI: https://doi.org/10.2105/AJPH.2024.307749

ORCID iD:

Tori L. Cowger https://orcid.org/0000-0001-5359-8155

CONTRIBUTORS

T. L. Cowger, M. T. Sharp, and J. D. Hart drafted the initial version of the article. T. L. Cowger, M. T. Sharp, J. D. Hart, and S. Nair conceptualized, analyzed, and interpreted the data. All authors drafted revisions to the article and approved the final version.

ACKNOWLEDGMENTS

Funding for Boston Public Health Commission's (BPHC's) wastewater epidemiology program comes from the American Rescue Plan Act of 2021.

We thank the Infectious Disease Bureau, Office of Public Health Preparedness and Response, and Informatics Team at BPHC, especially Sreedevi Ravi and Tahir Arif, for their assistance with data collection and analysis of COVID-19 clinical indicators and programmatic support. We thank our partners at Boston Water and Sewer Commission for their assistance with selecting sampling sites and programmatic support and collaboration that makes the program possible. We also thank our partners at Biobot Analytics and Flow Assessment Services for their assistance with sample collection, laboratory processing, data management and analysis, and programmatic support.

CONFLICTS OF INTEREST

The authors have no conflicts of interest to declare.

HUMAN PARTICIPANT PROTECTION

Data for this study were de-identified and collected and analyzed as part of routine public health practice and therefore did not require institutional review board oversight or approval.

REFERENCES

1. Boston Public Health Commission. Health of Boston 2023: the provisional mortality and life expectancy report. 2023. Available at: https://www.boston.gov/sites/default/files/file/2023/05/HOB_Mortality_LE_2023_FINAL_May12.pdf. Accessed July 8, 2024.
2. Njoku AU. COVID-19 and environmental racism: challenges and recommendations. *Eur J Environ Public Health*. 2021;5(2):em0079. https://doi.org/10.21601/ejeph/10999
3. Johns Hopkins Bloomberg School of Public Health. How COVID-19 created a "watershed" moment for wastewater surveillance. May 13, 2022. Available at: https://publichealth.jhu.edu/2022/how-covid-19-created-a-watershed-moment-for-wastewater-surveillance. Accessed May 3, 2024.
4. Alonso C, Keppard B, Bates S, Cortez D, Amaya F, Dinakar K. The Chelsea Project: turning research and wastewater surveillance on COVID-19 into health equity action, Massachusetts, 2020–2021. *Am J Public Health*. 2023;113(6):627–630. https://doi.org/10.2105/AJPH.2023.30725
5. Anderson LB, Ness HD, Holm RH, Smith T. Wastewater-informed digital advertising as a COVID-19 geotargeted neighborhood intervention: Jefferson County, Kentucky, 2021–2022. *Am J Public Health*. 2024;114(1):34–37. https://doi.org/10.2105/AJPH.2023.307439
6. Massachusetts Water Resources Authority. Wastewater COVID-19 tracking. July 5, 2024. Available at: https://www.mwra.com/biobot/biobotdata.htm. Accessed May 3, 2024.
7. Arcaya MC, Ellen IG, Steil J. Neighborhoods and health: interventions at the neighborhood level could help advance health equity. *Health Aff (Millwood)*. 2024;43(2):156–163. https://doi.org/10.1377/hlthaff.2023.01037
8. City of Boston. Permits for street work; conditions thereof. Vol. 11-6.9. Available at: https://codelibrary.amlegal.com/codes/boston/latest/boston_ma/0-0-0-9607. Accessed May 3, 2024.
9. Xiao A, Wu F, Bushman M, et al. Metrics to relate COVID-19 wastewater data to clinical testing dynamics. *Water Res*. 2022;212:118070. https://doi.org/10.1016/j.watres.2022.118070
10. Wolfe MK. Invited perspective: the promise of wastewater monitoring for infectious disease surveillance. *Environ Health Perspect*. 2022;130(5):51302. https://doi.org/10.1289/EHP11151
11. Keshaviah A, Huff I, Hu XC, et al. Separating signal from noise in wastewater data: an algorithm to identify community-level COVID-19 surges in real time. *Proc Natl Acad Sci U S A*. 2023;120(31):e2216021120. https://doi.org/10.1073/pnas.2216021120
12. Korfmacher KS, Harris-Lovett S. Invited perspective: implementation of wastewater-based surveillance requires collaboration, integration, and community engagement. *Environ Health Perspect*. 2022;130(5):51304. https://doi.org/10.1289/EHP11191

The Influence of a COVID-19 Vaccine Mandate on Vaccination Rates in a University Setting

Elisabeth Brandstetter Figueroa, MPH, Bruno Bohn, PhD, MPH, J. Michael Oakes, PhD, and Ryan T. Demmer, PhD, MPH

See also Notes From the Field, pp. 1202–1231.

We surveyed (September 9–17, 2021) students, staff, and faculty at the University of Minnesota, a large, highly vaccinated university, to evaluate whether the COVID-19 vaccine mandate increased self-reported vaccine uptake. Vaccine mandates have the potential to improve public health but should consider the context of implementation and costs associated with infringements on personal choice. Policymakers need to be equipped with data to inform decisions about vaccine mandates in light of contextual factors and potential backlash affecting public health interventions. (*Am J Public Health*. 2024;114(11):1222–1227. https://doi.org/10.2105/AJPH.2024.307804)

AJPH November 2024, Vol. 114, No. 11

The administration of COVID-19 vaccines to those aged 16 years and older began in December 2020 under US Food and Drug Administration (FDA) emergency use authorization. On August 23, 2021, the COMIRNATY COVID-19 vaccine received full approval from the FDA, demonstrating that it met rigorous safety, manufacturing, and effectiveness standards. This official regulatory approval removed legal barriers that had previously barred workplace entities from requiring their employees to be vaccinated.

INTERVENTION AND IMPLEMENTATION

Shortly after the full approval of the COMIRNATY COVID-19 vaccine, the University of Minnesota joined more than 800 US private and public colleges and universities in mandating students, staff, and faculty be fully vaccinated against COVID-19.[1,2] Members of the University of Minnesota community were required to submit proof of their vaccination status (or a religious or philosophical exemption from the requirement) after August 23 and before September 18 (faculty and staff) or October 9 (students) 2021.

PLACE, TIME, AND PERSONS

We administered an e-mail–distributed online survey to the University of Minnesota's five campuses between September 9 and 17, 2021, with a focus on COVID-19 vaccination initiation, barriers to vaccination, and perceptions and opinions of the vaccine mandate at the university. Potential participants were students (n = 57 846), staff (n = 13 800), and faculty (n = 3506).

Using stratified random sampling by campus and role to ensure sufficient representation of the university population at large, we invited 12 340 (16.4%) eligible individuals to participate. Sampling rates ranged from 11.4% on larger campuses to 100% on smaller campuses. Of these, 6288 (50.9%) responded, with response rates varying from 42.5% to 81.8% (Table A, available as a supplement to the online version of this article at http://www.ajph.org). We applied inverse probability of selection weights to each response based on role and campus. We present the results of the weighted pseudopopulation to better reflect the mandate's effect on the actual numbers of the greater university community members who were influenced.

Survey responses were anonymous. We obtained basic demographic information (age, campus affiliation, race/ethnicity, role, and sex) from the University of Minnesota's Office of Measurement Services. The Office of Measurement Services served to collect third-party data and preserve confidentiality of participants; the office decoupled identifying information from survey answers before they transferred the data to us.

Nearly half (49.1%) of the sample was aged 16 to 22 years, with 60.0% being women, 73.9% being White, and 14.6% reporting previous suspected or confirmed COVID-19 disease (Figure A, Table B, available as a supplement to the online version of this article at http://www.ajph.org).

PURPOSE

Quantitative evidence of the impact of vaccine mandates on COVID-19 vaccine rates in businesses, government settings, and educational facilities after implementation remains limited but is crucial for data-driven decision-making related to vaccine mandates during future pandemics and in response to future severe acute respiratory syndrome coronavirus 2 variants of concern. Previous studies have assessed COVID-19 vaccination attitudes and perceptions but have not quantified vaccine uptake owing to the mandate, especially in an educational setting.[3–7]

We aimed to describe the COVID-19 vaccination landscape among students, staff, and faculty; investigate self-reported vaccination pursuant to the mandate; and explore reasons for vaccination decisions.

EVALUATION AND ADVERSE EFFECTS

Participants self-reported their vaccination status at the time of the survey. We considered individuals who received at least one dose vaccinated, and we categorized those with unknown or missing vaccination status as unvaccinated. We performed all analyses using R Statistical Software version 4.1.0 (RStudio, Boston, MA).

Vaccination Rates

Approximately 93% of the University of Minnesota population had received at least one dose of an emergency use authorization–approved COVID-19 vaccine by September 2021, with individual campus rates ranging from 67% at campus B to 95% at campus A, reflecting the vaccination rates in their surrounding communities. We estimated the proportion of participants who had received at least one dose of a COVID-19 vaccine and compared relative proportions of vaccinated individuals using the two-sided Pearson χ^2 test with a second-order Rao-Scott correction for weighting. We computed *P* values with the Satterthwaite approximation, where statistical significance was determined by $P < .05$.

Vaccination rates were highest among faculty (98%) and lowest among students, 92% of whom reported at least one dose of the COVID-19 vaccine. Older participants were more likely to be vaccinated than were younger, with the proportion vaccinated ranging from 90% among those aged 16 to 22 years to 97% among those aged 60 years and older. More women were vaccinated than men (Figure 1).

We fit separate modified univariate Poisson regressions with robust SEs to estimate the unadjusted relative risks and 95% confidence intervals (CIs) of being vaccinated and being influenced by the mandate. We then added all univariate predictors (role, age group, sex, race/ethnicity, international status, and previous COVID-19 disease) to multivariate models to estimate adjusted relative risks (ARR) and corresponding 95% CIs.

After adjustment, each 10-year age increase was associated with 1.01 times greater probability of being vaccinated (95% CI = 1.00, 1.01), with the greatest adjusted probability in the 50 to 59 years and 60 years and older groups (ARR = 1.04; 95% CI = 1.01, 1.06 and ARR = 1.04; 95% CI = 1.01, 1.07, respectively) compared with those aged 16 to 22 years. Additionally, participants with a previously suspected or confirmed COVID-19 disease were less likely to be vaccinated than were their uninfected counterparts (ARR = 0.91; 95% CI = 0.88, 0.94; Table C, available as a supplement to the online version of this article at http://www.ajph.org).

Mandate Influence

We calculated Wald-based 95% CIs to determine proportions influenced by the mandate stratified by vaccination status at the time of the survey that accounted for survey weights. Among all members of the university community, the COVID-19 vaccine mandate was a contributing reason for vaccination for an estimated 1884 individuals. They represented 2.5% (95% CI = 1.9%, 3.1%) of the weighted university population or 29.5% (95% CI = 23.3%, 37.0%) of those who were not already vaccinated for other reasons (Figure 2).

After fitting a multivariable regression model, age, campus affiliation, and previous infection status were the greatest predictors of becoming vaccinated because of the mandate. In the adjusted model, individuals with previous suspected or confirmed COVID-19 were more likely to be vaccinated because of the mandate (ARR = 2.19; 95% CI = 1.48, 3.23) than were individuals without a known history of COVID-19. Finally, for every 10-year age increase, the mandate became less influential in the decision to vaccinate (ARR = 0.45; 95% CI = 0.26, 0.80; Table D, available as a supplement to the online version of this article at http://www.ajph.org).

Vaccine Acceptance, Hesitancy, and Refusal

Among those vaccinated before mandate implementation and across

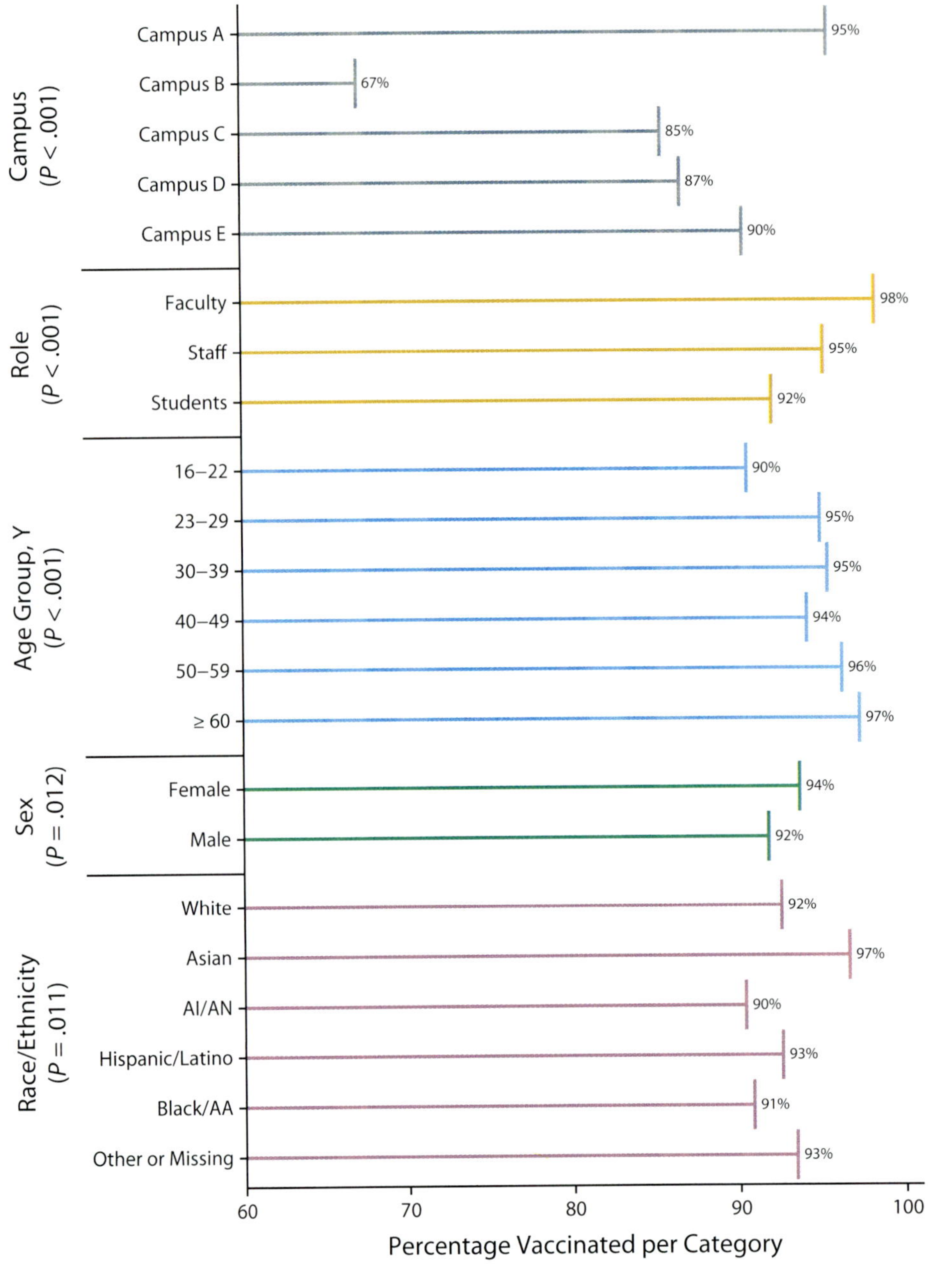

FIGURE 1— **Percentage of Individuals Vaccinated With at Least One Dose of an Emergency Use Authorization–Approved Vaccine by September 2021 Among Weighted Survey Population by Sociodemographic Characteristics: United States**

Note. AA = African American; AI/AN = American Indian/Alaska Native. Study population size was n = 75 152. We compared the relative proportions of vaccinated individuals for each sociodemographic characteristic (i.e., campus, role, age group, sex, and race/ethnicity) using the 2-sided Pearson χ^2 test with a second-order Rao-Scott correction for weighting. We computed *P* values with the Satterhwaite approximation, where statistical significance is denoted by *P* < .05.

demographic strata (n = 69 806), protecting self and others were the most frequently cited reasons for receiving the vaccine (89% and 88%, respectively; Figure B, available as a supplement to the online version of this article at http://www.ajph.org). As the university shifted back to in-person operations, many activities (e.g., athletic participation and attendance) were restricted to those with proof of vaccination. Continued participation in these activities had a slight influence on the decision to vaccinate among those aged 16 to 22 years (19%), students (17%), and

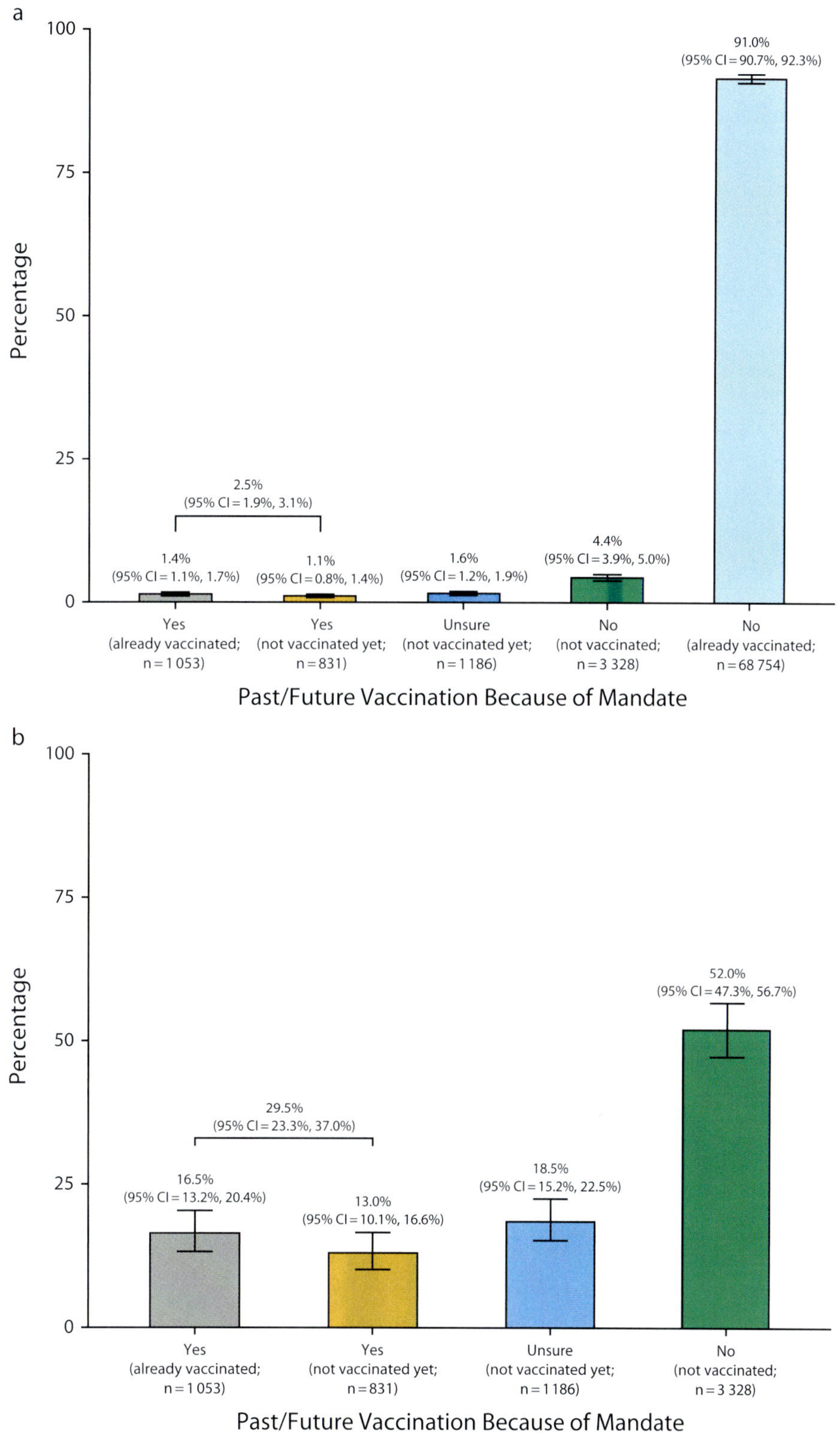

FIGURE 2— Proportions of Participants Reporting the Decision to Have Been Vaccinated or Become Vaccinated Because of the Upcoming Vaccine Mandate Among (a) the Total Weighted Survey Population (n = 75 152), and (b) Those Who Were Not Already Vaccinated for Other Reasons Before the Mandate Was Announced in the Weighted Survey Population (n = 6398): United States, September 2021

Note. CI = confidence interval. CI = Wald-based 95% confidence interval for proportion, accounting for sampling weights.

individuals at campus C (20%). A doctor's recommendation to vaccinate was also somewhat influential (37%), but full US FDA approval and incentives or rewards for receiving the vaccine were less commonly cited as motivators for vaccine acceptance (≤ 10%).

In the weighted sample, 4515 (6.0%) individuals would not or were unsure whether they would become vaccinated by the time of the mandate. Among 4387 individuals who provided a reason for hesitancy or refusal, vaccine safety concerns were most commonly cited (65%), particularly vaccine side effects (55%), the speed at which the vaccines were developed (48%), and infertility (25%; Table D, available as a supplement to the online version of this article at http://www.ajph.org). One third of those hesitant or refusing to be vaccinated felt that COVID-19 was not a threat to them, and 22% reported intentions to instead use other infection prevention measures (e.g., masking, social distancing). Religious (32%) and philosophical (27%) contraindications to vaccination also influenced the decision not to vaccinate. Peer perceptions, lack of perceived vaccine effectiveness, and difficulty accessing the vaccine were less commonly reported, and no respondents cited lack of vaccine access as a reason for not being vaccinated.

SUSTAINABILITY

Our findings indicate that students, staff, and faculty may have different motivations for becoming vaccinated and that COVID-19 vaccine mandates may be more effective in settings of lower baseline vaccine coverage (e.g., campus B, which had the lowest vaccination rate and greatest relative proportion of people who became vaccinated because of the mandate). Students who were admitted, staff who were hired, and faculty with tenure continued to vocalize strong opinions both for and against the COVID-19 vaccine at the time of mandate implementation.

Vaccination has demonstratively reduced the morbidity and mortality associated with COVID-19.[8] The strong potential for vaccine mandates to improve public health (i.e., vaccine effectiveness, herd immunity, and reduction in health care burden) should be weighed against the potential for infringement on personal choice related to health decisions and animosity toward public health policy. Institutional-level policies on vaccine mandates, particularly in the higher education setting, should be informed by a consideration of the spectrum of these contextual factors.

PUBLIC HEALTH SIGNIFICANCE

Understanding the effects of vaccine mandates on vaccination rates is important. If mandates do in fact have a strong influence on vaccine uptake, the potential benefit to public health is significant and may justify infringement on personal choice. However, vaccine mandates may also come at the cost of engendering resentment toward and intensifying distrust in public health policy. Therefore, decisions on vaccine mandates should be carefully considered and informed by data regarding their potential to reduce disease transmission and severity of disease. AJPH

ABOUT THE AUTHORS

Elisabeth Brandstetter Figueroa is with the Division of Epidemiology and Community Health, School of Public Health, University of Minnesota, Minneapolis. Bruno Bohn is with the Lifecourse Epidemiology of Adiposity and Diabetes Center, Department of Epidemiology, Colorado School of Public Health, University of Colorado, Anschutz Medical Campus, Aurora. J. Michael Oakes is with the Department of Population Health Sciences, School of Medicine, and the Office of Research and Technology Management, Case Western Reserve University, Cleveland, OH. Ryan T. Demmer is with the Division of Epidemiology, Department of Quantitative Health Sciences, College of Medicine and Science, Mayo Clinic, Rochester, MN, and the Division of Epidemiology and Community Health, School of Public Health, University of Minnesota, Minneapolis.

CORRESPONDENCE

Correspondence should be sent to Ryan T. Demmer, 200 First St SW, Rochester, MN 55905 (e-mail: demmer.ryan@mayo.edu). Reprints can be ordered at https://www.ajph.org by clicking the "Reprints" link.

PUBLICATION INFORMATION

Full Citation: Figueroa EB, Bohn B, Oakes JM, Demmer RT. The influence of a COVID-19 vaccine mandate on vaccination rates in a university setting. *Am J Public Health*. 2024;114(11):1222–1227.

Acceptance Date: July 10, 2024.

DOI: https://doi.org/10.2105/AJPH.2024.307804

ORCID iDs:

Elisabeth Brandstetter Figueroa https://orcid.org/0000-0003-0521-4131

Bruno Bohn https://orcid.org/0000-0001-8961-6968

Ryan T. Demmer https://orcid.org/0000-0003-3429-0379

CONTRIBUTORS

E. Brandstetter Figueroa performed the statistical analyses and wrote the first draft of the article. B. Bohn contributed to analysis. B. Bohn and J. M. Oakes provided critical review of the draft article. J. M. Oakes and R. T. Demmer contributed to study conceptualization, funding acquisition, and study design and implementation. R. T. Demmer led the study, supervised the analysis, and contributed to early and final drafts of the article.

ACKNOWLEDGMENTS

This research was funded by a grant from the University of Minnesota, Office for the Vice President of Research.

We are indebted to the contributions of the University of Minnesota's Office of Measurement Services for their contributions to survey development and distribution.

CONFLICTS OF INTEREST

The authors have no conflicts of interest to report.

HUMAN PARTICIPANT PROTECTION

This study was determined to be exempt from the institutional review board at the University of Minnesota (study ID 00013786).

REFERENCES

1. White House. Executive order on ensuring adequate COVID safety protocols for federal contractors. September 9, 2021. Available at: https://www.whitehouse.gov/briefing-room/presidential-actions/2021/09/09/executive-order-on-ensuring-adequate-covid-safety-protocols-for-federal-contractors. Accessed January 17, 2022.
2. Nadworny E, Dey S. Full FDA approval triggers more universities to require the COVID-19 vaccine. September 1, 2021. Available at: https://www.npr.org/2021/09/01/1031385629/full-fda-approval-triggers-more-universities-to-require-the-covid-19-vaccine. Accessed January 17, 2022.3.
3. Haeder SF. Joining the herd? US public opinion and vaccination requirements across educational settings during the COVID-19 pandemic. *Vaccine*. 2021;39(17):2375–2385. https://doi.org/10.1016/j.vaccine.2021.03.055
4. Kecojevic A, Basch CH, Sullivan M, Chen YT, Davi NK. COVID-19 vaccination and intention to vaccinate among a sample of college students in New Jersey. *J Community Health*. 2021;46(6):1059–1068. https://doi.org/10.1007/s10900-021-00992-3
5. Silva J, Bratberg J, Lemay V. COVID-19 and influenza vaccine hesitancy among college students. *J Am Pharm Assoc (2003)*. 2021;61(6):709–714.e1. https://doi.org/10.1016/j.japh.2021.05.009
6. Graupensperger S, Abdallah DA, Lee CM. Social norms and vaccine uptake: college students' COVID vaccination intentions, attitudes, and estimated peer norms and comparisons with influenza vaccine. *Vaccine*. 2021;39(15):2060–2067. https://doi.org/10.1016/j.vaccine.2021.03.018
7. Elliott L, Yang K. Vaccine acceptance and hesitancy among college students in Nevada: a state-wide cross-sectional study. *Vaccines (Basel)*. 2022;10(1):105. https://doi.org/10.3390/vaccines10010105
8. Polack FP, Thomas SJ, Nicholas K, et al. Safety and efficacy of the BNT162b2 mRNA COVID-19 vaccine. *N Engl J Med*. 2020;383(27):2603–2615. https://doi.org/10.1056/NEJMoa2034577

Automated Opt-Out Hepatitis C Testing to Reduce Missed Screening Opportunities in the Emergency Department

Heather Sperring, MS, Glorimar Ruiz-Mercado, MD, Brian J. Yun, MD, MBA, MPH, David Twitchell, PharmD, MBA, Bhavesh Shah, RPh, BCOP, and Elissa M. Schechter-Perkins, MD, MPH

See also Notes From the Field, pp. 1202–1227.

We evaluated the impact of implementing automated hepatitis C (HCV) opt-out screening in the emergency department of an urban, academic medical center with high HCV prevalence, in the context of a longstanding HCV opt-in screening model. We compared nine-month periods before and after implementation. HCV testing increased by 502%, and active HCV infection identification increased by 212%. Settings where there is great opportunity for HCV diagnosis, such as emergency department settings, should consider opt-out HCV screening models. (*Am J Public Health*. 2024;114(11):1228–1231. https://doi.org/10.2105/AJPH.2024.307783)

AJPH November 2024, Vol. 114, No. 11

Hepatitis C virus (HCV) is the most commonly reported bloodborne infection, and there are an estimated 2.4 million people in the United States living with HCV.[1] Although HCV has become a treatable disease, roughly 75% of those infected are unaware that they have the virus.[2] Because emergency department (ED) patients are found to have a higher prevalence of HCV compared with the general population, the ED has become a focal point for HCV screening.[3,4] This higher prevalence can be attributed to the greater proportion of patients at risk for HCV in the ED, including people who inject drugs.

INTERVENTION AND IMPLEMENTATION

Boston Medical Center (BMC) is an urban, academic facility located in Boston, Massachusetts. BMC is the largest essential hospital in New England, and its patients are disproportionately impacted by substance use. Boston Emergency Medical Services, the municipal emergency medical services provider for the city of Boston, transports 34% of their patients with drug-related illnesses to BMC, and BMC's ED receives more than 140 000 visits per year.[5] For these reasons, BMC's ED has made longstanding and continuously improving efforts to identify individuals with HCV and link them to care.

Previously, the BMC ED team collaborated with in-hospital laboratory partners to move reflex testing in house and decrease time to result delivery. Concurrently, we implemented in our electronic health record (EHR) a best-practice advisory (BPA) that recommends providers to order opt-in HCV laboratory tests for patients having other laboratory tests ordered and meeting HCV screening criteria.[6] In accordance with US Preventive Services Task Force and Centers for Disease Control and Prevention screening guidelines, the BPA was activated for patients with no previous HCV antibody (Ab) test in the EHR for once-lifetime screening for all patients and every six months for patients at increased risk for HCV.[7,8] Patients with increased risk for HCV were defined as those who had documented substance use disorder in their problem list within the EHR.

These interventions greatly increased HCV screening in the ED, from approximately 18 tests per month before the BPA to approximately 1269 tests per month, a 6950% initial increase in testing. However, the effects waned over time beyond that initial period, to an average of 246 tests per month immediately before the automated order intervention. The additional steps required of providers to add the test order to the patient laboratory tests still led to missed screening opportunities because of the already fast-paced and high-workload environment of an ED. For this reason, we considered options to remove the provider burden barrier to widespread HCV testing with the aim of increasing overall HCV screening and identification of active HCV infections in the ED.

PLACE, TIME, AND PERSONS

As a quality improvement project to improve HCV screening in the ED and reduce missed opportunities for screening, we enhanced our EHR system by transitioning from an existing automated opt-in HCV testing BPA to an automatic electronic order of HCV testing (opt-out) upon any phlebotomy order placed in the ED. This EHR update triggers HCV laboratory test orders to be added automatically when providers are ordering other blood sampling for patients meeting our HCV screening criteria and automatically, without additional manual chart review, excludes those who have an HCV test result in our EHR within the last six months. To implement these changes, we worked closely with hospital leadership, ED clinicians, information technologists, and our internal laboratory. Clinician and leadership buy-in were essential to moving the proposed intervention forward. In addition to those participating in the implementation, we also worked closely with our program's data manager, HCV patient navigators, and HCV pharmacists to ensure all HCV testing would be captured and newly identified HCV-positive patients would receive follow-up, connected to appropriate care and treatment.

We collected HCV laboratory test results daily through an existing EHR report, and compared testing and result data for a period of nine months before automatic order implementation to nine months after implementation, December 21, 2021, to June 20, 2023. We included patients aged 18 years and older with HCV Ab labs through the ED. We de-duplicated testing data and excluded patients previously identified by our program as HCV-positive. We collected test dates and results for all included HCV Ab labs and additionally collected HCV RNA laboratory test results for those testing Ab-positive. All positive HCV laboratory tests in our medical system are flagged by the laboratory to our HCV patient navigators daily. The navigators attempt to contact all patients with active HCV infections to arrange linkage to HCV care.

PURPOSE

Our aim with this intervention was to remove the provider burden barrier that we had been experiencing with our already-established HCV opt-in model, with the goal of increasing HCV screening and identification in our ED.

EVALUATION AND ADVERSE EFFECTS

In our nine-month preintervention period, there were 2211 unique HCV Ab tests. Of those, 211 (9.5%) were HCV Ab–positive, and of the HCV Ab–positive patients, 85 (40.3%) had active HCV infections. In the nine months following the implementation of opt-out testing, there were 13 318 HCV Ab tests. Of those, 746 (5.6%) were Ab-positive, and of the HCV Ab–positive patients, 265 (35.5%) had active infections. Overall, there was a 502% increase in the number of HCV tests in the nine months following opt-out HCV screening compared with the nine months before. For the same time periods, HCV Ab–positive tests increased by 253%, and identification of active HCV infections increased by 212%. The percentage of active infections among all tested decreased, likely secondary to more patients without risk factors being tested after the intervention; however, the overall number of infections detected was notably higher. Figure 1 shows the change in HCV testing, Ab-positive identification, and RNA-positive identification over time for our project period. The percentage of patients with active HCV infection linked to outpatient HCV care increased after the intervention, from 21.1% before the intervention to 27.5% after the intervention.

Transitioning from an opt-in testing based on a BPA-driven HCV screening model to an opt-out, automatic-order HCV screening model was effective at increasing HCV screening, identifying HCV Ab–positive patients, and identifying active HCV infections. Automatic ordering of tests reduces clinician workload and removes barriers to universal HCV screening. Increasing screening reduces missed opportunities for diagnosing HCV infections in the ED and provides more patients with the information they need to access HCV treatment. Opt-out screening should be considered where there is great opportunity for HCV diagnosis, such as in ED settings. Our institution had sufficient navigator and clinic capacity to continue to link newly diagnosed patients to outpatient HCV care, even with the increased volume of cases. Institutions implementing or activating a similar screening model in the ED should make sure they also dedicate appropriate resources to connecting patients to care and treatment,

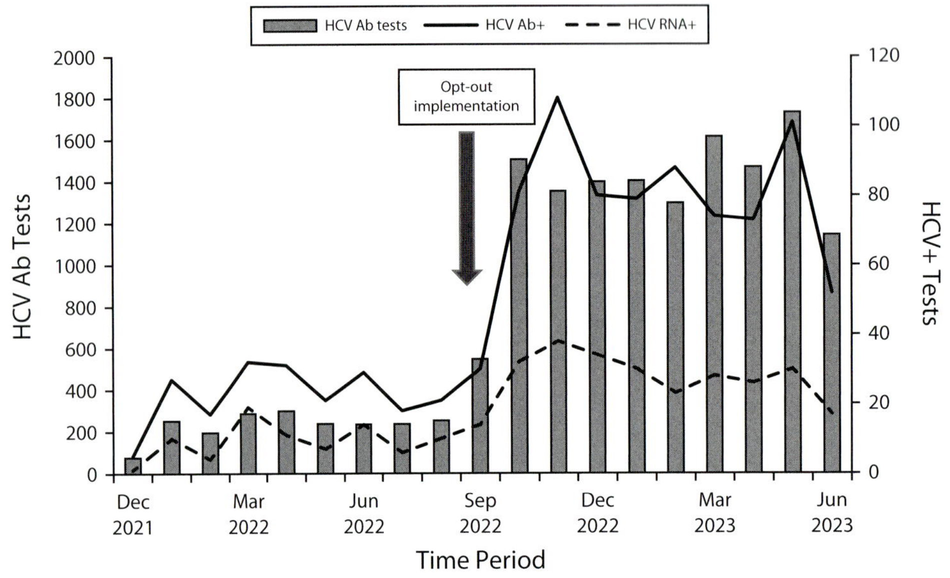

FIGURE 1— Best-Practice Advisory Versus Automatic Screening for Hepatitis C at an Urban Essential Emergency Department: Boston, MA, 2021–2023

Note. Ab = antibody; HCV = hepatitis C virus.

because recent Centers for Disease Control and Prevention reports show that there are major gaps in treatment, with only one in six patients with Medicaid and one in three with commercial insurance achieving viral clearance.[9]

SUSTAINABILITY

Our intervention is very sustainable because, once implemented, the HCV opt-out screening system will continue to work automatically without any further intervention from providers. This model is self-sustaining.

PUBLIC HEALTH SIGNIFICANCE

Universal screening is essential to meeting the public health goal of ending the spread of HCV. Opt-out screening for HCV in settings with great opportunity for HCV diagnosis are effective in increasing screening and increasing diagnosis of active HCV infections, making it a useful model for bringing us closer to this goal. AJPH

ABOUT THE AUTHORS

Heather Sperring and Glorimar Ruiz-Mercado are with the Department of Medicine, Section of Infectious Diseases, Boston Medical Center, Boston, MA. Brian J. Yun and Elissa M. Schechter-Perkins are with the Department of Emergency Medicine, Boston University Chobanian and Avedisian School of Medicine, Boston. David Twitchell and Bhavesh Shah are with the Department of Pharmacy, Boston Medical Center.

CORRESPONDENCE

Correspondence should be sent to Heather Sperring, 850 Harrison Ave, Boston, MA 02118 (e-mail: heather.sperring@bmc.org). Reprints can be ordered at https://www.ajph.org by clicking the "Reprints" link.

PUBLICATION INFORMATION

Full Citation: Sperring H, Ruiz-Mercado G, Yun BJ, Twitchell D, Shah B, Schechter-Perkins EM. Automated opt-out hepatitis C testing to reduce missed screening opportunities in the emergency department. *Am J Public Health*. 2024;114(11):1228–1231.

Acceptance Date: June 26, 2024.

DOI: https://doi.org/10.2105/AJPH.2024.307783

ORCID iD:

Heather Sperring https://orcid.org/0000-0002-1347-5748

CONTRIBUTORS

H. Sperring contributed to formal analysis, data curation, and writing the original draft. G. Ruiz-Mercado and D. Twitchell reviewed and edited the article and contributed to project administration. B. J. Yun and B. Shah reviewed and edited the article. E. Schechter-Perkins contributed to supervision, reviewing and editing the article, and conceptualization.

ACKNOWLEDGMENTS

H. Sperring, G. Ruiz-Mercado, and E. M. Schechter-Perkins are partially funded by a Frontlines of Communities in the United States (FOCUS) grant from Gilead Sciences that supports HIV, hepatitis C virus, and hepatitis B virus screening and linkage to care.

Note. Gilead Sciences had no role in the development of this article.

CONFLICTS OF INTEREST

The authors report no conflicts of interest.

HUMAN PARTICIPANT PROTECTION

This project was undertaken as a quality improvement initiative at Boston Medical Center and, as such, was exempt from institutional review board approval per their policies.

REFERENCES

1. Centers for Disease Control and Prevention. Hepatitis C. June 14, 2021. Available at: https://www.cdc.gov/hepatitis/hcv/index.htm. Accessed August 10, 2023.

2. American Liver Foundation. Hepatitis C Information Center. May 23, 2022. Available at: https://liverfoundation.org/liver-diseases/viral-hepatitis/hepatitis-c. Accessed August 10, 2023.
3. Jones AT, Moreno-Walton L, Tran T, et al. Emergency department versus community screening on hepatitis C follow-up care. *Am J Emerg Med.* 2022;56:151–157. https://doi.org/10.1016/j.ajem.2022.03.041
4. Galbraith JW. High prevalence of hepatitis C infection among adult patients at four urban emergency departments—Birmingham, Oakland, Baltimore, and Boston, 2015–2017. *MMWR Morb Mortal Wkly Rep.* 2020;69(19):569–574. https://doi.org/10.15585/mmwr.mm6919a1
5. Boston Medical Center. Substance use disorders. Available at: https://www.bmc.org/addiction/about. Accessed August 10, 2023.
6. Schechter-Perkins EM, Miller NS, Hall J, et al. Implementation and preliminary results of an emergency department nontargeted, opt-out hepatitis C virus screening program. *Acad Emerg Med.* 2018;25(11):1216–1226. https://doi.org/10.1111/acem.13484
7. Centers for Disease Control and Prevention. Clinical screening and diagnosis for hepatitis C. July 13, 2023. Available at: https://www.cdc.gov/hepatitis/hcv/management.htm. Accessed August 10, 2023.
8. Owens DK, Davidson KW, Krist AH, et al.; US Preventive Services Task Force. Screening for hepatitis C virus infection in adolescents and adults: US Preventive Services Task Force recommendation statement. *JAMA.* 2020;323(10):970–975. https://doi.org/10.1001/jama.2020.1123
9. Wester C, Hepatitis C. Virus clearance cascade—United States, 2013–2022. *MMWR Morb Mortal Wkly Rep.* 2023;72(26):716–720. https://doi.org/10.15585/mmwr.mm7226a3

Four Models of Wastewater-Based Monitoring for SARS-CoV-2 Complementing Individual Screening in Jail Settings

Shanika S. Kennedy, MPH, Lindsay B. Saber, MPH, Victoria M. Brown, MPH, Rachel A. Boehm, MPH, Amadin A. Olotu, MBBS, MPH, Jeffery Osei, MD, MPH, Jacob A. Pluznik, MPH, Lindsey R. Riback, MPH, Ebrima Sidibeh, MHS, MPH, Beth Jordan, MD, Eleni O'Donovan, MD, Anilkumar Mangla, PhD, MPH, MS, Christine Nzokou, MPH, Tracey L. Elam, EdD, MS, Jane Gubser, PsyD, Peter J. Koutoujian, JD, MPA, Kashif A. Siddiqi, MBA, MS, Steven Wilensky, JD, Victoria L. Phillips, PhD, Alysse G. Wurcel, MD, MS, Chad J. Zawitz, MD, Matthew J. Akiyama, MD, MSc, and Anne C. Spaulding, MD, MPH

See also Holm and Smith, p. 1156.

AJPH November 2024, Vol. 114, No. 11

Objectives. To describe 4 unique models of operationalizing wastewater-based surveillance (WBS) for severe acute respiratory syndrome coronavirus 2 (SARS-CoV-2) in jails of graduated sizes and different architectural designs.

Methods. We summarize how jails of Cook County, Illinois (average daily population [ADP] 6000); Fulton County, Georgia (ADP 3000); Middlesex County, Massachusetts (ADP 875); and Washington, DC (ADP 1600) initiated WBS between 2020 and 2023.

Results. Positive signals for SARS-CoV-2 via WBS can herald a new onset of infections in previously uninfected jail housing units. Challenges implementing WBS included political will and realized value, funding, understanding the building architecture, and the need for details in the findings.

Conclusions. WBS has been effective for detecting outbreaks of SARS-CoV-2 in different sized jails, those with both dorm- and cell-based architectural design.

Public Health Implications. Given its effectiveness in monitoring SARS-CoV-2, WBS provides a model for population-based surveillance in carceral facilities for future infectious disease outbreaks. (*Am J Public Health*. 2024;114(11):1232–1241. https://doi.org/10.2105/AJPH.2024.307785)

Severe acute respiratory syndrome coronavirus 2 (SARS-CoV-2) transmission spiked early in carceral populations[1] because of congregate living, poor ventilation, and frequent cellblock transfers.[2–4] Since before the COVID-19 pandemic, the United States has led the world in incarceration.[5] Jails (short-term correctional facilities) averaged 11 million admissions yearly,[6] representing 7 to 8 million individuals, when accounting for repeat admissions.[7] By January 2023, COVID-19 had caused 3181 deaths in US prisons and jails.[8] Surveillance and interventions to decrease COVID-19 incidence and mortality in custody populations are crucial. A safe custodial environment is a human right, and carceral health affects community health.[9]

Centers for Disease Control and Prevention (CDC) guidance on the management of COVID-19 in homeless service sites and in correctional and detention facilities initially focused on individual testing, quarantine, isolation, and mitigation. Revisions added wastewater-based surveillance (WBS) as another mitigation strategy.[10] WBS consists of testing wastewater to identify pathogens, which can then be linked to a population source. This surveillance strategy can act as an early warning signal and guide targeted routine diagnostic tests to identify individual cases: WBS complements individual surveillance.

Because the virus persists in fecal matter, WBS is a practical method of mass surveillance. WBS has proven useful for infections that spread rapidly or start with either no or nonspecific symptoms.[11] These characteristics align with SARS-CoV-2. College dormitory studies confirmed WBS as a sensitive, low-cost, noninvasive surveillance tool for early detection of SARS-CoV-2 at an institutional level.[12–15]

Guidance for operationalizing WBS in carceral settings is sparse and needs to consider facility architecture (cells vs dorm rooms), size, and sewer system configuration. To evaluate the acceptability of WBS for COVID-19, we conducted qualitative studies with individuals who experienced incarceration during the COVID-19 pandemic. After finding that WBS was highly acceptable,[16,17] we initiated regular WBS at Fulton County Jail (FCJ) in Atlanta, Georgia, and tested the correlation of the proportion of the population infected with SARS-CoV-2 and the level of virus in the wastewater.[18] We report on the expanded operationalization of WBS at 4 US jails to demonstrate its wider feasibility and associated effectiveness outcomes.

METHODS

Four jail systems participated in this study: Cook County Jail (CCJ), Chicago, Illinois; FCJ, Atlanta, Georgia; Middlesex Jail and House of Correction (MJHOC), North Billerica, Massachusetts; and the District of Columbia Jail (DCJ), Washington, DC. Each secured funding and was willing to engage in an implementation study to assess the feasibility of WBS for SARS-CoV-2 surveillance and implementation outcomes. One or more authors participated in WBS at each site.

We explored and compared funding, starting points, jail architecture, sample collection processes, and laboratory methods.

Funding, Starting Points, and Laboratory Linkage

Our study included jails of different sizes, architectural designs, sewer system configurations, and funding levels (Table 1). Each jail used external laboratories for wastewater testing.

CCJ in Chicago, Illinois, used a citywide project monitoring wastewater for SARS-CoV-2 starting November 2020. We included all 16 housing buildings in the CCJ compound in this project and tested them biweekly. A private, quickly mobilized funding source supported CCJ and other Chicago Department of Public Health sites. The University of Illinois at Chicago processed the specimens.

FCJ in Atlanta, Georgia, had WBS funding from federal sources via a private company. Emory University received a subcontract in 2021 to pilot test wastewater at points around the city of Atlanta. Subsequently, Emory University received another grant from a private foundation to demonstrate the efficiency of self-collected nasal swabbing of jail residents, to correlate individual testing with WBS, and to interview relevant stakeholders. Funding was time limited.

MJHOC, the smallest jail included in this study, is ranked as a medium-sized jail by national standards.[19] The sheriff's office provided funding. Biobot Analytics (Cambridge, MA) performed WBS laboratory analysis. MJHOC began weekly sampling of wastewater in April 2021 and continued to fund surveillance through the first half of 2024.

The Washington, DC, Department of Health established WBS at DCJ via federal funding in 2020. The DC Department of Health initially delayed mobilization of funds and commencement of WBS in the jail. There has been a lag in providing feedback of WBS results to jail clinicians. DC Department of Health contracted with EA/Ecological Analysts Engineering (Hunt Valley, MD) for sample collection, and the District of Columbia Public Health Lab (Washington, DC) provided analysis. Sampling at DCJ began in March 2023. Long-term surveillance is expected to continue.

Wastewater Collection and Laboratory Methods

Two principal methods of wastewater sampling are grab samples and Moore swabs: a snapshot and a longitudinal measurement of viral signals, respectively. These 2 collection methods are analogous to a finger-stick blood glucose (single point) measurement and a hemoglobin A1C (period) measurement for monitoring blood glucose in diabetic patients. Moore swabs are 4″ × 4″ gauze squares made from a 48-inch–long gauze strip Z-folded to be 12 ply, then tied in the middle with a fishing line (Figure 1). These are dropped in sewer lines for 24 to 48 hours. Wastewater laboratory analysis provides a semiquantitative measurement of virus in the sample.[20,21] Results are presented as cycle thresholds, which are higher with decreasing concentrations of viral RNA. This semiquantitative measurement provides a rough comparison of relative levels of virus over time. WBS can also monitor for the presence of specific gene sequences associated with new variants.[20,21]

Operations and Jail Structure

For CCJ, University of Illinois at Chicago School of Public Health researchers

TABLE 1— Preliminary Characteristics of WBS Methods Among Enrolled Jails: 4 US Jails, 2020–2024

Jail: ADP, 2020	Change Goal	No. of Buildings (No. of Manholes per Building)	Housing Configuration	WBS in Place? Frequency?	Private or Public Funder? Grant Recipients?	Lab for Specimens	Health Care Provider	Specificity of WW Sample to Case Location	How Has WBS Related to Individual Testing?	Championing to Sustain?	Funding Duration	Internal Data Sharing
CCJ: 6000	Refinement: increase efficiency, automation, and throughput; move on to other infectious disease surveillance	16 (1–4)	Mix of single cell units (few), 2-person cells, 4-person cells, dorms holding ~40, 1 large 250-person dorm	Multiple (20) collection points 1–2 times/wk	Public and private funding; began with private funding by Chicago area philanthropy foundation. Replaced with funding from Chicago Department of Public Health after 1 y	University of Illinois, Chicago, IL	Public sector	Data from facilities management moderately successful; occasions of discordant results	Pinpointed site of outbreak; could limit where testing is needed (e.g., maximum-security unit)	Medical sees a need; custody also champions it; has helped set up mpox; may add influenza	Ongoing as of 2024	Via data analyst (sheriff's office) and infection control department
FCJ: 3000	Refinement: consistent collection schedule with high throughput	1 main/2 satellite (6 in main jail, 1 in small satellite, 2 in larger satellite)	Predominately 2-person cells	Multiple (≥ 8) collections points; once weekly	Public funder (National Institutes of Health) recipient: private business, to academic institution	Rollins School of Public Health, Atlanta, GA	Private, for-profit	Clarified during study	WBS results inform intensity of testing; individual testing less frequent when/where WW without virus	Sheriff's office requested additional funding from department of health	Concluded	Disjointed; tried to coordinate
DCJ: 1600	Introduce system: singular collection site	2 main (4)	Predominately 2-person cells	One collection point	Public funder (Centers for Disease Control and Prevention); recipient: Department of Health	DC Department of Health, Washington, DC	Community FQHC site	Schematic map available	Pilot phase	Yes; DC Department of Health is using the experience of employing granular data in schools to inform jail WBS	Ongoing as of 2024	Data shared internally with department of health
MJHOC: 825	Sustain collection: explore expanding to more than 1 collection point	1 main (1)	Mix of single cell units, 2-person cells; dorms holding ~60 persons	Single collection point once a week with a 2-d turnaround	County funded through the sheriff's office annual budget	Biobot Analytics, Cambridge, MA	Hybrid model; health services are provided by a contracted vendor and in-house public sector health care employees	Not applicable	Viral load monitored by health services	Initiative of sheriff's office	Concluded in midyear of 2024	Data shared internally weekly

Note. ADP = average daily population; FQHC = federally qualified health center; WBS = wastewater-based surveillance; WW = wastewater. The 4 US jails were Cook County Jail (CCJ), Chicago, IL; Fulton County Jail (FCJ), Atlanta, GA; Middlesex Jail and House of Correction (MJHOC), North Billerica, MA; and the District of Columbia Jail (DCJ), Washington, DC.

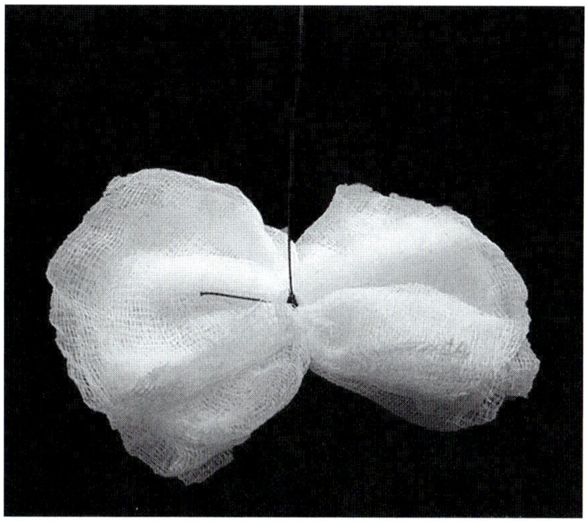

FIGURE 1— Moore Swab: A 4″ × 4″ Gauze Square, Tied Together With Fishing Line, Which Is Suspended in Wastewater for 24 Hours

Source. Saber et al.[18]

tested wastewater samples as part of a larger SARS-CoV-2 surveillance project with the Discovery Partners Institute (Chicago, IL).[22] Testing involved collecting grab and Moore samples. We identified more than 30 possible collection sites during the initial site visit to the multibuilding CCJ complex (Figure 2). The leader of CCJ's infection control team selected which sites to monitor weekly. Initially, 6 sites were tested biweekly, with periodic adjustments based on disease activity. Collection site selection was initially based on confirmed clinical activity or suspicion of new infections to validate the connection between wastewater readings and cases. Subsequently, the strategy shifted to focus on the areas where suspicion of infection was low to provide an early warning of new outbreaks. For buildings in which known cases were rare and the wastewater remained negative, CCJ minimized active surveillance of individuals.

For FCJ, in April 2021, the Emory University Center for Global Safe Water, Sanitation, and Hygiene performed a pilot wastewater collection at the jail. Its environmental microbiology laboratory followed the RNA extraction and real-time quantitative polymerase chain reaction (PCR) protocol for analyzing specimens previously used in university dorm testing.[20,23] Afterward, starting in June 2021, a jail representative collected regular weekly water samples. We collected Moore swabs retrieved after 24-hour placement, grab samples of 40 mL of wastewater, or both weekly, rotating between 11 accessible manholes on the property (Figure 2b; see Supplemental Figure A [available as a supplement to the online version of this article at http://www.ajph.org] for more details on specific site processing). The semiquantitative results were reported the following day.[24]

The main FCJ complex consists of a 7-floor structure with 2 towers, both of which contain 6 housing units (Figure 2; Supplemental Figure B [available as a supplement to the online version of this article at http://www.ajph.org]). Initially, we could not locate FCJ's sewage system blueprints. We poured tracer dye (EcoClean Solutions, Copiague, NY) into the plumbing system at various source locations, with study staff stationed at manholes relaying when color appeared, which gave us a preliminary indication of wastewater flow. Locating plumbing blueprints in October 2022 confirmed the findings. By early 2023, dye studies demonstrated the precise flow patterns (Supplemental Figure B). With future outbreaks of pathogens that can be tracked in wastewater, the precise origin can thus be narrowed down to a specific housing area in 1 of the towers.

At MJHOC, we sampled wastewater from the single facility manhole site weekly using an automated sampler (Figure 2).[25] The commercial laboratory Biobot Analytics (Cambridge, MA) analyzed specimens and delivered the results electronically to the sheriff's office 48 hours later. Increased viral concentrations in the wastewater prompted the infectious disease consultant and jail staff to meet to discuss enhanced individual testing and mitigation.

At the DC jail, the DC Department of Health used an automatic sampler and selected a single site for collection near the infirmary and a housing unit for mid- to long-term residents (Figure 2). At the time of this report, how DCJ would use the WBS data to inform clinical care was still under consideration.

RESULTS

We have demonstrated the feasibility of using WBS to guide dynamic COVID-19 response protocols that included resident and staff testing in the jails. Three jails used WBS to help guide clinical care.

Individual Testing Procedures

When WBS was established, the CCJ compared results with a rapid PCR

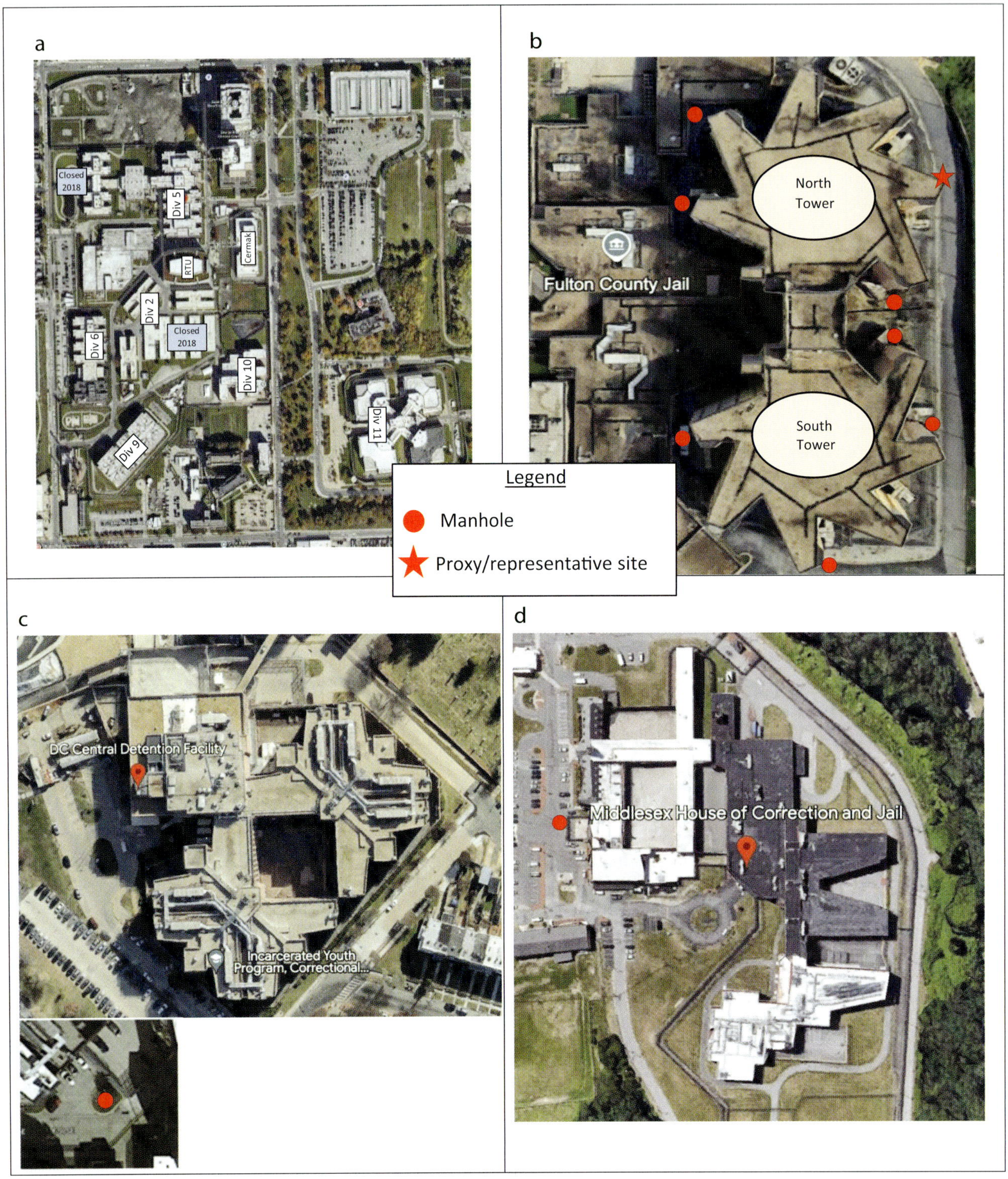

FIGURE 2— **Aerial Photographs, With Locations of Housing Units and Manhole Points, of Jails in (a) Cook County, IL; (b) Fulton County, GA; (c) Middlesex County, MA; and (d) Washington, DC: 2020–2024**

Note. Cook County Jail provided residential housing across 16 buildings. Each had its own wastewater-based sampling site. Specific locations are not shared because of security concerns. Proxy/representative site at Fulton County Jail represents sampling site that pools wastewater from the majority of housing sites in the jail.

(IDNow, Abbot Laboratories, Abbot Park, IL) test at intake and in the urgent care unit. To screen housing units after exposure, before medical procedures, or before prison transfer, staff collected swabs from individuals for laboratory-based PCR testing, which was performed at the John H. Stroger Jr. Hospital (Chicago, IL). Before the Omicron variant emerged, entrants were quarantined in intake housing, and PCR testing was used to clear them for transfer to the general population. This procedure was revised as CDC guidelines evolved.

FCJ conducted opt-out rapid testing of individuals at intake as well as point-of-care testing for suspected cases in the population using point-of-care antigen tests (BinaxNow, Abbot Laboratories, Chicago IL, through January 2022; then QuickVue, QuidelOrtho, San Diego, CA, from February 2022 onward). A team from Rollins School of Public Health performed periodic mass testing. The Gates Foundation suggested that random population testing be done via self-collected SteriPack nasal swabs (SteriPack USA, Lakeland, FL), collection devices for molecular diagnostic testing (Supplemental Figure C, available as a supplement to the online version of this article at http://www.ajph.org). Before piloting this strategy, the Emory team held 3 focus groups of recently released individuals from local jails to gauge acceptability; these groups specifically endorsed this collection strategy.[16]

Once mass testing began, the Emory team developed a tracking system to study the relationship between SARS-CoV-2 diagnostic test positivity rates and the signal strength in wastewater.[18] Specimens collected at FCJ were tested by Northwell Health Laboratory, which used an LGC Biosearch Technologies SARS-CoV-2 ultrahigh-throughput end-point reverse transcription PCR test (Middlesex, UK) with 100% sensitivity. Jail medical staff could access results the next day. The individual test positivity rates and the cycle threshold of SARS-CoV-2 in the wastewater were correlated (Figure 3).[18]

Testing individuals for SARS-CoV-2 at MJHOC started with PCR testing in April 2020. In November 2021, PCR testing was replaced by rapid antigen testing. The DC Department of Corrections procedures for screening, isolation, and quarantine followed the CDC guidelines as they evolved.[26]

Adding Individual Testing

Targeted testing can follow a newly positive wastewater signal. The number of possible wastewater collection points, shown in Table 1, is proportional to the size of each jail. With 1 collection point, the readings are akin to a community viral load. However, when wastewater can be collected from multiple collection sites and the source is known to originate from a particular location in the jail, 1 or more positive signals informed the jail to consider testing where there may be highest risk of infection or spread. When positive sites were widespread, negative sites signaled where cases were not occurring and, therefore, resources could be spared. CCJ demonstrated the most progress in using WBS to locate and respond to outbreaks identified by WBS at various jail housing units. Once the Omicron variant of SARS-CoV-2 was widespread in the community at large, wastewater was consistently positive in most buildings. This guided the jail to focus on monitoring for clinical illness through nurse-led symptom checks.

Multiple Wastewater Collection Sites

At CCJ, each manhole access point drains from a single living unit. This permitted infection control teams to plan for optimal isolation housing configurations and identify zones that did not require targeted testing. In October 2021, SARS-CoV-2 was detected in the wastewater from the maximum-security living unit after prolonged negative results. At the time, no individuals were being monitored for infection. The infection control team interpreted the newly positive WBS readings as a harbinger of undetected infection in this unit. They preemptively notified custody staff that new isolation beds were necessary. Transfers out of the building halted to prevent exporting cases without proactive testing. Three days after the WBS signal appeared, clinical cases were diagnosed in the building. This early warning spared staff from scrambling for isolation beds and facilitated the prompt application of infection control measures.

Since the summer of 2021, wastewater results have been shared weekly with health care leadership at FCJ. For the entire duration of WBS, the jail population exceeded its capacity of 2688 persons, limiting their ability to isolate and quarantine infected and exposed populations. WBS spurred testing and led to isolation and quarantine as space permitted. Approaches were different during 2 periods.

Period 1 was from summer 2021 to summer 2022. In summer 2021, wastewater was clear of SARS-CoV-2 for several weeks. Health care staff identified no active cases. Later, the wastewater tested positive, preceding the detection of infected individuals in the population. Because WBS could not pinpoint which

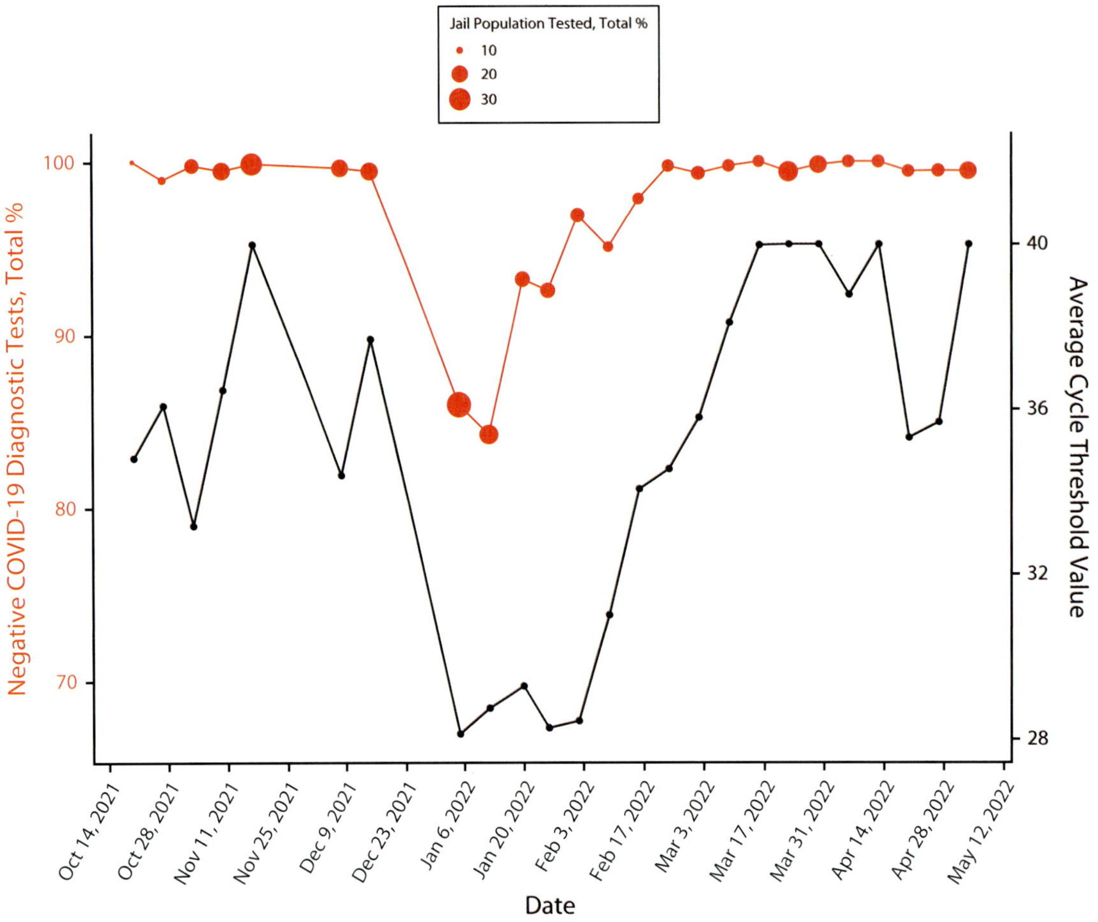

FIGURE 3— Comparison of Wastewater and Diagnostic Results With Population Percentage: Fulton County Jail, GA, 2021–2022

Source. Saber et al.[18]

Note. Average cycle threshold refers to the number of cycles needed to detect a florescent signal in a real-time polymerase chain reaction test as a result of detection of amplified nucleic acid (RNA or DNA). It is inversely proportional to the amount of RNA in the initial sample. With increasing percentages of negative tests (fewer people infected, less RNA) the cycle threshold increases as more cycles are required to amplify it to detectable levels.

housing units had infected individuals, mass testing occurred beginning October 2021. This supplemented ongoing, opt-out antigen testing of entrants and symptomatic individuals. Throughout 2022, the team increasingly understood the source of cases leading to positive wastewater sites (Supplement B).

Period 2 began in fall 2022. Locating the jail's blueprints (Supplements A and B) permitted the Emory team to map plumbing lines. There are 42 housing units in the north tower and 36 in the south tower. Sewer mapping helped narrow down the source site to 7 housing units (or 14 in the case where 2 spokes of a tower drained into 1 site). The week of October 17, wastewater was positive in the North 5 manhole but negative at North 6, prompting screening in units 500 and 600 of the north tower. A cluster of 4 cases was found on the second floor of the north tower in the 500-housing block and no cases in the latter.

DISCUSSION

As jails around the country ramped up WBS for SARS-CoV-2, we learned that facilities of different sizes found WBS effective for monitoring new outbreaks. We have described 4 jail systems that established WBS systems and used the results to mitigate outbreaks. The average daily population of these jails varied widely, from less than 1000 to several thousand individuals, affording a view of WBS operations across a broad range of jail average daily population sizes (Table 1). Each of these programs had unique, innovative approaches to WBS; they also had challenges to overcome, such as funding issues that delayed the Washington, DC, rollout.

WBS can indicate the emergence of infection after a period of no activity. In CCJ, we observed a lead time on identification of an emerging outbreak, which allowed advance preparation of mitigation practices. The duration of lead time can change with SARS-CoV-2 variants. This effect of a lead time was observed in CCJ, a large jail, and in MJHOC, a smaller one, in August 2021, with the emergence of the Delta strain of SARS-CoV-2 (Supplement D, available as a supplement to the online version of this article at http://www.ajph.org). This highlights that WBS can serve as an early warning system for disease detection in multiple jail settings. WBS also functions as a collective signal on behalf of individuals who are unable or reluctant to self-report or self-identify because of barriers faced in jail (e.g., difficulty accessing health services, stigma, mistrust of providers, concerns surrounding isolation).

In larger jails, with multiple collection points corresponding to separate housing units, WBS may offer the added benefit of knowing where to focus, conserving resources. In CCJ, results streamlined resource use by indicating the areas without virus. These areas did not require surveillance testing or advance preparation of quarantine or isolation beds. Conversely, when a jail lacked these features (e.g., MJHOC), mass testing became necessary. Nevertheless, WBS still gave a lead time, which enabled a quicker response.

In jails with numerous prospective collection points but limited knowledge of the source living unit, a delineating step may be introduced. FCJ demonstrated the usefulness of dye testing to confirm wastewater flow, which consequently led to more accurate localization of infections and targeted nasal testing. MJHOC and DCJ used automatic samplers for obtaining samples for WBS. The advantage of this technology is more regulated, periodic sampling of the wastewater, removing the need to use Moore swabs.

When WBS indicates infection, a strategy of focused testing can enhance case-finding efficiency. However, administering an increased volume of individual tests may be labor intensive. In its protocol for follow-up individual testing, FCJ demonstrated that numerous nasal swabs could be collected quickly using barcode scanning to register specimens. The process for developing this strategy for FCJ is discussed in Supplement C. We believe that combining automatic sampling and establishing clear links between collection sites and housing units for precise infection locations will be the most favorable future practice.

We discovered that, aside from jail size, each site's architectural features had implications for WBS. Configurations of jails varied from a collection of independent buildings, towers with multiple wings, and a singular structure. Each configuration posed different challenges. One such challenge was access to critical points of the drainage lines and interpretation of results obtained from such sites. CCJ had housing units in separate smaller buildings, making it easier to access points in the drainage system that corresponded to separate housing units (each manhole access point drains from a single living unit), compared with the high towers of FCJ. FCJ had a complex interconnecting drainage system that had some drains flowing into others. A knowledge of the direction of flow was also needed to interpret which housing units were associated with positive results from manholes. The pattern of which manholes yielded wastewater suggestive of SARS-CoV-2 indicated the locations of infection (Supplement B). Across the project, residents were housed in dorms, double occupancy cells, single occupancy cells, or mixed housing. Diversity in housing is important to consider when planning testing and other mitigation strategies.

A fundamental component underlying successful implementation of WBS in jails is support from various stakeholders, which will be the focus in future steps of our study. Across the country, early attitudes toward SARS-CoV-2 case finding varied. They ranged from withholding testing of asymptomatic persons, even with known exposure,[27] to aggressive identification of all cases and transparently posting results.[28] Cooperation between entities included interjail cooperation and communication between custody officials and respective medical operations.

FCJ and MJHOC operated with contracted medical vendors that approved surveillance activity. External jail support included close relationships between jail staff and academic institutions, such as the University of Illinois in Chicago, Emory University, Montefiore Medical Center/Albert Einstein College of Medicine, and Tufts University. Funding entities made study activities possible, as WBS was not yet considered standard population-level surveillance practice. Former jail residents were important to implementing the surveillance project, as their participation was necessary for calibrating individual testing logistics. The diversity represented in our study's stakeholders was key to its success. Increased participation and awareness between different entities strengthened the process overall.

Our study results suggest that WBS could be a useful population-level system for other emerging infectious diseases, such as mpox, polio, and tuberculosis. Wastewater was archived at CCJ and FCJ starting in May 2022 at the onset of the mpox outbreak. Validation of mpox detection in wastewater has since been demonstrated.[29] CCJ observed 2 confirmed cases of mpox[30] but did not detect the virus in the weekly wastewater samples archived from the same period. Reasons for missing mpox virus in the wastewater could include waning viral shedding by the day that virus was collected. CCJ has also used WBS for influenza, respiratory syncytial virus, and hepatitis A.

WBS opens the possibility of surveillance for noninfectious agents, such as opioids and other illicit drugs.[31] Detection of substances in a sample representing the aggregate of the jail wastewater can provide public health data on what substances are present. Determining the precise location to narrow the search to a single housing unit could lead to an individual's entrapment. Opinions of persons with lived experience of incarceration, correctional medicine experts, and others are mixed: some support such a move; others believe it may erode residents' trust in WBS programs. Although targeted searches could save resources and better prevent overdose-associated morbidity and mortality, it could lead to associating WBS with punishment rather than health promotion.

We have demonstrated that WBS can serve as an early warning system for disease detection in carceral settings. Its potential to assist corrections and public health agencies with outbreak mitigation is enormous. The application needs to be thoughtful, and input from a wide range of stakeholders, including those with lived experience of incarceration, could be useful when deciding its scope. Supplemental Figure E (available as a supplement to the online version of this article at http://www.ajph.org) provides a flowchart on operationalizing WBS using lessons learned in this project. With all voices at the table planning its implementation, the new technology could change the landscape of infection control in carceral settings and other congregate environments. AJPH

ABOUT THE AUTHORS

Shanika S. Kennedy, Lindsay B. Saber, Victoria M. Brown, Rachel A. Boehm, Amadin A. Olotu, Jeffery Osei, Jacob A. Pluznik, Ebrima Sidibeh, Victoria L. Phillips, and Anne C. Spaulding are with the Rollins School of Public Health, Emory University, Atlanta, GA. Lindsey R. Riback and Matthew J. Akiyama are with the Albert Einstein College of Medicine, New York, NY. Beth Jordan is with the DC Department of Corrections, Washington, DC. Eleni O'Donovan is with Unity Healthcare, Washington, DC. Anilkumar Mangla and Christine Nzokou are with the DC Department of Health, Washington, DC. Tracey L. Elam is with the Fulton County Sheriff's Office, Atlanta, GA. Jane Gubser, Steven Wilensky, and Chad J. Zawitz are with the Cook County Department of Corrections, Chicago, IL. Peter J. Koutoujian and Kashif A. Siddiqi are with the Middlesex Sheriff's Office, Billerica, MA. Alysse G. Wurcel is with Tufts Medicine, Boston, MA.

CORRESPONDENCE

Correspondence should be sent to Anne Spaulding, MD, MPH, Emory University, 1518 Clifton Rd NE, Atlanta, GA 30322 (e-mail: aspauld@emory.edu). Reprints can be ordered at https://www.ajph.org by clicking the "Reprints" link.

PUBLICATION INFORMATION

Full Citation: Kennedy SS, Saber LB, Brown VM, et al. Four models of wastewater-based monitoring for SARS-CoV-2 complementing individual screening in jail settings. *Am J Public Health*. 2024;114(11):1232–1241.

Acceptance Date: June 30, 2024.

DOI: https://doi.org/10.2105/AJPH.2024.307785

ORCID iD:

Anne C. Spaulding https://orcid.org/0000-0002-0281-0248

CONTRIBUTORS

S. S. Kennedy, L. B. Saber, V. M. Brown, R. A. Boehm, A. Mangla, B. Jordan, E. O'Donovan, V. L. Phillips, A. G. Wurcel, C. J. Zawitz, M. J. Akiyama, and A. C. Spaulding conceptualized the study, developed the design, analyzed and interpretated the data, and wrote the initial draft of the article. J. Osei, E. Sidibeh, and C. Nzokou analyzed and interpreted the data. T. L. Elam, J. Gubser, P. J. Koutoujian, K. A. Siddiqi, and S. Wilensky conceptualized the study and assisted in the design development. All authors revised the article and approved the final draft.

ACKNOWLEDGMENTS

This work was funded by the Gates Foundation (grant INV-035562, 64986), the Walder Foundation, the Centers for Disease Control and Prevention, and a National Institute on Drug Abuse, National Institutes of Health, Rapid Acceleration of Diagnostics Underserved Populations Program cooperative agreement (U01 DA056000) with Emory University).

We extend our thanks to all participating jails' sheriff's offices and collaborating institutions.

CONFLICTS OF INTEREST

A. J. Wurcel has received funding from the Massachusetts Sheriff Association. C. J. Zawitz has received funding from serving on Gilead Sciences Speaker's Bureau. M. J. Akiyama reports grants from NIDA, NIH (K99/R00 DA043011; DP2 DA053730), the National Institute on Minority Health and Health Disparities (R01 MD016744), the National Institute of Allergy and Infectious Diseases (P30 AI124414), and investigator-initiated funding paid to his institution from Gilead Sciences and Abbvie. A. C. Spaulding has received in the past 3 years funding through her university from Health Resource Services Administration and Health Through Walls, and internal funding from Emory University. She has personally received consulting fees from the Medical Association of Georgia and funding for travel from the Infectious Disease Society of America.

HUMAN PARTICIPANT PROTECTION

The study described in this article did not constitute human participant research according to criteria followed by the Emory University institutional review board.

REFERENCES

1. Marusinec R, Brodie D, Buhain S, et al. Epidemiology of coronavirus disease 2019 at a county jail—Alameda County, California, March 2020–March 2021. *J Public Health Manag Pract*. 2022;28(1):50–59. https://doi.org/10.1097/PHH.0000000000001453
2. Lofgren ET, Lum K, Horowitz A, Mabubuonwu B, Meyers K, Fefferman NH. Carceral amplification of COVID-19: impacts for community, corrections officer, and incarcerated population risks. *Epidemiology*. 2022;33(4):480–492. https://doi.org/10.1097/EDE.0000000000001476
3. Centers for Disease Control and Prevention. Network characteristics and visualization of COVID-19 outbreak in a large detention facility in the United States—Cook County, Illinois, 2020.

MMWR Morb Mortal Wkly Rep. 2020;69(44): 1625–1630. https://doi.org/10.15585/mmwr.mm6944a3

4. Centers for Disease Control and Prevention. Outbreak of SARS-CoV-2 B. 1.617. 2 (Delta) variant infections among incarcerated persons in a federal prison—Texas, July–August 2021. *MMWR Morb Mortal Wkly Rep.* 2021;70(38):1349–1354. https://doi.org/10.15585/mmwr.mm7038e3
5. Institute for Crime & Justice Policy Research. World prison brief. Available at: https://www.prisonstudies.org. Accessed December 2, 2023.
6. Minton TD, Zeng Z. Jail inmates in 2020—statistical tables. December 14, 2021. Available at: https://bjs.ojp.gov/library/publications/jail-inmates-2020-statistical-tables#additional-details-0. Accessed August 29, 2022.
7. Spaulding AC, Seals RM, Page MJ, Brzozowski AK, Rhodes W, Hammett TM. HIV/AIDS among inmates of and releasees from US correctional facilities, 2006: declining share of epidemic but persistent public health opportunity. *PLoS One.* 2009;4(11):e7558. https://doi.org/10.1371/journal.pone.0007558
8. UCLA Law. COVID behind bars data project. Available at: https://uclacovidbehindbars.org. Accessed November 2, 2022.
9. Akiyama MJ, Spaulding AC, Rich JD. Flattening the curve for incarcerated populations—COVID-19 in jails and prisons. *N Engl J Med.* 2020;382(22): 2075–2077. https://doi.org/10.1056/NEJMp2005687
10. Centers for Disease Control and Prevention. Guidance on management of COVID-19 in homeless service sites and in correctional and detention facilities. Available at: https://www.cdc.gov/coronavirus/2019-ncov/community/homeless-correctional-settings.html. Accessed January 30, 2024.
11. Daughton CG. Wastewater surveillance for population-wide COVID-19: the present and future. *Sci Total Environ.* 2020;736:139631. https://doi.org/10.1016/j.scitotenv.2020.139631
12. Betancourt WQ, Schmitz BW, Innes GK, et al. COVID-19 containment on a college campus via wastewater-based epidemiology, targeted clinical testing and an intervention. *Sci Total Environ.* 2021;779:146408. https://doi.org/10.1016/j.scitotenv.2021.146408
13. Gibas C, Lambirth K, Mittal N, et al. Implementing building-level SARS-CoV-2 wastewater surveillance on a university campus. *Sci Total Environ.* 2021;782:146749. https://doi.org/10.1016/j.scitotenv.2021.146749
14. Harris-Lovett S, Nelson KL, Beamer P, et al. Wastewater surveillance for SARS-CoV-2 on college campuses: initial efforts, lessons learned, and research needs. *Int J Environ Res Public Health.* 2021;18(9):4455. https://doi.org/10.3390/ijerph18094455
15. Karthikeyan S, Nguyen A, McDonald D, et al. Rapid, large-scale wastewater surveillance and automated reporting system enable early detection of nearly 85% of COVID-19 cases on a university campus. *mSystems.* 2021;6(4):e0079321. https://doi.org/10.1128/msystems.00793-21
16. González-Montalvo MDM, Dickson PF, Saber LB, et al. Opinions of former jail residents about self-collection of SARS-CoV-2 specimens, paired with wastewater surveillance: a qualitative study rapidly examining acceptability of COVID-19 mitigation measures. *PLoS One.* 2023;18(5): e0285364. https://doi.org/10.1371/journal.pone.0285364
17. Riback LR, Dickson P, Ralph K, et al. Coping with COVID in corrections: a qualitative study among the recently incarcerated on infection control and the acceptability of wastewater-based surveillance. *Health Justice.* 2023;11(1):5. https://doi.org/10.1186/s40352-023-00205-0
18. Saber LB, Kennedy SS, Yang Y, et al. Correlation of SARS-CoV-2 in wastewater and individual testing results in a jail, Atlanta, Georgia, USA. *Emerg Infect Dis.* 2024;30(suppl 1):S21. https://doi.org/10.3201/eid3013.230775
19. Zeng Z, Minton TD. Census of jails, 2005–2019—statistical tables. October 2021. Available at: https://www.ojp.gov/library/publications/census-jails-2005-2019-statistical-tables. Accessed April 22, 2023.
20. Liu P, Ibaraki M, VanTassell J, et al. A sensitive, simple, and low-cost method for COVID-19 wastewater surveillance at an institutional level. *Sci Total Environ.* 2022;807(pt 3):151047. https://doi.org/10.1016/j.scitotenv.2021.151047
21. Chen Y, Chen L, Deng Q, et al. The presence of SARS-CoV-2 RNA in the feces of COVID-19 patients. *J Med Virol.* 2020;92(7):833–840. https://doi.org/10.1002/jmv.25825
22. Owen C, Wright-Foulkes D, Alvarez P, et al. Reduction and discharge of SARS-CoV-2 RNA in Chicago-area water reclamation plants. *FEMS Microbes.* 2022;3:xtac015. https://doi.org/10.1093/femsmc/xtac015
23. VanTassell J, Raymond J, Wolfe MK, Liu P, Moe C. Wastewater sample collection—Moore swab and grab sample methods. Available at: https://www.protocols.io/view/wastewater-sample-collection-moore-swab-and-grab-s-81wgb6djnlpk/v1. Accessed August 29, 2022.
24. Sablon O, VanTassell J, Raymond J, Wolfe MK, Liu P, Moe C. Nanotrap KingFisher concentration/extraction & MagMAX KingFisher extraction protocol. Available at: https://www.protocols.io/view/nanotrap-kingfisher-concentration-extraction-amp-m-bp2l61ke5vqe/v1.2021. Accessed August 28, 2024.
25. Curtis A. Middlesex Sheriff's Office using wastewater analysis to monitor for COVID. Available at: https://www.lowellsun.com/2021/05/10/middlesex-sheriffs-office-using-wastewater-analysis-to-monitor-for-presence-of-coronavirus-at-facility. Accessed August 28, 2024.
26. Epting ME, Pluznik JA, Levano SR, et al. Aiming for zero: reducing transmission of COVID-19 in the D.C. Department of Corrections. Available at: https://einstein.elsevierpure.com/en/publications/aiming-for-zero-reducing-transmission-of-coronavirus-disease-2019. Accessed August 28, 2024.
27. Rankin W. Lawsuit alleges Clayton Jail indifferent to pandemic spread. *Atlanta Journal Constitution.* Available at: https://www.ajc.com/news/atlanta-news/lawsuit-alleges-clayton-jail-indifferent-to-pandemic-spread/6UWIHUL3UZCVPGVUMJYXTWDIAY. Accessed 7 December 2022.
28. California Department of Corrections and Rehabilitation. Population COVID-19 tracking. Available at: https://www.cdcr.ca.gov/covid19/population-status-tracking. Accessed December 7, 2022.
29. Wolfe MK, Yu AT, Duong D, et al. Use of wastewater for mpox outbreak surveillance in California. *N Engl J Med.* 2023;388(6):570–572. https://doi.org/10.1056/NEJMc2213882
30. Centers for Disease Control and Prevention. Monkeypox case investigation—Cook County Jail, Chicago, Illinois, July–August 2022. *MMWR Morb Mortal Wkly Rep.* 2022;71(40):1271–1277. https://doi.org/10.15585/mmwr.mm7140e2
31. van Dyken E, Thai P, Lai FY, et al. Monitoring substance use in prisons: assessing the potential value of wastewater analysis. *Sci Justice.* 2014;54(5): 338–345. https://doi.org/10.1016/j.scijus.2014.06.006

Health Care Delivery Site– and Patient-Level Factors Associated With COVID-19 Primary Vaccine Series Completion in a National Network of Community Health Centers

Rachel Gold, PhD, MPH, Anna Steeves-Reece, PhD, MPH, MA, Aileen Ochoa, MPH, Jee Oakley, MPH, Rose Gunn, MA, Shuling Liu, PhD, Brigit A. Hatch, MD, Sean T. O'Leary, MD, Christine I. Spina, MSPH, Treasure Allen, MPH, and Erika K. Cottrell, PhD, MPP

See also Hechter, p. 1146.

AJPH November 2024, Vol. 114, No. 11

Objectives. To assess multilevel factors associated with variation in COVID-19 vaccination rates in a US network of community health centers.

Methods. Using multilevel logistic regression with electronic health record data from ADVANCE (Accelerating Data Value Across a National Community Health Center Network; January 1, 2022–December 31, 2022), we assessed associations between health care delivery site–level (n = 1219) and patient-level (n = 1 864 007) characteristics and COVID-19 primary vaccine series uptake.

Results. A total of 1 337 440 patients completed the COVID-19 primary vaccine series. Health care delivery site characteristics were significantly associated with lower series completion rates, including being located in non-Medicaid expansion states and isolated or rural communities and serving fewer patients. Patient characteristics associated with significantly lower likelihood of completing the vaccine series included being Black/African American or American Indian/Alaska Native (vs White), younger age, lower income, being uninsured or publicly insured (vs using private insurance), and having fewer visits.

Conclusions. Both health care delivery site– and patient-level factors were significantly associated with lower COVID-19 vaccine uptake. Community health centers have been a critical resource for vaccination during the pandemic. (*Am J Public Health*. 2024;114(11):1242–1251. https://doi.org/10.2105/AJPH.2024.307773)

The introduction of COVID-19 vaccines in December 2020 was critical to reducing morbidity and mortality from COVID-19.[1] Yet by the end of the federal public health emergency in May 2023,[2] only 70% of the US population had completed the COVID-19 primary vaccination series.[3] Differences in rates of COVID-19 vaccination are known to follow racial/ethnic, socioeconomic, geographic, and political affiliation lines.[4] Less is known about the associations between health care delivery site–level factors and vaccination rates. In particular, there is little knowledge about patterns of COVID-19 vaccine uptake in settings that serve patients regardless of ability to pay: community health centers (CHCs), including federally qualified health centers, rural health centers, and similar care delivery sites.

CHCs provide comprehensive primary care—including COVID-19 vaccines—to low-income populations, whose members are at elevated risk for developing severe illness from COVID-19.[5] COVID-19 vaccine distribution in CHCs has been reported by patient race and ethnicity,[6] but to our knowledge no studies have examined health care delivery site–level factors associated with variation in COVID-19 vaccination in the CHC setting.

Understanding the multilevel factors driving COVID-19 vaccination patterns is necessary to inform future efforts to increase uptake of COVID-19 and other vaccines across the United States. We describe health care delivery site– and patient-level characteristics associated with COVID-19 vaccination across a national network of CHCs to provide knowledge that could inform future vaccination efforts in CHC-served populations.

METHODS

OCHIN is a nonprofit health equity innovation center serving a national network of health care delivery site members located in 34 states. Its members share a single instance of the Epic electronic health record (EHR).[7] The majority of the network is composed of CHCs. We used data from the OCHIN Epic EHR that was collected as part of routine clinical care and then made research ready and housed in the Accelerating Data Value Across a National Community Health Center Network, a member of the Patient-Centered Outcomes Research Network.[8]

Measures

Our analyses included patients who had 1 or more in-person visits at 1 of 1219 OCHIN health care delivery sites between January 1, 2022, and December 31, 2022. If a patient visited more than 1 care delivery site, we attributed them to the first site visited during the analysis period. We excluded from analysis patients who were younger than 6 months at their first visit in 2022, who had a recorded allergy to a COVID-19 vaccine, or who visited only a mobile health care delivery site.

The primary outcome was completion of the COVID-19 primary vaccine series by the end of 2022, defined according to the Centers for Disease Control and Prevention's interim COVID-19 immunization schedule for those aged 6 months and older.[9] The primary series completion definition included COVID-19 vaccines administered at OCHIN health care delivery sites or as recorded in the EHR of OCHIN via CHC queries to states' immunization information systems. Such queries are either conducted via automated nightly bulk requests or initiated by the health system in accordance with a patient visit.

We considered diverse health care delivery site–level variables shown to be associated with variation in other measures of CHC care quality.[10,11] These were whether the CHC was in a state that had adopted Medicaid expansion, whether it was in an accountable care organization,[12] the total number of patients served, urban versus rural designation per rural–urban commuting area code,[13] whether it was a school-based health center, and whether it was above the mean for all sites for percentage of staff in several specialties: pediatricians, family medicine physicians, or internal medicine physicians.

The patient-level variables were sex, race, ethnicity, total number of health care delivery site visits, household federal poverty level (FPL) as defined by the 2021–2022 US Census Bureau, insurance payor, and age at the time of first visit in 2022, as well as the documented presence of conditions that increase the risk of severe illness from COVID-19 (i.e., diabetes mellitus, immunosuppression, chronic kidney disease, chronic neurologic disease, chronic cardiovascular disease, chronic liver disease, chronic pulmonary disease).[14] We determined the presence of these conditions based on whether the patient had relevant problem list codes[15] in the 2 years before either their first COVID-19 vaccine dose or, for those without a COVID-19 vaccine, their first visit in 2022. We included overweight and obesity indicators based on patient body mass index. We included smoking status based on structured EHR data. We assessed all of these variables because they have been shown to be associated with variation in receipt of preventive care in CHC patients.

Statistical Analysis

We stratified all analyses by "new patients" (no visits before January 2021) and "established patients" (≥ 1 visit before January 2021) based on the assumption that many new patients visited these health care delivery sites solely to receive a COVID-19 vaccine and would differ from patients who went for additional reasons. We compared the characteristics of new and established patients by using the χ^2 test.

To determine the unadjusted association between each independent variable and the outcome of interest, we conducted bivariate analyses by using the χ^2 test. We determined multicollinearity to be low using the calculated variance inflation factor. Next, we used multilevel logistic regression to investigate factors associated with the probability of completing a COVID-19 primary vaccine series among patients nested in health care delivery sites. The model accounted for the hierarchical data structure using a random intercept for site-level effects, and we fitted it using PROC GLIMMIX in SAS version 9.4 (SAS Institute, Cary, NC), with a binary distribution and a logit link function.[16]

AJPH November 2024, Vol. 114, No. 11

We modeled random intercepts for health care delivery sites using a compound symmetry covariance structure to account for clustering among patients in the same site. This approach allowed us to estimate the effect of patient- and site-level factors on the probability of completing a COVID-19 primary vaccine series, while accounting for the complex data structure and the variation among health care delivery sites. We used the missing indicator method to account for missing covariate data. We conducted a sensitivity analysis limited to persons with complete data (Table A, available as a supplement to the online version of this article at http://www.ajph.org). We conducted all analyses with SAS.

TABLE 1— Health Care Delivery Site Characteristics in a US Network: 2022

Site Characteristic	No. (%)
Total health care delivery sites	1219 (100.0)
In an accountable care organization	194 (15.9)
In a Medicaid expansion state	981 (80.5)
School-based health center	153 (12.6)
RUCA classification	
Urban	998 (81.9)
Large rural	114 (9.4)
Small rural	51 (4.2)
Isolated	50 (4.1)
Missing	6 (0.5)
Total patients quartiles	
1–93 (Q1)	303 (24.9)
94–495 (Q2)	307 (25.2)
496–1994 (Q3)	311 (25.5)
> 1994 (Q4)	298 (24.5)
No. family medicine physicians above OCHIN's mean %	474 (38.9)
No. internal medicine physicians above OCHIN's mean %	293 (24.0)
No. pediatricians above OCHIN's mean %	256 (21.0)

Note. OCHIN = Oregon Community Health Information Network; RUCA = rural–urban commuting area codes.

RESULTS

We describe health care delivery site characteristics, including patient characteristics, in this study's national network of community-based health care delivery sites, and the results of multilevel regression analyses of associations between these characteristics and the outcomes of interest.

Health Care Delivery Site and Patient Characteristics

Health care delivery site (n = 1219) and patient (n = 1 864 007) characteristics are described in Tables 1 and 2, respectively. There was considerable heterogeneity in terms of sites' size, with 25% of sites serving 93 or fewer total patients and 25% serving more than 1994 total patients in 2022. Most (81%) sites were located in a Medicaid expansion state, 16% were affiliated with an accountable care organization, and 13% were school-based health centers. Regarding staff composition, 21% of sites had greater than the health care delivery site mean percentage of pediatricians, 39% had greater than the mean percentage of family physicians, and 24% had greater than the mean percentage of internal medicine physicians.

The majority of included patients were aged 30 years or older (61%) and female (58%) (Table 2). Less than 1% (0.7%) of patients were Native Hawaiian or other Pacific Islander, 1% were American Indian or Alaska Native (AI/AN), 7% were Asian, 16% were Black/African American, 58% were White, and 1% had more than 1 race listed; 40% were Hispanic/Latino. Most (79%) patients had household incomes at less than 185% of the FPL, 53% were Medicaid beneficiaries, and 18% were uninsured. The majority (70%) of patients had 4 or more total OCHIN health care delivery site visits. By chronic condition category, 5% had diabetes mellitus, 1% immunosuppression, 1% chronic kidney disease, 1% chronic neurologic disease, 2% chronic cardiac disease, 1% chronic liver disease, and 5% chronic pulmonary disease; 16% were overweight, 25% were obese, and 10% were smokers.

As of December 31, 2022, 1 337 440 patients in this national network had received a COVID-19 primary vaccine series (72% of those seen during the analysis period). This rate was higher for new (89%) than established (60%) patients ($P \le .001$). Many patient-level characteristics were significantly different between the new and established patients, and new patients had notably more missing data for ethnicity, race, and FPL.

TABLE 2— Descriptive Characteristics for New, Established, and All Patients in a US Network: 2022

Characteristic	New Patients, No. (%)	Established Patients, No. (%)	P[a]	All Patients, No. (%)
Total	761 260 (40.8)	1 102 747 (59.2)		1 864 007 (100.0)
COVID-19 vaccine series completion	680 895 (89.4)	656 545 (59.5)	≤ .001	1 337 440 (71.8)
Age			≤ .001	
6 mo–4 y	5 464 (0.7)	105 285 (9.6)		110 749 (5.9)
5–11 y	45 385 (6.0)	108 668 (9.9)		154 053 (8.3)
12–17 y	72 480 (9.5)	102 278 (9.3)		174 758 (9.4)
18–29 y	150 414 (19.8)	137 602 (12.5)		288 016 (15.5)
30–49 y	230 635 (30.3)	289 013 (26.2)		519 648 (27.9)
50–64 y	158 055 (20.8)	223 461 (20.3)		381 516 (20.5)
65–74 y	65 025 (8.5)	95 411 (8.7)		160 436 (8.6)
≥ 75 y	33 802 (4.4)	41 029 (3.7)		74 831 (4.0)
Sex			≤ .001	
Female	319 808 (42.0)	462 353 (41.9)		782 161 (42.0)
Male	440 722 (57.9)	639 866 (58.0)		1 080 588 (58.0)
Missing	730 (0.1)	528 (0.1)		1258 (0.1)
Race			≤ .001	
American Indian/Alaska Native	10 297 (1.4)	10 820 (1.0)		21 117 (1.1)
Asian	58 542 (7.7)	74 127 (6.7)		132 669 (7.1)
Native Hawaiian/other Pacific Islander	4 450 (0.6)	7 872 (0.7)		12 322 (0.7)
Black/African American	88 399 (11.6)	214 019 (19.4)		302 418 (16.2)
White	431 523 (56.7)	646 656 (58.6)		1 078 179 (57.8)
≥ 1 race	7 398 (1.0)	14 627 (1.3)		22 025 (1.2)
Missing	160 651 (21.1)	134 626 (12.2)		295 277 (15.8)
Hispanic/Latino			≤ .001	
No	376 260 (49.4)	617 518 (56.0)		993 778 (53.3)
Yes	312 644 (41.1)	432 543 (39.2)		745 187 (40.0)
Missing	72 356 (9.5)	52 686 (4.8)		125 042 (6.7)
Federal poverty level,[b] %			≤ .001	
< 50	330 218 (43.4)	475 001 (43.1)		805 219 (43.2)
50–< 100	112 724 (14.8)	234 259 (21.2)		346 983 (18.6)
100–< 130	51 558 (6.8)	94 274 (8.6)		145 832 (7.8)
130–< 185	67 655 (8.9)	106 882 (9.7)		174 537 (9.4)
≥ 185	84 388 (11.1)	129 280 (11.7)		213 668 (11.5)
Missing	114 717 (15.1)	63 051 (5.7)		177 768 (9.5)
Payor type			≤ .001	
Medicaid	367 259 (48.2)	625 211 (56.7)		992 470 (53.2)
Medicare	75 256 (9.9)	127 758 (11.6)		203 014 (10.9)
Other public	4 046 (0.5)	7 949 (0.7)		11 995 (0.6)
Private	147 068 (19.3)	167 551 (15.2)		314 619 (16.9)
Uninsured	167 631 (22.0)	174 278 (15.8)		341 909 (18.3)
Patient visits			≤ .001	
1–3	473 341 (62.2)	88 699 (8.0)		562 040 (30.2)
4–16	260 177 (34.2)	567 619 (51.5)		827 796 (44.4)
> 16	27 742 (3.6)	446 429 (40.5)		474 171 (25.4)

Continued

TABLE 2— Continued

Characteristic	New Patients, No. (%)	Established Patients, No. (%)	P[a]	All Patients, No. (%)
Chronic health condition			≤ .001	
Diabetes	13 701 (1.8)	75 733 (6.9)		89 434 (4.8)
Immunosuppression	3 828 (0.5)	22 459 (2.0)		26 287 (1.4)
Chronic kidney disease	2 439 (0.3)	19 548 (1.8)		21 987 (1.2)
Chronic neurologic disease	1 990 (0.3)	17 150 (1.6)		19 140 (1.0)
Chronic cardiac disease	4 713 (0.6)	32 673 (3.0)		37 386 (2.0)
Chronic liver disease	2 641 (0.4)	14 033 (1.3)		16 674 (0.9)
Chronic pulmonary disease	13 008 (1.7)	70 754 (6.4)		83 762 (4.5)
Overweight	73 418 (9.6)	223 584 (20.3)		297 002 (15.9)
Obesity	112 354 (14.8)	352 193 (31.9)		464 547 (24.9)
Current or former smoker	15 635 (2.1)	172 930 (15.7)		188 565 (10.1)

[a]P values generated from the χ^2 test of independence. The P values and χ^2 test of independence compare new patients with established patients.
[b]Defined by the 2021–2022 US Census Bureau depending on last date of patient federal poverty level assessment.

Multilevel Logistic Regression Analysis

Health care delivery site location in a non-Medicaid expansion state was associated with lower likelihood of COVID-19 primary vaccine series completion for both new (AOR [adjusted odds ratio] = 0.85; 95% CI [confidence interval] = 0.77, 0.95; P = .004) and established (AOR = 0.39; 95% CI = 0.34, 0.45; P ≤ .001) patients (Table 3).

Sites in isolated (AOR = 0.65; 95% CI = 0.51, 0.83; P ≤ .001), small rural (AOR = 0.68; 95% CI = 0.52, 0.89; P = .004), and large rural (AOR = 0.73; 95% CI = 0.62, 0.86; P ≤ .001) communities had lower likelihoods of primary series completion than did sites in urban communities, among established patients only. Sites serving a smaller patient population had lower likelihood of primary series completion than did the largest sites for both new (AOR = 0.80; 95% CI = 0.68, 0.94; P = .006) and established (AOR = 0.60; 95% CI = 0.50, 0.73; P ≤ .001) patients.

Sites with less than the mean percentage of certain clinician types had lower COVID-19 vaccination rates in 2 instances: those with less than the mean percentage of pediatricians (among new patients: AOR = 0.88; 95% CI = 0.80, 0.97; P ≤ .001) and those with less than the mean percentage of family physicians (among established patients: AOR = 0.85; 95% CI = 0.76, 0.95; P = .003).

Multiple patient-level characteristics were associated with COVID-19 primary vaccine series completion among both new and established patients. Hispanic/Latino patients had a higher likelihood of vaccination than did non-Hispanic/Latino patients (new patients: AOR = 1.14; 95% CI = 1.11, 1.16; P ≤ .001; established patients: AOR = 1.50; 95% CI = 1.48, 1.52; P ≤ .001). Black/African American patients (new: AOR = 0.93; 95% CI = 0.91, 0.96; P ≤ .001; established: AOR = 0.90; 95% CI = 0.89, 0.91; P ≤ .001) and AI/AN patients (new: AOR = 0.90; 95% CI = 0.83, 0.97; P = .007; established: AOR = 0.92; 95% CI = 0.88, 0.97; P ≤ .001) had lower likelihoods of primary series completion than did White patients. Asian patients (new: AOR = 1.12; 95% CI = 1.08, 1.17; P ≤ .001; established: AOR = 2.92; 95% CI = 2.84, 3.00; P ≤ .001) had a higher likelihood than did White patients.

Younger patients generally had lower likelihoods of primary series completion than did patients 75 years or older, except among new patients aged 50 to 64 years (AOR = 1.15; 95% CI = 1.09, 1.21; P ≤ .001) and 65 to 74 years (AOR = 1.17; 95% CI = 1.10, 1.23; P ≤ .001), who had a higher likelihood of primary series completion than did patients 75 years or older.

Established patients at less than 50% of the FPL (AOR = 0.70; 95% CI = 0.68, 0.71; P ≤ .001), 50% to less than 100% of the FPL (AOR = 0.76; 95% CI = 0.75, 0.77; P ≤ .001), 100% to less than 130% of the FPL (AOR = 0.83; 95% CI = 0.81, 0.85; P ≤ .001), and 130% to less than 185% of the FPL (AOR = 0.86; 95% CI = 0.84, 0.88; P ≤ .001) were less likely to be vaccinated than were those at 185% or more of the FPL. New patients at less than 50% of the FPL were also less likely to be vaccinated than were those at 185% or higher of the FPL (AOR = 0.82; 95% CI = 0.79, 0.84; P ≤ .001).

TABLE 3— Factors Associated With the Probability of Completing a Primary COVID-19 Vaccine Series in New and Established Patients in a US Network: 2022

Factor	New Patients (n = 761 260), AOR (95% CI)	Established Patients (n = 1 102 747), AOR (95% CI)
Health care delivery site variables		
Not in an ACO (ref: in an ACO)	0.90 (0.80, 1.00)	1.01 (0.87, 1.16)
Not in a Medicaid expansion state (ref: expansion state)	0.85 (0.77, 0.95)	0.39 (0.34, 0.45)
SBHC (ref: not SBHC)	1.09 (0.94, 1.26)	0.92 (0.78, 1.09)
RUCA classification		
Urban (Ref)	1	1
Isolated	1.00 (0.81, 1.24)	0.65 (0.51, 0.83)
Small rural	0.87 (0.72, 1.06)	0.68 (0.52, 0.89)
Large rural	0.91 (0.79, 1.04)	0.73 (0.62, 0.86)
Unknown	0.84 (0.47, 1.50)	1.13 (0.55, 2.34)
Total patients quartiles		
> 1994 (Q4) (Ref)	1	1
496–1994 (Q3)	0.99 (0.89, 1.09)	0.88 (0.77, 1.00)
94–495 (Q2)	0.93 (0.82, 1.04)	0.89 (0.76, 1.04)
1–93 (Q1)	0.80 (0.68, 0.94)	0.60 (0.50, 0.73)
No. family medicine physicians below OCHIN's mean %	0.93 (0.86, 1.01)	0.85 (0.76, 0.95)
No. internal medicine physicians below OCHIN's mean %	1.00 (0.91, 1.09)	0.96 (0.85, 1.09)
No. pediatricians below OCHIN's mean %	0.88 (0.80, 0.97)	0.91 (0.80, 1.03)
Patient-level variables		
Age		
≥ 75 y (Ref)	1	1
6 mo–4 y	0.03 (0.03, 0.04)	0.01 (0.01, 0.01)
5–11 y	0.37 (0.35, 0.39)	0.10 (0.10, 0.10)
12–17 y	0.66 (0.62, 0.70)	0.31 (0.30, 0.32)
18–29 y	0.58 (0.55, 0.61)	0.32 (0.31, 0.33)
30–49 y	0.83 (0.79, 0.87)	0.43 (0.42, 0.44)
50–64 y	1.15 (1.09, 1.21)	0.73 (0.71, 0.75)
65–74 y	1.17 (1.10, 1.23)	0.94 (0.91, 0.97)
Male (ref: female)	0.96 (0.94, 0.97)	0.96 (0.95, 0.97)
Race		
White (Ref)	1	1
Native Hawaiian/other Pacific Islander	1.06 (0.96, 1.18)	1.01 (0.95, 1.07)
American Indian/Alaska Native	0.90 (0.83, 0.97)	0.92 (0.88, 0.97)
Asian	1.12 (1.08, 1.17)	2.92 (2.84, 3.00)
Black/African American	0.93 (0.91, 0.96)	0.90 (0.89, 0.91)
> 1 race	1.16 (1.07, 1.26)	0.98 (0.94, 1.02)
Unknown	0.92 (0.90, 0.94)	1.05 (1.04, 1.07)
Hispanic/Latino (ref: not Hispanic/Latino)	1.14 (1.11, 1.16)	1.50 (1.48, 1.52)
Federal poverty level,[a] %		
≥ 185 (Ref)	1	1
< 50	0.82 (0.79, 0.84)	0.70 (0.68, 0.71)
50– < 100	0.96 (0.93, 1.00)	0.76 (0.75, 0.77)
100– < 130	1.01 (0.97, 1.05)	0.83 (0.81, 0.85)

Continued

TABLE 3— Continued

Factor	New Patients (n = 761 260), AOR (95% CI)	Established Patients (n = 1 102 747), AOR (95% CI)
130– < 185	1.02 (0.98, 1.06)	0.86 (0.84, 0.88)
Unknown	0.79 (0.76, 0.82)	0.75 (0.73, 0.77)
Payor type		
Private (Ref)	1	1
Medicaid	0.82 (0.80, 0.84)	0.56 (0.56, 0.57)
Medicare	1.23 (1.18, 1.28)	0.86 (0.84, 0.88)
Other public	0.76 (0.68, 0.85)	0.65 (0.62, 0.69)
Uninsured	0.73 (0.71, 0.75)	0.60 (0.59, 0.61)
Patient visits		
1–3 (Ref)	1	1
4–16	1.65 (1.62, 1.68)	1.53 (1.50, 1.56)
> 16	2.34 (2.22, 2.47)	2.28 (2.23, 2.32)
Chronic health condition		
Diabetes (ref: no diabetes)	0.96 (0.90, 1.01)	1.81 (1.77, 1.85)
Immunosuppression (ref: no immunosuppression)	0.71 (0.64, 0.78)	1.47 (1.42, 1.53)
CKD (ref: No CKD)	0.80 (0.70, 0.91)	1.16 (1.12, 1.21)
CND (ref: no CND)	0.84 (0.72, 0.97)	1.33 (1.28, 1.39)
CCD (ref: No CCD)	0.84 (0.77, 0.93)	1.24 (1.20, 1.27)
CLD (ref: No CLD)	1.18 (1.03, 1.36)	1.40 (1.33, 1.46)
CPD (ref: no CPD)	0.96 (0.91, 1.01)	1.47 (1.44, 1.50)
Overweight (ref: not overweight)	0.20 (0.19, 0.20)	0.72 (0.71, 0.73)
Obesity (ref: not obese)	0.23 (0.22, 0.23)	0.80 (0.79, 0.80)
Current or former smoker (Ref: not current/former smoker)	0.64 (0.61, 0.67)	0.74 (0.73, 0.75)

Note. ACO = accountable care organization; AOR = adjusted odds ratio; CI = confidence interval; CCD = chronic cardiac disease; CKD = chronic kidney disease; CLD = chronic liver disease; CND = chronic neurologic disease; CPD = chronic pulmonary disease; RUCA = rural–urban commuting area codes; SBHC = school-based health center. The table presents the results of our multilevel logistic regression analysis.
[a]Defined by the 2021–2022 US Census Bureau depending on last date of patient federal poverty level assessment.

Medicaid beneficiaries (new: AOR = 0.82; 95% CI = 0.80, 0.84; $P \le .001$; established: AOR = 0.56; 95% CI = 0.56, 0.57; $P \le .001$) and uninsured patients (new: AOR = 0.73; 95% CI = 0.71, 0.75; $P \le .001$; established: AOR = 0.60; 95% CI = 0.59, 0.61; $P \le .001$) were less likely to complete the series than were those with private insurance.

Patients with more visits had a higher likelihood of vaccination completion; for example, those with 4 to 16 visits compared with 1 to 3 visits (new: AOR = 1.65; 95% CI = 1.62, 1.68; $P \le .001$; established: AOR = 1.53; 95% CI = 1.50, 1.56; $P \le .001$). Patients with indicators for overweight (new: AOR = 0.20; 95% CI = 0.19, 0.20; $P \le .001$; established: AOR = 0.72; 95% CI = 0.71, 0.73; $P \le .001$), obesity (new: AOR = 0.23; 95% CI = 0.22, 0.23; $P \le .001$; established: AOR = 0.80; 95% CI = 0.79, 0.80; $P \le .001$), and smoking (new: AOR = 0.64; 95% CI = 0.61, 0.67; $P \le .001$; established: AOR = 0.74; 95% CI = 0.73, 0.75; $P \le .001$) were less likely to have completed a primary series than were patients without those indicators.

Among established patients, those with chronic disease indicators were consistently more likely than were those without these indicators to be vaccinated; for example, patients with diabetes mellitus (AOR = 1.81; 95% CI = 1.77, 1.85; $P \le .001$) and chronic pulmonary disease (AOR = 1.47; 95% CI = 1.44, 1.50; $P \le .001$). There was no such pattern among new patients.

DISCUSSION

The majority (72%) of patients in this national sample of community-based health center sites completed a COVID-19 primary vaccine series by the end of 2022—greater than the completion rate for the total US population (69%) at that time.[17] Vaccination rates among new patients were considerably higher than were those among established patients (89% vs 60%, respectively). This suggests that many of the new patients established care with these sites primarily to access COVID-19 vaccines once they became widely available in January 2021. It also underscores previous findings that community-based health centers may have been critical vaccination access points during the pandemic.[18]

The factors that appear to have influenced the 60% completion rate among established patients, which was substantially lower than the US rate of 69%, are as follows. Several health care delivery site– and patient-level characteristics were associated with primary series completion, with important implications. First, sites in non-Medicaid expansion states had lower vaccination rates. It is possible that the financial challenges that community-based health centers in nonexpansion states faced during the pandemic[19] created barriers to prioritizing COVID-19 vaccination. Another possible explanation is that state leadership priorities influenced both whether a state expanded Medicaid and their emphasis on and support for COVID-19 vaccination.[20]

The finding that health care delivery sites in rural areas had lower primary series completion is corroborated by the literature.[21] Several studies indicate that vaccine hesitancy and misinformation is greater in rural areas.[22] Evidence also suggests that insufficient rural vaccine access influenced COVID-19 vaccination rates, at least earlier in the pandemic.[23]

Primary series completion rates were consistently higher among older populations, likely because of earlier availability of the vaccine and a higher risk of severe illness from COVID-19 for older people.[24] This result may also reflect concerns about vaccine safety and effectiveness among younger people.[25]

The findings that Black/African American patients had lower rates of series completion than did White patients, that Asian patients had higher rates than did White patients, and that Hispanic/Latino patients had higher rates than did patients who were not Hispanic/Latino, are similar to rates seen in national data.[26] These patterns are concerning given COVID-19's impact on Black/African American communities. Several studies indicate that lower vaccination rates among Black/African American populations may have been driven by individuals' past experiences of structural racism when engaging with the health care system rather than by vaccine hesitancy per se.[23]

Lower COVID-19 vaccination rates were also seen among AI/AN patients than among White patients, unlike in national data.[26] This difference may reflect the fact that federal Indian Health Services are not required to submit vaccination data to state-level immunization information systems, which may have affected the completeness of analysis data for AI/AN patients.[27] Further research is needed to understand this finding.

Patients with lower incomes had lower overall COVID-19 vaccination rates than did those with higher incomes, and Medicaid-insured and uninsured patients were also less likely to be vaccinated than were those with private insurance.[28] These results align with previous research that showed lower vaccination rates among persons in socioeconomically disadvantaged populations, Medicaid beneficiaries, and the uninsured.[29] The associations between overweight and obesity and smoking status with lower vaccination rates may also reflect these socioeconomic differences, as both are associated with income.[30,31]

Patients with more visits and those with chronic diseases had higher vaccine completion rates. These findings may reflect the importance of long-term patient–provider relationships: established patients with chronic conditions have better relationships with their providers than do those who do not, and trust in one's provider is correlated with higher vaccine uptake.[32] This finding may also reflect that patients with chronic diseases were more likely to need multiple visits to their local health care delivery site, yielding more opportunities for vaccination.

Limitations

Health care delivery site characteristics that we were unable to assess are likely associated with COVID-19 vaccine uptake in community-based health care settings (e.g., having community health workers or vaccine champions). Assessing this was beyond the scope of our analyses.[33] We were not able to detail vaccine series completion by vaccine type; future analyses might assess whether this affects series completion. The data also had a considerable amount of missingness for certain patient-level characteristics (e.g., ethnicity, race, FPL), a common EHR data limitation. Sensitivity analysis results (Table A) suggest that this did not affect study outcomes. The data lacked detail for variables that would have yielded more informative results if disaggregated (e.g., the Asian race category).[34]

Still, EHR data have strengths (e.g., detailed clinical information, more representative than administrative claims limited to a single payor)[35] that support this review of community-based health center data and its contribution to the literature.

It is also possible that vaccine administration data were incomplete, as clinics had to request vaccination data from the immunization information systems and some may not have done so systematically. This is especially likely for vaccines received at federal agencies (e.g., the Department of Veterans Affairs, the Department of Defense, and Indian Health Services), which are not required to share vaccination data with state-level immunization information systems.[27]

There are also limitations to the interpretation of results involving new patients. It is likely that many of those in this category accessed a study clinic for the primary purpose of vaccination, as hypothesized. However, it is also likely that some percentage of new patients came to the clinic to receive a full range of medical care and thus might have been more appropriately included in the established patient group.

Conclusions

Our results indicate that CHCs may have been a critical resource for vaccination in their communities during the pandemic, especially for new patients. Both health care setting– and patient-level factors were associated with lower COVID-19 vaccine uptake in this setting (i.e., in terms of Medicaid nonexpansion and in rural vs urban areas). Additional resources for interventions and policies at the health care delivery site, state, and national levels are likely needed to improve rates of COVID-19 vaccine uptake in the United States. Our results provide useful information for policy development seeking to improve rates of other vaccinations, as well as future COVID-19 boosters. AJPH

ABOUT THE AUTHORS

Rachel Gold, Anna Steeves-Reece, Aileen Ochoa, Jee Oakley, Rose Gunn, Brigit A. Hatch, Treasure Allen, and Erika K. Cottrell are with the Research Division, OCHIN, Inc. Portland, OR. Shuling Liu is with the Department of Family Medicine, Oregon Health & Science University, Portland. Sean T. O'Leary and Christine I. Spina are with the Adult and Child Center for Health Outcomes Research and Delivery Science University of Colorado Anschutz Medical Campus, Aurora.

CORRESPONDENCE

Correspondence should be sent to Rachel Gold, PhD, MPH, Kaiser Permanente, Center for Health Research, 3800 N Interstate Ave, Portland, OR 97227 (e-mail: Rachel.Gold@kpchr.org). Reprints can be ordered at https://www.ajph.org by clicking the "Reprints" link.

PUBLICATION INFORMATION

Full Citation: Gold R, Steeves-Reece A, Ochoa A, et al. Health care delivery site– and patient-level factors associated with COVID-19 primary vaccine series completion in a national network of community health centers. *Am J Public Health*. 2024; 114(11):1242–1251.

Acceptance Date: June 17, 2024.

DOI: https://doi.org/10.2105/AJPH.2024.307773

ORCID iDs:

Rachel Gold https://orcid.org/0000-0001-6326-5012

Aileen Ochoa https://orcid.org/0009-0005-3553-1615

Brigit A. Hatch https://orcid.org/0000-0002-1828-7279

Erika K. Cottrell https://orcid.org/0000-0003-0481-4485

CONTRIBUTORS

R. Gold, A. Steeves-Reece, B. A. Hatch, S. T. O'Leary, and A. Ochoa conceptualized the study and conducted the analyses. R. Gold, A. Steeves-Reece, and J. Oakley drafted the article. All authors participated in data interpretation and revised the article for intellectual content.

ACKNOWLEDGMENTS

This work was conducted with the Accelerating Data Value Across a National Community Health Center Network (ADVANCE) Clinical Research Network. ADVANCE is led by Oregon Community Health Information Network in partnership with Health Choice Network, Fenway Health, and Oregon Health & Science University. ADVANCE is funded through the Patient-Centered Outcomes Research Institute (contract RI-OCHIN 01-MC).

We would like to thank Brenda McGrath, Teresa Schmidt and Fran Biel from OCHIN, and Peter Thomas Baltrus from the Morehouse School of Medicine for providing editorial feedback and edits.

CONFLICTS OF INTEREST

The authors have no known competing financial interests or personal relationships that could have appeared to influence the work reported in this article.

HUMAN PARTICIPANT PROTECTION

This study was approved by the Advarra institutional review board.

REFERENCES

1. Mohammed I, Nauman A, Paul P, et al. The efficacy and effectiveness of the COVID-19 vaccines in reducing infection, severity, hospitalization, and mortality: a systematic review. *Hum Vaccin Immunother*. 2022;18(1):2027160. https://doi.org/10.1080/21645515.2022.2027160
2. Centers for Disease Control and Prevention. End of the federal COVID-19 public health emergency (PHE) declaration. https://archive.cdc.gov/#/details?q=End%20of%20the%20federal%20COVID-19%20public%20health%20emergency%20(PHE)%20declaration&start=0&rows=10&url=https://www.cdc.gov/coronavirus/2019-ncov/your-health/end-of-phe.html. Accessed August 23, 2024.
3. Centers for Disease Control and Prevention. COVID-19 update for the United States. Available at: https://covid.cdc.gov/covid-data-tracker/#vaccinations_vacc-people-booster-percent-pop5. Accessed August 23, 2024.
4. Nguyen KH, Anneser E, Toppo A, Allen JD, Parott JS, Corlin L. Disparities in national and state estimates of COVID-19 vaccination receipt and intent to vaccinate by race/ethnicity, income, and age group among adults ≥ 18 years, United States. *Vaccine*. 2022;40(1):107–113. https://doi.org/10.1016/j.vaccine.2021.11.040
5. Crane JT, Fabi R, Pacia D, Neuhaus CP, Berlinger N. "We're here to take care of our community": lessons learned from the US Federal Health Center COVID-19 vaccine program. *Health Promot Pract*. 2024;25(1):137–144. https://doi.org/10.1177/15248399221151178
6. Corallo B, Artiga S, Tolbert J. Are health centers facilitating equitable access to COVID-19 vaccinations? A June 2021 update. June 2, 2021. Available at: https://www.kff.org/coronavirus-covid-19/issue-brief/are-health-centers-facilitating-equitable-access-to-covid-19-vaccinations-a-june-2021-update. Accessed August 23, 2024.
7. Oregon Community Health Information Network. Our members. Available at: https://ochin.org/network/members. Accessed August 23, 2024.
8. DeVoe JE, Gold R, Cottrell E, et al. The ADVANCE network: accelerating data value across a national community health center network. *J Am Med Inform Assoc*. 2014;21(4):591–595. https://doi.org/10.1136/amiajnl-2014-002744

9. Centers for Disease Control and Prevention. Interim COVID-19 immunization schedule for persons 6 months of age and older. 2024. Available at: https://www.cdc.gov/vaccines/covid-19/downloads/covid-19-immunization-schedule-ages-6months-older.pdf. Accessed August 23, 2024.
10. Hatch BA, Tillotson CJ, Huguet N, Hoopes MJ, Marino M, DeVoe JE. Use of a preventive index to examine clinic-level factors associated with delivery of preventive care. *Am J Prev Med.* 2019;57(2):241–249. https://doi.org/10.1016/j.amepre.2019.03.016
11. Angier HE, Marino M, Springer RJ, Schmidt TD, Huguet N, DeVoe JE. The Affordable Care Act improved health insurance coverage and cardiovascular-related screening rates for cancer survivors seen in community health centers. *Cancer.* 2020;126(14):3303–3311. https://doi.org/10.1002/cncr.32900
12. Centers for Medicare & Medicaid Services. Accountable care organization participants. January 2023. Available at: https://data.cms.gov/medicare-shared-savings-program/accountable-care-organization-participants/data. Accessed August 23, 2024.
13. Rural Health Research Center. Map classifications. Available at: https://depts.washington.edu/uwruca/ruca-maps.php. Accessed August 23, 2024.
14. Centers for Disease Control and Prevention. Underlying medical conditions associated with higher risk for severe COVID-19: information for healthcare professionals. August 2023. Available at: https://archive.cdc.gov/#/details?q=Underlying%20medical%20conditions%20associated%20with%20higher%20risk%20for%20severe%20COVID-19:%20information%20for%20healthcare%20professionals&start=0&rows=10&url=https://www.cdc.gov/coronavirus/2019-ncov/hcp/clinical-care/underlyingconditions.html. Accessed August 23, 2024.
15. Centers for Disease Control and Prevention. Risk factors for severe COVID-19 outcomes among persons aged ≥ 18 years who completed a primary COVID-19 vaccination series—465 health care facilities, United States, December 2020–October 2021. *MMWR Morb Mortal Wkly Rep.* 2022;71(1):19–25. https://doi.org/10.15585/mmwr.mm7101a4
16. Schabenberger O. Introducing the GLIMMIX procedure for generalized linear mixed models. *SUGI 30 Proceedings.* 2005;196:1–20. Available at: https://support.sas.com/resources/papers/proceedings/proceedings/sugi30/196-30.pdf. Accessed August 23, 2024.
17. Centers for Disease Control and Prevention. Trends in number of COVID-19 vaccinations in the US. Available at: https://data.cdc.gov/Vaccinations/COVID-19-Vaccination-Trends-in-the-United-States-N/rh2h-3yt2/about_data. Accessed August 23, 2024.
18. Cole MB, Raifman JR, Assoumou SA, Kim JH. Assessment of administration and receipt of COVID-19 vaccines by race and ethnicity in US federally qualified health centers. *JAMA Netw Open.* 2022;5(1):e2142698. https://doi.org/10.1001/jamanetworkopen.2021.42698
19. Morrison D, Schwartz KA, Wolcott L. COVID-19 reflections: we are not OK: safety net primary care access in a non-expansion state amid COVID-19. *N C Med J.* 2022;83(3):194–196. https://doi.org/10.18043/ncm.83.3.194
20. Hu S, Xiong C, Li Q, Wang Z, Jiang Y. COVID-19 vaccine hesitancy cannot fully explain disparities in vaccination coverage across the contiguous United States. *Vaccine.* 2022;40(37):5471–5482. https://doi.org/10.1016/j.vaccine.2022.07.051
21. Centers for Disease Control and Prevention. Disparities in COVID-19 vaccination coverage between urban and rural counties—United States, December 14, 2020–January 31, 2022. *MMWR Morb Mortal Wkly Rep.* 2022;71(9):335–340. https://doi.org/10.15585/mmwr.mm7109a2
22. Kearney A, Lopes L, Washington I, Valdes I, Yilma H, Hamel L. Addressing misinformation in rural communities: snapshot from the KFF health misinformation tracking poll pilot. Available at: https://www.kff.org/coronavirus-covid-19/poll-finding/addressing-misinformation-in-rural-communities-snapshot-from-the-kff-health-misinformation-tracking-poll-pilot. Accessed August 23, 2024.
23. Hernandez I, Dickson S, Tang S, Gabriel N, Berenbrok LA, Guo J. Disparities in distribution of COVID-19 vaccines across US counties: a geographic information system–based cross-sectional study. *PLoS Med.* 2022;19(7):e1004069. https://doi.org/10.1371/journal.pmed.1004069
24. Teo SP. Review of COVID-19 vaccines and their evidence in older adults. *Ann Geriatr Med Res.* 2021;25(1):4–9. https://doi.org/10.4235/agmr.21.0011
25. Lee YM, Simonovich SD, Li S, et al. Motivators and barriers to COVID-19 vaccination in young adults living in the USA. *Clin Nurs Res.* 2023;32(6):971–982. https://doi.org/10.1177/10547738231177331
26. Centers for Disease Control and Prevention. Percent of people receiving COVID-19 vaccine by race/ethnicity and date administered, United States. Available at: https://covid.cdc.gov/covid-data-tracker/#datatracker-home. Accessed August 23, 2024.
27. US Department of Health and Human Services. Challenges with vaccination data hinder state and local immunization program efforts to combat COVID-19. Available at: https://oig.hhs.gov/oei/reports/OEI-05-22-00010.asp#:~:text=As%20of%20December%202021%2C%20nearly,DoD)%2C%20and%2For%20the. Accessed August 23, 2024.
28. Medicaid and CHIP Payment and Access Commission. *Report to Congress on Medicaid and CHIP.* March 2022. Available at: https://www.macpac.gov/wp-content/uploads/2022/03/March-2022-Report-to-Congress-on-Medicaid-and-CHIP.pdf. Accessed August 23, 2024.
29. Gertz A, Rader B, Sewalk K, Brownstein JS. Emerging socioeconomic disparities in COVID-19 vaccine second-dose completion rates in the United States. *Vaccines (Basel).* 2022;10(1):121. https://doi.org/10.3390/vaccines10010121
30. Casetta B, Videla AJ, Bardach A, et al. Association between cigarette smoking prevalence and income level: a systematic review and meta-analysis. *Nicotine Tob Res.* 2017;19(12):1401–1407. https://doi.org/10.1093/ntr/ntw266
31. Levine JA. Poverty and obesity in the US. *Diabetes.* 2011;60(11):2667–2668. https://doi.org/10.2337/db11-1118
32. Viskupič F, Wiltse DL, Meyer BA. Trust in physicians and trust in government predict COVID-19 vaccine uptake. *Soc Sci Q.* 2022;103(3):509–520. https://doi.org/10.1111/ssqu.13147
33. Smith DO, Wennerstrom A. To strengthen the public health response to COVID-19, we need community health workers. May 6, 2020. Available at: https://www.healthaffairs.org/content/forefront/strengthen-public-health-response-covid-19-we-need-community-health-workers. Accessed August 23, 2024.
34. Kalyanaraman Marcello R, Dolle J, Tariq A, et al. Disaggregating Asian race reveals COVID-19 disparities among Asian American patients at New York City's public hospital system. *Public Health Rep.* 2022;137(2):317–325. https://doi.org/10.1177/00333549211061313
35. Savitz ST, Savitz LA, Fleming NS, Shah ND, Go AS. How much can we trust electronic health record data? *Healthc (Amst).* 2020;8(3):100444. https://doi.org/10.1016/j.hjdsi.2020.100444

Trends in Nonfatal Overdose Rates Due to Alcohol and Prescription and Illegal Substances in Colombia, 2010–2021

Julian Santaella-Tenorio, DVM, DrPH, Jhoan S. Zapata-López, MSc, Thiago M. Fidalgo, MD, PhD, Vítor S. Tardelli, MD, PhD, Luis E. Segura, MD, DrPH, Magdalena Cerda, DrPH, and Silvia S. Martins, MD, PhD

See also Diaz-Moreno and Rojas, p. 1151, and Friedman, p. 1153.

Objectives. To examine drug overdoses in Colombia by type of substance, sex, age, and intent using data from a health surveillance system from 2010 to 2021.

Methods. We characterized data by year, type of substance, and sociodemographic variables. We calculated age-adjusted overdose rates by substance type, sex, age groups, and intent. We used Poisson regression models to examine trend differences across sex and age groups.

Results. Age-adjusted rates of drug overdoses increased from 8.51 to 40.52 per 100 000 during 2010 to 2021. Men, compared with women, had higher overdose rates for every substance, except for opioids and psychotropics. Drug overdose rates involving cannabis and stimulants increased steadily until 2017 but decreased afterward. Overdose rates involving psychotropic medication increased greatly during 2018 to 2021, mainly because of intentional overdoses in young women.

Conclusions. Overdoses involving illegal drugs decreased in recent years in Colombia; however, the continuous increase in intentional psychotropic overdose rates highlights the need for prevention efforts to curb this trend. Health surveillance systems are an important tool that can guide overdose prevention efforts in countries with limited data resources. (*Am J Public Health*. 2024;114(11):1252–1260. https://doi.org/10.2105/AJPH.2024.307786)

Substance use and related disorders remain a major concern and an important challenge for public health. Worldwide, the prevalence of people with past-year use of any psychoactive substance increased from 5% in 2010 to 5.6% in 2020.[1] Approximately 13.6% of people using substances in 2020 met criteria for a substance use–related disorder.[1] Addressing substance use challenges, including the emergence of novel drugs and of polysubstance use, is a complex task that requires a good understanding of the magnitude of the problem and the burden it imposes on populations and the health system (e.g., stigmatization, substance-related disorders, overdoses, and drug trafficking–related violence). However, for many countries in Latin America, it is often difficult to obtain continuous and reliable information on drug use patterns and related problems.

In Colombia, results from the 2019 National Survey on Substance Use (CNSSU, *Estudio Nacional de Consumo de Sustancias Psicoactivas de Colombia, 2019*),[2] indicate that substance use has increased for most substances in the country in the past 3 decades, with only a small reduction in the prevalence of alcohol, cannabis, and cocaine use in 2019 compared with the prevalence in 2013.[2] However, because this survey is conducted only every 5 to 6 years, it is difficult to know how substance use patterns are evolving over time and if they are affected by national or local legislation. Survey data also likely underestimate the prevalence of drug use given that it is a household survey that excludes populations with high risk of drug use (e.g., homeless and incarcerated populations). In addition, mortality data can only provide limited information on the substances involved in overdoses given that only a small proportion of all suspected overdose cases get tested for multiple drugs (in Colombia, the protocol requires cases to be tested for alcohol but not for other substances unless this is requested by a prosecutor or legal authority).[3]

Alternatively, electronic records from emergency departments (EDs) can provide important information on nonfatal overdoses, given that it includes information from clinical notes, self-reports from patients and from those witnessing the event, and toxicological data in some cases.[4] Surveillance of nonfatal overdoses based on ED records can inform public health prevention efforts by providing not only information about the substances more frequently causing overdoses in a region but also information on possible changes in polysubstance use patterns, on the introduction of new drugs and changes in the composition of drugs, and on other factors that can influence overdose risks.[5–7] Although data from ED visits and hospitalization discharges are regularly used in high-income countries to better understand the factors associated with drug overdoses,[4,6,7] these data are not usually available or not frequently used for this purpose in Latin American countries.[8,9]

In 2007, Colombia initiated a national public health surveillance system (SIVIGILA)[10] an electronic system of health events that includes the mandatory reporting of drug and alcohol overdoses treated at health institutions. A previous study using SIVIGILA data shows that the rate of overdoses attributable to all types of prescription drugs increased from 10.2 to 22.9 per 100 000 from 2008 to 2015[11] and also that overdoses attributable to illegal drugs increased from 8.1 to 14.7 per 100 000 inhabitants from 2011 to 2015.[11] A recent report also shows the total number of overdoses attributable to illegal drugs increased by 41% from 2020 to 2023.[12] However, to date, there are no studies in Colombia examining trends in overdose rates attributable to specific drug types, including prescription drugs with addictive potential (e.g., tranquilizers, sedatives, or opioids), or examining overdose rates by sex, age, or intent. This information is important to guide public health efforts to prevent overdoses in specific groups of the population.

Given this gap in knowledge, in this study, we used SIVIGILA data on drug overdoses to examine annual trends in overdose rates from 2010 to 2021, by type of substance, sex, age group, and intent. We also aimed to describe sociodemographic characteristics associated with these events.

METHODS

In this retrospective data analysis, we used information from the SIVIGILA from 2010 to 2021.[10] The SIVIGILA is a mandatory notification system of health events that have been selected by the government as relevant or burdensome and that includes multiple infectious diseases (e.g., tuberculosis, malaria, and dengue), cancer, congenital defects, and also overdoses or intoxications attributable to pesticides, medications, and illegal substances. Health personnel from all emergency departments, hospitals, clinics, and other health care facilities must notify SIVIGILA of all overdoses attributable to these substances using a standardized form that includes information about the type of substance(s) causing the overdose, sociodemographic characteristics of the patient, the place where the event occurred, and the date and circumstances surrounding the event. From 2010 to 2017, SIVIGILA required the notification of all overdoses using a single notification form. Starting in 2018, SIVIGILA required that intentional overdoses (e.g., suicide intent) should be reported separately from unintentional overdoses, using a specific form for suicide attempts. In this study we merged the 2018–2021 data on intentional overdoses to the 2018–2021 data with unintentional overdoses, so data from 2018 to 2021 were comparable to data from previous years (2010–2017). Because data from SIVIGILA are based on overdose cases treated in health care facilities, a patient with multiple overdose visits can be included multiple times in analyses. Multiple visits for the same overdose were removed from the data to avoid counting the same event multiple times.

Information on the substance(s) reported in the clinical report was used to group overdoses by substance type in the following categories: hallucinogens; stimulants (including prescription stimulants, cocaine, and methamphetamine); opioids (including prescription opioids, heroin, methadone, and buprenorphine); inhalants; tranquilizers, sedatives, and antidepressants; cannabis (including smoked and ingested edibles, food with cannabis, and cannabis oils); scopolamine (*Brugmansia* spp); and alcohol. Appendix Table A (available as a supplement to the online version of this article at https://ajph.org) shows a list of the substances that were included in each category.

Sociodemographic variables included sex, age, place of residence (urban and rural), affiliation to the health system (contributive [individuals or families who work and can contribute to the system with monthly payments], subsidized [individuals or families in poverty, who are in a vulnerable situation and cannot financially contribute to the system], special or exception [those in the military forces, the national police, or other public organizations], and educational level [elementary or middle school, high school, and college or higher]). SIVIGILA data also include information on whether the overdose resulted in hospitalization (yes or no) and the final outcome (dead or alive).

Overdoses occurring among individuals aged 10 years and older were characterized by year, by sociodemographic variables, by whether the event resulted in hospitalization, and by the final outcome (dead or alive). We also identified the most frequent combinations of multiple substances across the study period and the number of overdoses caused by these combinations.

We calculated age-adjusted rates of overdoses per year and for each substance group using annual populations available from the 2018 census that includes projected estimates for years 2019 to 2021 and annual revised counts for the 2010–2017 period.[13] We examined trends in overdose rates by sex, age, type of substance, and intent (the latter only in 2018–2021, given the changes in the SIVIGILA protocol starting in 2018). We also tested if overdose rate trends differed across sex and age groups using Poisson regression models with the total population as an offset and interaction terms between year and sex and year and age groups. We conducted all analyses in Stata version 18 (StataCorp LP, College Station, TX).[14]

RESULTS

The SIVIGILA data (2010–2021) included 127 087 substance use–related overdoses among people aged 10 years and older, of which 54.2% occurred in males, 75.3% in persons aged 10 to 34 years, 71.5% in people with at least some high school education or higher, and 51.1% and 37.9% among people affiliated as contributive and as subsidized, respectively, in the health system (Table 1). In addition, most of these overdoses occurred in urban areas (90.0%), 55.7% resulted in hospitalization, and 0.3% resulted in death (Table 1). The most frequently reported substances were tranquilizers, sedatives, or antidepressants (42.9%); cannabis (16.4%); stimulants (15.7%); alcohol (15.6%); and opioids (5.8%; Table 1). The majority (95.2%) of stimulant overdoses were attributable to cocaine, while opioid overdoses were mostly attributable to prescription opioids (73.8%). Although most overdoses were attributable to a single type of substance, overdoses involving both stimulants and cannabis, and also stimulants and alcohol, were frequently reported (Appendix Table B).

The age-adjusted rate of drug overdoses in SIVIGILA increased from 8.5 to 40.5 per 100 000 from 2010 to 2021, a 355.6% increase ($P < .01$; Appendix Table C). Overdose rates involving tranquilizers, sedatives, and antidepressants and those involving opioids increased over the study period, growing at a faster rate after 2018 (Figure 1). Drug overdoses involving cannabis and stimulants also increased until 2017 but decreased afterward. Overall, overdoses attributable to other substances were more stable, including those involving alcohol, which increased until 2014 and remained stable afterward (Figure 1).

Trend Rates by Sex

Drug overdose rates increased faster in men than women up to 2017; however, they increased faster in women from 2018 to 2021 ($P < .01$; Figure 2). While intentional overdoses increased from 2018 to 2021 for both sex groups, they increased faster in women (Appendix Figure A). Among women, the sharpest increase in overdose rates were for tranquilizers, sedatives, or antidepressants, which increased faster from 2018 to 2021 (from 12.3 to 33.3 per 100 000, respectively; Appendix Figure B.a). Most overdoses involving tranquilizers, sedatives, or antidepressants in women were intentional (in 2021 intentional overdoses were 18.36 times more frequent than unintentional overdoses involving these medications). Also in women, overdoses involving the use of cannabis and stimulants slightly increased until 2018, decreasing afterward, and overdoses involving opioids increased steadily after 2016 (Appendix Figure B.a). Overdoses involving prescription opioids were the most frequent opioids reported in opioid overdoses in 2017 to 2021 (5.4 times more frequently reported than other opioids in 2018–2021; data not shown).

Among men, overdoses involving cannabis and stimulants increased up to 2017 and decreased at a similar rate from 2018 to 2021. Also, although overdose rates attributable to tranquilizers, sedatives, or antidepressants were relatively stable up to 2016, they doubled from 2016 to 2021 (from 6.9 to 13.7 per 100 000; Appendix Figure B.b). Most of these overdoses involving tranquilizers, sedatives, or antidepressants were intentional, which were 5.2 times more frequent than unintentional overdoses in 2021). Overall, men had higher rates of overdoses for every type of substance, except for opioids and tranquilizers, sedatives, and antidepressants, which in 2021 were 1.8 and 2.4 times higher in women, respectively (Appendix Table C and Figures B.a and B.b).

TABLE 1— Characteristics of Substance Overdose Events in SIVIGILA: Colombia, 2010–2021

Characteristic	SIVIGILA (n = 127 087), No. (%)
Hospitalization	
Yes	70 817 (55.7)
No	56 270 (44.3)
Final condition	
Alive	126 727 (99.7)
Dead	346 (0.3)
Sex	
Women	58 213 (45.8)
Men	68 874 (54.2)
Age, y	
10–19	39 699 (31.2)
20–34	56 074 (44.1)
35–54	23 910 (18.8)
≥ 55	7 404 (5.8)
Location where the overdose occurred	
Urban	114 410 (90.0)
Rural	12 677 (10.0)
Affiliation with the health system[a]	
Contributive	64 919 (51.1)
Subsidized	48 164 (37.9)
Special or exception	4 417 (3.5)
No insurance	8 653 (6.8)
Other	934 (0.7)
Education	
Elementary or middle school	29 912 (23.5)
High school	70 694 (55.6)
College or higher	20 241 (15.9)
No information	6 211 (4.9)
Type of substance[b]	
Hallucinogens	1 923 (1.5)
Stimulants	19 908 (15.7)
Opioids	7 315 (5.8)
Inhalants	917 (0.7)
Tranquilizers, sedatives, or antidepressants	54 521 (42.9)
Cannabis	20 773 (16.4)
Scopolamine	6 125 (4.8)
Alcohol	19 879 (15.6)

Note. SIVIGILA is the National Public Health Surveillance System from Colombia, an electronic system of prioritized health events that includes the mandatory reporting of drug and alcohol overdoses treated at health institutions.

[a]Affiliation with the health system includes the following categories: (a) contributive (individuals or families who work and can contribute to the system with monthly payments), (b) subsidized (individuals or families in poverty, who are in a vulnerable situation and cannot financially contribute to the system), and (c) special or exception (applies to individuals in the military forces, the National Police, in public universities, or in some other public organizations).

[b]The percentage for the different substances does not add up to 100%, given that 1 event may include multiple substances.

Trend Rates by Age

Drug overdose rates increased across all age groups, although they increased faster in those aged 10 to 19 and 20 to 34 years ($P < .01$; Figure 3). During 2018 to 2021, those aged 10 to 19 and 20 to 34 years experienced the sharpest increases in overdose rates compared with older age groups. In these younger groups, intentional overdoses (Appendix Figure C) and overdoses involving tranquilizers, sedatives, or antidepressants (Appendix Figures D.a and D.b) increased faster than in older groups. Among those aged 10 to 19 years, overdose rates attributable to cannabis also increased greatly until 2018 and then decreased steadily until 2021 (Appendix Figure D.a). In those aged 20 to 34 years, overdoses attributable to cannabis and stimulants followed a similar trend, increasing until 2017 and then decreasing in later years (Appendix Figure D.b). In addition, in those aged 10 to 19 and 20 to 34 years, the overdose rates involving the use of opioids started to increase after 2017, with prescription opioids being the opioids more frequently reported in these overdoses in 2017 to 2021 (3.6 times compared with other opioids; data not shown). In older adults (ages 34–54 and ≥ 55 years), overdose rates were relatively stable over the study period, except for overdose rates attributable to tranquilizers, sedatives, or antidepressants, which increased after 2018 (Appendix Figures D.c and D.d). Overall, drug overdose rates were lower among older adults (ages 35–54 and ≥ 55 years) compared with younger groups ($P < .01$; Appendix Table C and Figures D.a–D.d).

DISCUSSION

Our study is the first, to our knowledge, to describe national trends in overdose

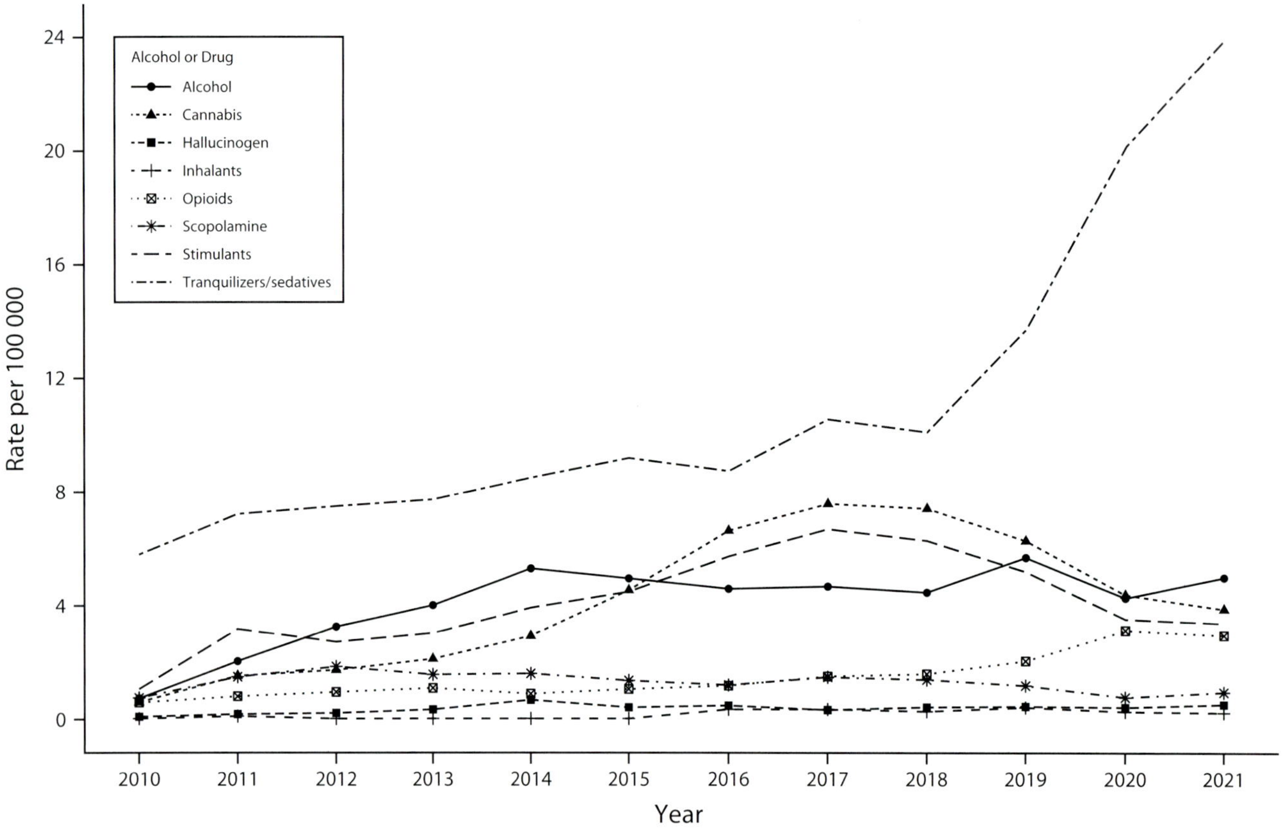

FIGURE 1— Age-Adjusted Rates of Drug and Alcohol Overdoses per 100 000 by Type of Substance: Colombia, 2010–2021

Note. Substance categories are not mutually exclusive, given that some overdoses involved multiple substances.

rates involving substances with psychoactive potential, including prescribed and illegal substances and alcohol, across different population groups in Colombia. Our results provide evidence of increases in overdose rates over the study period, in both women and men, that were more pronounced in adolescents and young adults. While overdose rates involving cannabis and stimulants decreased after 2018, the increase in intentional overdose rates involving tranquilizers, sedatives, or antidepressants among young women (aged ≤34 years) during the 2018–2021 period raises concerns about suicidal behavior in this population.

We observed that intentional overdose rates involving tranquilizers, sedatives, or antidepressants increased over time, with sharper increases in young women starting in 2018 and through the first years of the COVID-19 pandemic. Evidence shows that the pandemic contributed to higher levels of distress and mental health problems including depression and anxiety in Colombia,[15] similar to other countries,[16,17] and also higher prescription rates and use of tranquilizers, sedatives, and antidepressants.[18–22] In Colombia, during the pandemic, women, compared with men, experienced higher levels of anxiety, sadness, and difficulties with sleep.[15] Also, the 2019 CNSSU survey on psychoactive drug use shows that the prevalence of tranquilizer use without a prescription was similar among women and men (0.6%) and was higher among those aged 34 years or younger.[2] It is possible that higher levels of distress, along with higher availability of psychotropic medication (with or without a prescription), which can potentially serve as means of suicide, played a role in the occurrence of intentional overdoses involving these drugs in recent years. Although more research on risk factors, motivations for use, and sources of these medications is needed to improve harm-reduction interventions and policies, suicide risk screening and access to complementary mental health care addressing suicidal ideation or behavior may improve health outcomes among individuals being prescribed these medications and those

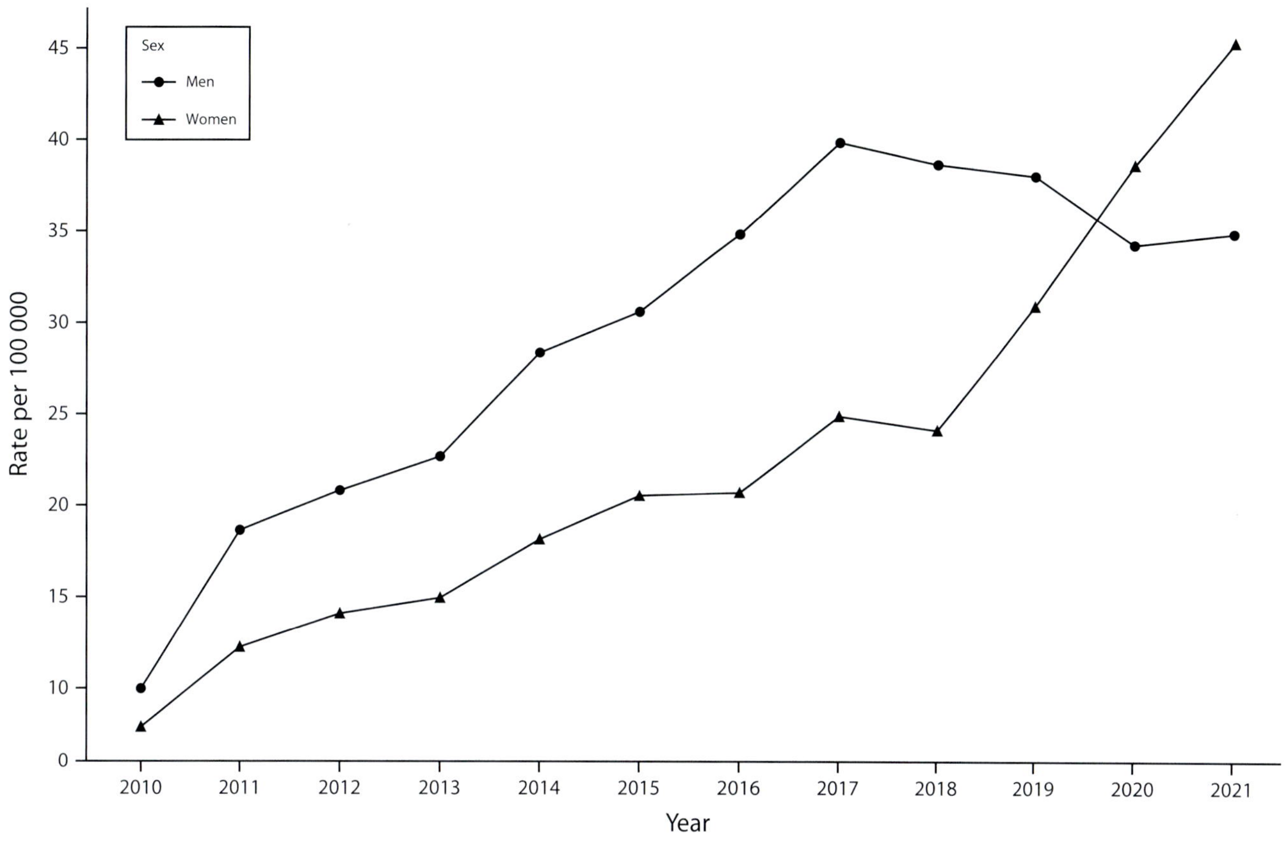

FIGURE 2— **Age-Adjusted Rates of Drug and Alcohol Overdoses per 100 000 by Sex: Colombia, 2010–2021**

having recently experienced an overdose.[23]

In addition, opioid overdose rates also increased after 2017, also mainly attributable to increases in overdoses involving prescription opioids among young women. In Colombia, 2 main factors may have contributed to low rates of opioid overdoses during 2010 to 2017. First, the prevalence of past-year nonmedical use of prescription opioids and use of heroin (0.3% and 0.02%, respectively in 2019)[2] has been traditionally low compared with the prevalences in other countries in North America (e.g., in the United States, the prevalence of past-year nonmedical use of prescription opioids use and of use of heroin was 3.5% and 0.3%, respectively).[24] Second, prior studies in Colombia show that codeine and tramadol, generally prescribed at low or intermediate doses (i.e., less than 50 morphine milligram equivalents per day),[25–27] are the most common opioids used for pain management in the country. In addition, preferences for other drugs such as cocaine and cannabis may also explain the low rate of opioid overdoses.[2] Despite the low rates compared with other countries, the observed increase in these overdose rates after 2018 highlights the need to continue surveillance efforts that can track if this trend continues to evolve and to identify timely interventions that can shift the trend.

We also observed that, among those aged 34 years or younger, overdose rates involving stimulants (mostly cocaine) and cannabis initially increased then later decreased after 2018. Results from the CNSSU survey[2] show that the past-year prevalence of use of most substances (including cannabis, cocaine, and tranquilizers) increased from 2008 to 2013 across all age groups; however, in 2019, the prevalence of cannabis and cocaine use decreased among adolescents and young adults (ages 18–24 years) and remained stable among older adults.[2] It is possible that this decrease in the prevalence of cannabis and stimulant use in younger populations is in part responsible for the observed reduction in overdoses involving these substances in adolescents and young adults after 2018. However, reductions in these overdose rates may be also related to

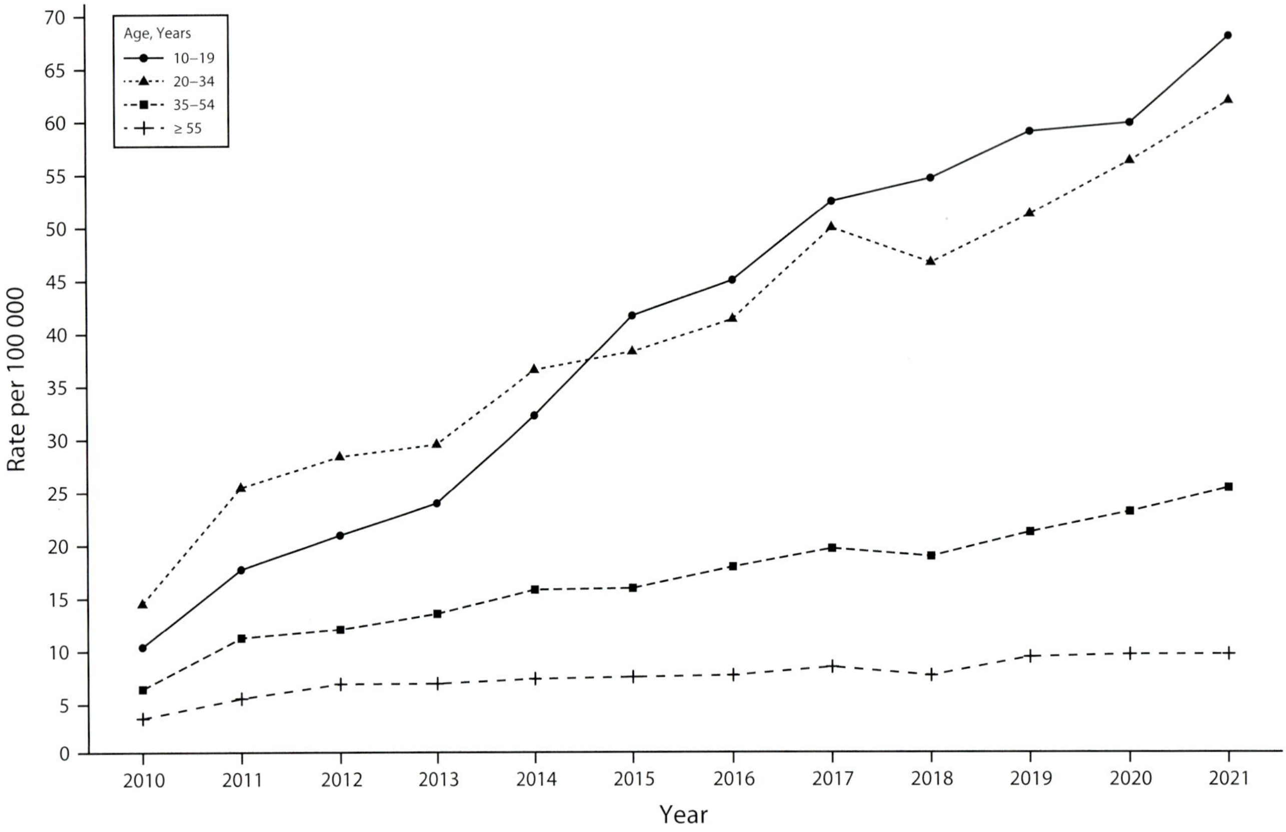

FIGURE 3— **Rates of Drug and Alcohol Nonfatal Overdoses per 100 000 by Age Group: Colombia, 2010–2021**

changes in consumption patterns that are less likely to result in overdose. The lack of data on drug consumption behavior in SIVIGILA prevent us from examining this, but future national surveys could explore consumption patterns in young populations to identify the potential factors behind these changes in overdose rates. In addition, mobility restrictions during the COVID-19 pandemic could have impacted the access to certain drugs, such as cocaine and cannabis, especially among youths, which in turn would have influenced the risk of overdose in this population. The pandemic also limited access to health services, which may have resulted in some individuals experiencing an overdose not being able to reach health institutions, where SIVIGILA data are generated.

Over the past 3 decades, Colombia has transitioned to a human rights and public health–approach regulatory framework regarding substance use, an approach that is aligned with the United Nations Office on Drugs and Crime guidelines[28] emphasizing the promotion of prevention measures and early intervention, treatment, care, and social rehabilitation for people using drugs.[28] These principles have been ratified by recent legislation mandating the development of strategic interventions or programs to reduce substance use and related risks, and to provide integral care based on harm-reduction approaches and on actions that facilitate the integral rehabilitation and social inclusion of people using drugs according to their needs.[29] Although these changes have resulted in improved access to substance use treatment in recent years,[30] it is estimated that only 10% of those in need (e.g., with substance use dependence) actually receive treatment.[30] Our findings suggest that additional prevention efforts are necessary, including harm-reduction and community-based programs, and better access to treatment services that can reduce the risk of overdose in the population.

Limitations

Our study results should be examined considering the following limitations. First, SIVIGILA overdose case definitions relied on discharge diagnosis, which vastly rely on information provided by the person experiencing the overdose or his or her companions, as only in few cases is laboratory testing performed. Although it is possible that stigmatization and fear of facing legal consequences can make some people reluctant to disclose the use of illegal substances to health personnel, we believe this behavior may be limited by the need of receiving appropriate treatment. Nevertheless, this could result in an underestimation of overdose rates.

Second, the observed increase in overdose rates may be attributable to the maturation of the surveillance system and improvements in case collection, especially during the first years of the study period when the system became more strictly regulated.

Third, SIVIGILA changed its data-collection methodology starting in 2018, requiring health institutions to submit all events with suicide intent separately from unintentional events. This could result in abrupt changes, from 2017 to 2018, in the rate of overdoses involving certain drugs, such as those frequently used in suicide attempts (e.g., tranquilizers, sedatives, or antidepressants). However, this change does not explain the increase in overdoses involving tranquilizers, sedatives, or antidepressants observed from 2018 to 2021.

Fourth, overdoses not treated at health facilities are not included in the SIVIGILA data; therefore, our estimates are likely underestimating the true rates of nonfatal overdose rates in the country.

Fifth, the patients' personal information was removed from the data; therefore, our models did not address correlations for repeated measurements, which we believe could have resulted in more conservative *P* values for the group comparisons.

Finally, data restrictions limited us from getting access to more recent SIVIGILA data that could inform if observed trends in drug overdose rates continued after the COVID-19 pandemic.

Conclusions

Our findings provide important novel information about the magnitude of the drug overdose problem in Colombia from 2010 to 2021. Our results show that overdose rates greatly increased in both women and men, and in adolescents and young adults. While overdoses involving cannabis and stimulants increased up to 2018 and decreased afterward, overdose rates involving tranquilizers, sedatives, or antidepressants continued to increase, accelerating in 2018 to 2021, mainly attributable to a sharp increase in intentional overdoses among young women. SIVIGILA data provide the most reliable drug overdose data in the country, which can be used to study drug overdose trends and the burden that overdoses pose on the Colombian population and the country's health system. This surveillance system methodology can be an important tool to track drug overdoses and to generate information for public health prevention efforts in other countries with limited resources. AJPH

ABOUT THE AUTHORS

Julian Santaella-Tenorio is with Departamento de Salud Pública y Epidemiología, Pontificia Universidad Javeriana, Cali, Colombia. Jhoan S. Zapata-López is with Escuela Nacional del Deporte, Facultad de Salud y Rehabilitación, Cali. Thiago M. Fidalgo is with Department of Psychiatry, Escola Paulista de Medicina, Universidade Federal de São Paulo, São Paulo, Brazil. Vítor S. Tardelli is with Translational Addictions Research Laboratory, Centre for Addiction and Mental Health, University of Toronto, Toronto, ON, Canada. Luis Segura and Silvia Martins are with the Mailman School of Public Health, Epidemiology Department, Columbia University, New York, NY. Magdalena Cerda is with Center for Opioid Epidemiology and Policy, Department of Population Health, NYU Grossman School of Medicine, New York, NY.

CORRESPONDENCE

Correspondence should be sent to Julian Santaella-Tenorio, Departamento de Salud Pública y Epidemiología, Pontificia Universidad Javeriana, Calle 18 #118-250, Cali, Colombia (e-mail: julian.santaella@javerianacali.edu.co). Reprints can be ordered at https://www.ajph.org by clicking the "Reprints" link.

PUBLICATION INFORMATION

Full Citation: Santaella-Tenorio J, Zapata-López JS, Fidalgo TM, et al. Trends in nonfatal overdose rates due to alcohol and prescription and illegal substances in Colombia, 2010–2021. *Am J Public Health*. 2024;114(11):1252–1260.

Acceptance Date: June 30, 2024.

DOI: https://doi.org/10.2105/AJPH.2024.307786

ORCID iDs:

Julian Santaella-Tenorio https://orcid.org/0000-0003-3060-5994

Jhoan S. Zapata-López https://orcid.org/0000-0002-5841-9387

Thiago M. Fidalgo https://orcid.org/0000-0003-3555-5228

Vítor S. Tardelli https://orcid.org/0000-0001-6040-7708

Luis E. Segura https://orcid.org/0000-0002-2299-9295

Magdalena Cerda https://orcid.org/0000-0001-8441-7046

CONTRIBUTORS

J. Santaella-Tenorio, J. S. Zapata-López, and S. Martins developed the design and conceptualization of the study. J. Santaella-Tenorio and J. S. Zapata-López collected and analyzed the data, interpreted the results, and wrote the original draft of the article. T. M. Fidalgo, V. Tardelli, L. Segura, M. Cerda, and S. Martins contributed to the interpretation of results and helped draft the article.

ACKNOWLEDGMENTS

This study was supported by Columbia University President's Global Innovation Fund and NYU Grossman School of Medicine. Thiago M. Fidalgo was funded by the National Council for Scientific and Technological Development (CNPq; grant #313241/2022-8).

We would like to thank the Colombia National Institute of Medicine for providing access to SIVIGILA data.

CONFLICTS OF INTEREST

The authors declare no conflicts of interest.

HUMAN PARTICIPANT PROTECTION

This study was conducted according to the principles expressed in the Declaration of Helsinki and based on Resolution 8430 of 1993 of the Colombian Ministry of Health and Social Protection.
This study involved analysis of routinely collected surveillance anonymized data and, thus, did not require ethical review.

REFERENCES

1. The United Nations Office on Drugs and Crime. *World Drug Report 2022*. 2022. Available at: https://www.unodc.org/unodc/en/data-and-analysis/world-drug-report-2022.html. Accessed October 19, 2023
2. Ministerio de Justicia y del Derecho – Observatorio de Drogas de Colombia. National Study of Psychoactive Substance Use, Colombia 2019 [in Spanish]. 2019. Available at: https://www.minjusticia.gov.co/programas-co/ODC/Paginas/Publicaciones-ODC.aspx. Accessed September 25, 2023.
3. Ministerio de Justicia y del Derecho, Gobierno de Colombia. Psychoactive Substance Use–Related Mortality Study [in Spanish]. 2022. Available at: https://www.minjusticia.gov.co/programas-co/ODC/Documents/Publicaciones/Consumo/Estudios/Nacionales/informe%20de%20resultados.pdf. Accessed August 26, 2023.
4. Jones NR, Hickman M, Larney S, et al. Hospitalisations for non-fatal overdose among people with a history of opioid dependence in New South Wales, Australia, 2001–2018: findings from the OATS retrospective cohort study. *Drug Alcohol Depend*. 2021;218:108354. https://doi.org/10.1016/j.drugalcdep.2020.108354
5. Hoots BE. Opioid overdose surveillance: improving data to inform action. *Public Health Rep*. 2021;136(1 suppl):5S–8S. https://doi.org/10.1177/00333549211020275
6. Hoots B, Vivolo-Kantor A, Seth P. The rise in non-fatal and fatal overdoses involving stimulants with and without opioids in the United States. *Addiction*. 2020;115(5):946–958. https://doi.org/10.1111/add.14878
7. Liu S, O'Donnell J, Gladden RM, McGlone L, Chowdhury F. Trends in nonfatal and fatal overdoses involving benzodiazepines—38 states and the District of Columbia, 2019–2020. *MMWR Morb Mortal Wkly Rep*. 2021;70(34):1136–1141. https://doi.org/10.15585/mmwr.mm7034a2
8. Colledge S, Peacock A, Leung J, et al. The prevalence of non-fatal overdose among people who inject drugs: a multi-stage systematic review and meta-analysis. *Int J Drug Policy*. 2019;73:172–184. https://doi.org/10.1016/j.drugpo.2019.07.030
9. Martins SS, Sampson L, Cerda M, Galea S. Worldwide prevalence and trends in unintentional drug overdose: a systematic review of the literature. *Am J Public Health*. 2015;105(11):e29–e49. https://doi.org/10.2105/AJPH.2015.302843
10. Instituto Nacional de Salud de Colombia. Portal of the National Public Health Surveillance System [in Spanish]. Available at: https://www.ins.gov.co/Direcciones/Vigilancia/Paginas/SIVIGILA.aspx. Accessed August 20, 2023.
11. Muñoz Guerrero MN, Díaz Criollo SM, Martinez Duran ME. Epidemiological profile of intoxications due to chemical substances, Colombia, 2008–2015 [in Spanish]. *Informe Quincenal Epidemiológico Nacional (IQEN)*. 2017;2(2):26–48.
12. Instituto Nacional de Salud de Colombia. Protocol for acute intoxications due to chemical substances [in Spanish]. Versión 7. April 23, 2024. https://doi.org/10.33610/YIHX9176.
13. Departamento Administrativo Nacional de Estadística. Projections and retro-projections of the national population 1950–2019 and 2020–2070 based on the 2018 National Census [in Spanish]. Available at: https://www.dane.gov.co/index.php/estadisticas-por-tema/demografia-y-poblacion/proyecciones-de-poblacion. Accessed August 22, 2023.
14. *Stata Statistical Software: Release 18*. College Station, TX: StataCorp LLC; 2023.
15. Ospina N, Chávez K. Mental health in Colombia, a study of the pandemic effects [in Spanish]. Departamento Administrativo Nacional de Estadística. 2021. Available at: https://www.dane.gov.co/files/investigaciones/notas-estadisticas/ago-2021-nota-estadistica-salud-mental-en-colombia-analisis-efectos-pandemia.pdf. Accessed September 22, 2023.
16. Ettman CK, Abdalla SM, Cohen GH, Sampson L, Vivier PM, Galea S. Prevalence of depression symptoms in US adults before and during the COVID-19 pandemic. *JAMA Netw Open*. 2020;3(9):e2019686. https://doi.org/10.1001/jamanetworkopen.2020.19686
17. COVID-19 Mental Disorders Collaborators. Global prevalence and burden of depressive and anxiety disorders in 204 countries and territories in 2020 due to the COVID-19 pandemic. *Lancet*. 2021;398(10312):1700–1712. https://doi.org/10.1016/S0140-6736(21)02143-7
18. Del Fiol FS, Bergamaschi CC, Lopes LC, Silva MT, Barberato-Filho S. Sales trends of psychotropic drugs in the COVID-19 pandemic: a national database study in Brazil. *Front Pharmacol*. 2023;14:1131357. https://doi.org/10.3389/fphar.2023.1131357
19. Estrela M, Silva TM, Gomes ER, et al. Prescription of anxiolytics, sedatives, hypnotics and antidepressants in outpatient, universal care during the COVID-19 pandemic in Portugal: a nationwide, interrupted time-series approach. *J Epidemiol Community Health*. 2022;76(4):335–340. https://doi.org/10.1136/jech-2021-216732
20. Levaillant M, Wathelet M, Lamer A, Riquin E, Gohier B, Hamel-Broza JF. Impact of COVID-19 pandemic and lockdowns on the consumption of anxiolytics, hypnotics and antidepressants according to age groups: a French nationwide study. *Psychol Med*. 2023;53(7):2861–2867. https://doi.org/10.1017/S0033291721004839
21. Sanborn M, Ali MM, Creedon TB. National trends in psychotropic medication prescribing before and during the COVID-19 pandemic. *Psychiatry Res*. 2023;325:115248. https://doi.org/10.1016/j.psychres.2023.115248
22. Tiger M, Wesselhoeft R, Karlsson P, et al. Utilization of antidepressants, anxiolytics, and hypnotics during the COVID-19 pandemic in Scandinavia. *J Affect Disord*. 2023;323:292–298. https://doi.org/10.1016/j.jad.2022.11.068
23. Goldman-Mellor S, Olfson M, Lidon-Moyano C, Schoenbaum M. Mortality following nonfatal opioid and sedative/hypnotic drug overdose. *Am J Prev Med*. 2020;59(1):59–67. https://doi.org/10.1016/j.amepre.2020.02.012
24. Substance Abuse and Mental Health Services Administration. *Key Substance Use and Mental Health Indicators in the United States: Results From the 2019 National Survey on Drug Use and Health* (HHS Publication No. PEP20-07-01-001, NSDUH Series H-55). Rockville, MD: Center for Behavioral Health Statistics and Quality. 2020. Available at: https://www.samhsa.gov/data. Accessed August 20, 2023.
25. Machado-Alba JE, Gaviria-Mendoza A, Vargas-Mosquera CA, Gil-Restrepo AF, Romero-Zapata LC. Opioid prescribing patterns and costs in a large group of patients in Colombia. *J Pain Palliat Care Pharmacother*. 2017;31(1):57–65. https://doi.org/10.1080/15360288.2016.1276504
26. Machado-Alba JE, Serna-Echeverri LS, Valladales-Restrepo LF, Machado-Duque ME, Gaviria-Mendoza A. Use of tramadol or other analgesics in patients treated in the emergency department as a risk factor for opioid use. *Pain Res Manag*. 2020;2020:8847777. https://doi.org/10.1155/2020/8847777
27. Valladales-Restrepo LF, Rubio-Londono S, Poveda-Martinez LF, Machado-Alba JE. Prescribing pattern of analgesics in Colombia. Are there differences between capital cities and municipalities? A cross-sectional study. *Drugs Real World Outcomes*. 2022;9(3):487–501. https://doi.org/10.1007/s40801-022-00318-2
28. Oficina de las Naciones Unidas contra la Droga y el Delito. Treatment and services for people with drug use–related disorders who are in contact with the justice system [in Spanish]. 2019. Available at: https://www.unodc.org/documents/UNODC_WHO_Alternatives_to_conviction_or_punishment_SP.pdf. Accessed October 19, 2023.
29. Ministerio de Salud y Protección Social. Integral policy for the prevention and treatment of substance use disorders [in Spanish]. Resolución 089 de 2019. 2019. Available at: https://www.minsalud.gov.co/sites/rid/Lists/BibliotecaDigital/RIDE/VS/PP/politica-prevencion-atencion-spa.pdf. Accessed May 1, 2024
30. Ministerio de Salud y Protección Social and Unión Temporal Sigma Dos—Bioestadística. *Evaluation and Situational Diagnosis of Substance Abuse Treatment Services in Colombia* [in Spanish]. 2016. Available at: http://www.odc.gov.co/Portals/1/publicaciones/pdf/consumo/estudios/nacionales/CO034492016_estudio_evaluacion_diagnostico_servicios_tratamiento_consumidor_sustancias.pdf. Accessed October 19, 2023.

Long COVID Among People With Preexisting Disabilities

Jean P. Hall, PhD, Noelle K. Kurth, MS, Lisa McCorkell, MPP, and Kelsey S. Goddard, PhD

Objectives. To document the prevalence of long COVID among a sample of survey respondents with long-term disabilities that existed before 2020 and to compare the prevalence among this group with that among the general population.

Methods. We conducted a cross-sectional, descriptive study using data from the 2022 National Survey on Health and Disability (n = 2262) and comparative data for the general population from the federal Household Pulse Survey (HPS).

Results. The prevalence of long COVID was higher among people with preexisting disabilities than in the general population (40.6% vs 18.9%).

Conclusions. People with preexisting disabilities experienced and continue to experience increased exposure to COVID-19 and barriers to accessing health care, COVID-19 vaccines, and COVID-19 tests. These barriers, combined with long-standing health disparities in this population, may have contributed to the greater prevalence of long COVID among people with disabilities.

Public Health Implications. The needs of people with disabilities must be centered in the response to the COVID-19 pandemic and future pandemics. (*Am J Public Health*. 2024;114(11):1261–1264. https://doi.org/10.2105/AJPH.2024.307794)

AJPH November 2024, Vol. 114, No. 11

At least 66 million adults in the United States, or 27% of the country's adult residents, experience disabilities.[1] People with disabilities are at higher risk for COVID-19 infection and severe acute illness than people without disabilities, and some evidence indicates that people with certain preexisting disabilities (e.g., type 2 diabetes, connective tissue disorders) may also be at increased risk for long COVID, broadly defined as symptoms that continue or develop after a COVID-19 infection and last for months or years or are lifelong.[2,3] Despite their increased risk, these individuals experience multiple barriers to accessing key mitigation techniques (e.g., personal protective equipment, tests, and vaccines) and receiving equitable treatment for COVID-19 infection.[4,5] These inequities may have further exacerbated the risk of developing long COVID among people with disabilities.[6]

Because disability measures were not routinely included in early pandemic surveillance efforts, and because such measures typically assess disability status only at the time a survey is being conducted, the experiences of people with preexisting disabilities who had COVID-19 and subsequently developed long COVID are not well known (with the exception of some of the specific disabilities just listed). Miller et al. reported post-COVID-19 conditions in late 2021 among a small sample of people with disabilities who tested positive for COVID-19 (n = 82) and found that 20% reported having at least 1 symptom 3 to 6 months after their initial infection, as compared with 6% of respondents without disabilities.[7] In our study, we used a larger national sample to examine the prevalence of long COVID among people with preexisting disabilities (Figure 1).

METHODS

We used data from the 2022 administration of the National Survey on Health and Disability (NSHD), a national online survey, to explore the prevalence of long COVID among adults aged 18 years or older with self-reported preexisting disabilities.[8] The 2022 NSHD was conducted from May 2 to September 2 with a total sample of 2725 respondents. Individuals responding

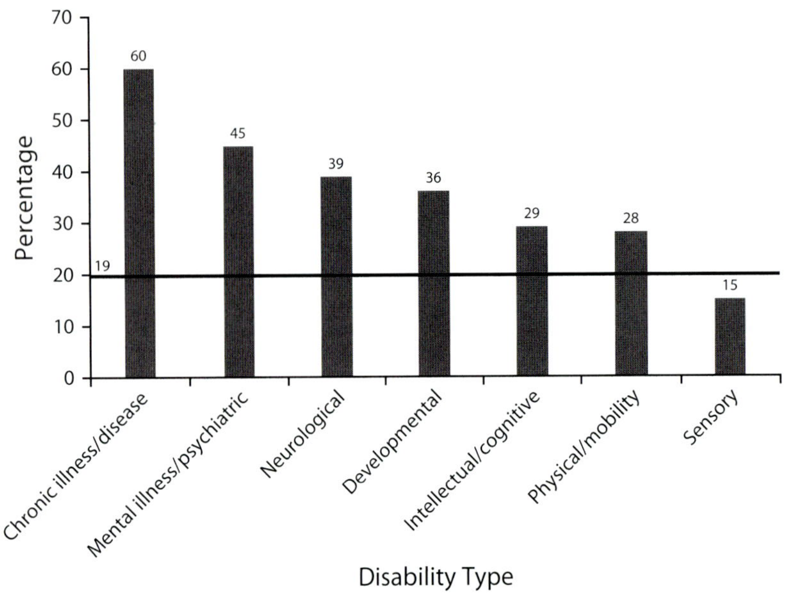

FIGURE 1— Prevalence of Long COVID Among NSHD Respondents Testing Positive for COVID-19 by Self-Reported Disability Type Relative to the General Population With a Suspected or Confirmed COVID-19 Infection: United States, 2022

Note. NSHD = National Survey on Health and Disability. Long COVID was determined according to whether respondents reported a positive COVID-19 test and had a positive response to the question "Have you experienced any COVID-19 symptoms for 3 months or longer following a suspected or confirmed COVID-19 infection—also known as long COVID? Examples of symptoms include fatigue or extreme tiredness, cognitive problems, abnormal heart rate, shortness of breath, loss of taste or smell, depression, or other mental health conditions." Disability type was determined via the question "Of the categories below, which one would you use to describe your main disability?" The prevalence of long COVID in the general population with a suspected or confirmed COVID-19 infection was 19%.

affirmatively to the disability screening question (Figure 1) were asked to describe their disability using an open-ended question, to provide the age of their disability onset, and to select 1 of 7 categories to characterize their primary condition.

The study sample included 2262 respondents whose disability onset occurred before the beginning of the pandemic in 2020 to ensure that the sample included only people who had an existing disability before contracting COVID-19 and long COVID. Within the sample of 2262 NSHD respondents with preexisting disabilities, we examined frequencies of those who reported a positive COVID-19 test (n = 581) and, among those who had a positive test, the number who reported symptoms lasting 3 or more months (long COVID; n = 236). Within the sample of respondents reporting long COVID symptoms, we explored the differential prevalence of long COVID among a variety of demographic and disability groups (Figure 1 and the Appendix, available as a supplement to the online version of this article at http://www.ajph.org).

The prevalence of long COVID among NSHD respondents was compared with the Household Pulse Survey (HPS) prevalence for the general population in June 2022, when long COVID questions were added to that instrument.[9,10] The HPS is a national, online, cross-sectional, multiagency federal survey designed to assess the effects of the coronavirus pandemic on the American public. The HPS asked 2 questions to assess the long COVID prevalence among respondents with a previous COVID-19 infection: "Did you have any symptoms lasting 3 months or longer that you did not have prior to having coronavirus or COVID-19? (long-term symptoms might include tiredness or fatigue; difficulty thinking, concentrating, forgetfulness, or memory problems [sometimes referred to as 'brain fog']; difficulty breathing or shortness of breath; joint or muscle pain; fast-beating or pounding heart [also known as heart palpitations]; chest pain; dizziness on standing; menstrual changes; changes to taste/smell; or inability to exercise)" and "Do you have symptoms now?"

RESULTS

Of the entire NSHD sample of people with preexisting disabilities (n = 2262), 10.4% (n = 236) reported having long COVID symptoms in summer 2022. This figure is substantially greater than the 7.5% of the general population reporting current long COVID symptoms in June 2022.[9] Among the 581 NSHD respondents with preexisting disabilities who reported testing positive for COVID-19, 40.6% (n = 236) reported experiencing COVID symptoms for 3 months or more (long COVID). This figure is substantially greater than the 18.9% of the general public who reported having had COVID-19 and currently having symptoms lasting 3 months or more in the HPS and also greater than the 35.1% of HPS respondents who reported ever having long COVID symptoms (Figure 1).[9,10]

A chi-square test showed significant differences ($P < .001$) in the prevalence of long COVID among respondents with different self-reported primary disability types. In particular, the prevalence of long COVID was highest among those with preexisting chronic illnesses (e.g., diabetes, asthma) and those with preexisting psychiatric disabilities (e.g., depression, anxiety) and lowest among those with sensory disabilities (e.g., blindness, deafness; Figure 1).

DISCUSSION

Although differences in questions used by the NSHD and HPS and their timing make direct comparisons difficult, it is clear that the prevalence of long COVID was higher in the NSHD sample of adults with preexisting disabilities than in the general population in 2022. In fact, the reported prevalence of long COVID in the NSHD sample may be artificially low as a result of the inaccessibility of COVID-19 tests for many people with disabilities to confirm a previous infection.[11]

With the exception of sensory disabilities, NSHD respondents with preexisting disabilities had a greater prevalence of long COVID than the general population across all age, gender, and race/ethnicity categories (Figure 1 and the Appendix). Interestingly, a recent study revealed lower reported levels of unmet need and forgone care during the pandemic among people with sensory disabilities than among people with other disabilities but still greater than among the general population.[4] Additional research is needed to understand the reasons for differences in long COVID prevalence by disability type and to develop appropriate interventions and support.

Despite repeated calls for better preparation to support them during a pandemic,[12] people with disabilities were and continue to be neglected, and systemic barriers exacerbate their increased risk for poor outcomes related to COVID-19. For example, people with disabilities were often not prioritized for COVID-19 vaccines, and many have been unable to access vaccination Web sites and administration sites.[5] In addition, many have been at increased risk of exposure because of their reliance on in-home help or because they live in congregate settings.[12] Once they contract the virus, people with disabilities are at greater risk for being refused treatment, developing severe symptoms, being hospitalized, and, as this study demonstrates, developing long COVID.[2,5]

Limitations of this study include differences in long COVID questions between the NSHD and the HPS as well as the relatively small sample sizes for each survey. A strength is the fact that the NSHD sample is specifically limited to respondents experiencing long-term disabilities that began before the pandemic, providing a unique opportunity to study long COVID outcomes among people with preexisting disabilities.

PUBLIC HEALTH IMPLICATIONS

The implications of this study are twofold. First, we must better document the prevalence of long COVID, possible contributing factors, and effects among people with varying preexisting disabilities so that adequate services and support are provided. Second, as the COVID-19 pandemic continues and as we prepare for future pandemics, we must center the needs of people with disabilities to create equitable policies and responses that result in better health outcomes for this health disparity population. AJPH

ABOUT THE AUTHORS

Jean P. Hall, Noelle K. Kurth, and Kelsey S. Goddard are with the Institute for Health and Disability Policy Studies, Life Span Institute, University of Kansas, Lawrence. Lisa McCorkell is with the Patient-Led Research Collaborative, Calabasas, CA.

CORRESPONDENCE

Correspondence should be sent to Jean P. Hall, PhD, Institute for Health and Disability Policy Studies, University of Kansas, 1000 Sunnyside Ave, Room 1052, Lawrence, KS 66045 (e-mail: jhall@ku.edu). Reprints can be ordered at https://www.ajph.org by clicking the "Reprints" link.

PUBLICATION INFORMATION

Full Citation: Hall JP, Kurth NK, McCorkell L, Goddard KS. Long COVID among people with preexisting disabilities. *Am J Public Health*. 2024;114(11):1261–1264.

Acceptance Date: July 7, 2024.

DOI: https://doi.org/10.2105/AJPH.2024.307794

ORCID iDs:

Jean P. Hall https://orcid.org/0000-0001-7236-1807

Noelle K. Kurth https://orcid.org/0000-0003-2525-3605

Lisa McCorkell https://orcid.org/0000-0002-3261-6737

Kelsey S. Goddard https://orcid.org/0000-0003-0477-3951

CONTRIBUTORS

J. P. Hall wrote the initial draft of the article. J. P. Hall, N. K. Kurth, and L. McCorkell conceptualized the study. J. P. Hall, N. K. Kurth, and K. S. Goddard acquired the data. N. K. Kurth analyzed the data. All of the authors interpreted the results and contributed to the final revision of the article.

ACKNOWLEDGMENTS

The National Survey on Health and Disability is administered by the University of Kansas Institute for Health and Disability Policy Studies and funded by the National Institute on Disability, Independent Living, and Rehabilitation Research (NIDILRR; project 90IFRE0050). The NIDILRR is part of the Administration for Community Living (ACL) of the US Department of Health and Human Services (HHS).

Note. The contents of this article do not necessarily represent the policies of the NIDILRR, ACL, or HHS, and endorsement by the federal government should not be assumed.

CONFLICTS OF INTEREST

The authors have no conflicts of interest to report.

HUMAN PARTICIPANT PROTECTION

This study was reviewed and approved by the University of Kansas institutional review board. All participants provided informed consent.

REFERENCES

1. Centers for Disease Control and Prevention (CDC). Disability and Health Data System.

Available at: https://www.cdc.gov/ncbddd/disabilityandhealth/dhds/index.html. Accessed February 23 2024.

2. Crook H, Raza S, Nowell J, Young M, Edison P. Long Covid—mechanisms, risk factors and management. *BMJ*. 2021;374(1648):n1648. https://doi.org/10.1136/bmj.n1648
3. Davis HE, McCorkell L, Vogel JM, Topol EJ. Long COVID: major findings, mechanisms and recommendations. *Nat Rev Microbiol*. 2023;21(3):133–146. https://doi.org/10.1038/s41579-022-00846-2
4. Akobirshoev I, Vetter M, Iezzoni LI, Rao SR, Mitra M. Delayed medical care and unmet care needs due to the COVID-19 pandemic among adults with disabilities in the US. *Health Aff (Millwood)*. 2022;41(10):1505–1512. https://doi.org/10.1377/hlthaff.2022.00509
5. Lund EM, Ayers KB. Ever-changing but always constant: waves of disability discrimination during the COVID-19 pandemic in the United States. *Disabil Health J*. 2022;15(4):101374. https://doi.org/10.1016/j.dhjo.2022.101374
6. Centers for Disease Control and Prevention (CDC). Long COVID or post-COVID conditions. Available at: https://www.cdc.gov/coronavirus/2019-ncov/long-term-effects/index.html. Accessed February 23, 2024.
7. Miller MJ, Feldstein LR, Holbrook J, et al. Post-COVID conditions and healthcare utilization among adults with and without disabilities—2021 Porter Novelli FallStyles survey. *Disabil Health J*. 2023;16(2):101436. https://doi.org/10.1016/j.dhjo.2022.101436
8. University of Kansas Institute for Health and Disability Policy Studies. NSHD background and overview. Available at: https://ihdps.ku.edu/nshd-background-and-overview. Accessed June 12, 2024.
9. Ford ND, Slaughter D, Edwards D, et al. Long COVID and significant activity limitation among adults, by age—United States, June 1–13, 2022 to June 7–19, 2023. *MMWR Morb Mortal Wkly Rep*. 2023;72(32):866–870. https://doi.org/10.15585/mmwr.mm7232a3
10. National Center for Health Statistics. Long COVID, Household Pulse Survey. Available at: https://www.cdc.gov/nchs/covid19/pulse/long-covid.htm. Accessed February 23, 2024.
11. Martin HR, Hu N, Liu Q, et al. Disability and COVID-19: challenges, testing, vaccination, and postponement and avoidance of medical care among minoritized communities. *Disabil Health J*. 2024;17(2):101571. https://doi.org/10.1016/j.dhjo.2023.101571
12. Campbell VA, Gilyard JA, Sinclair L, Sternberg T, Kailes JI. Preparing for and responding to pandemic influenza: implications for people with disabilities. *Am J Public Health*. 2009;99(suppl 2):S294–S300. https://doi.org/10.2105/AJPH.2009.162677

Cognitive Difficulty in Middle Eastern and North African Adults Living in the United States Compared With Other Racial and Ethnic Categories, 2017–2021

Tiffany B. Kindratt, PhD, MPH, and Alexandra Smith, MS

See also Schachter et al., p. 1158.

Objectives. To estimate the odds of having cognitive difficulties among Middle Eastern and North African (MENA) American adults and compare these odds with those of White, Black, Hispanic/Latino, Asian, American Indian or Alaska Native (AI/AN), and Native Hawaiian/Other Pacific Islander adults nationally and in the 4 states with the largest MENA populations (California, New York, Michigan, and Texas) after adjusting for sociodemographic factors.

Methods. We analyzed 2017–2021 American Community Survey data (aged ≥ 45 years; n = 7 284 988), comparing presence of cognitive difficulties by race/ethnicity.

Results. MENA adults had greater odds of reporting cognitive difficulties than did White (odds ratio [OR] = 1.49; 95% confidence interval [CI] = 1.42, 1.56), Black (OR = 1.20; 95% CI = 1.14, 1.26), Hispanic (OR = 1.46; 95% CI = 1.39, 1.53), Asian (OR = 1.31; 95% CI = 1.25, 1.38), and AI/AN (OR = 1.07; 95% CI = 1.01, 1.14) adults. In all 4 states, odds of having cognitive difficulties were higher among MENA than Asian adults. Other racial/ethnic comparisons differed by state.

Conclusions. A separate checkbox for MENA Americans approved by the Office of Management and Budget is important so health outcomes can be studied in more detail and funds can be allocated for research and resources at state and national levels. (*Am J Public Health*. 2024;114(11):1265–1274. https://doi.org/10.2105/AJPH.2024.307803)

Population research on disability has increased over the past 25 years to address the growing prevalence of disabilities and the aging of the US population.[1] In 2021, the national prevalence of any disability among all adults was 27.2%, which is higher (41.7%) when limited to adults aged 65 years and older.[2,3] National health surveys and other health surveillance systems measure 6 types of disability: hearing, vision, mobility, self-care, independent living, and cognition. The prevalence of cognitive disability in the United States, which is an indicator of Alzheimer's disease and related dementias, is 11.9% for adults aged 45 to 64 years and 9.5% for noninstitutionalized adults aged 65 years and older.[3] The proportion of older adults living with cognitive disabilities is expected to double by 2060, and large disparities exist by race/ethnicity.[4]

To uncover racial/ethnic health disparities, the US Office of Management and Budget's (OMB's) Statistical Policy Directive 15 requires that national health surveys include a minimum of 6 reporting categories for race/ethnicity. The categories for the 2020 decennial census have been collected since 1970.[5] Individuals were asked (1) to report whether they were of "Hispanic, Spanish or Latino origin,"[6] and (2) to select their race from the following groups: White, Black or African American (hereafter, Black), Asian, American Indian or Alaska Native (AI/AN), and Native Hawaiian or other Pacific Islander (NH/OPI).

AJPH November 2024, Vol. 114, No. 11

Research on racial/ethnic disparities in cognitive difficulties (also termed "cognitive limitations," "cognitive impairment," "cognitive disability," and "cognitive decline") usually accounts only for White, Black, Hispanic, and Asian Americans, which is often because of small sample sizes among other groups.[7] These reporting categories do not allow the assessment of disparities in all races/ethnicity, for example, Middle Eastern and North African (MENA) Americans are left out. In January 2023, the OMB published initial proposals to revise Statistical Policy Directive 15 to combine the 2 race and ethnicity questions into a single question and add a separate checkbox for MENA Americans.[8] An analysis of public comments demonstrated strong support for the addition of a separate MENA checkbox.[9]

Research to determine the suitability of the MENA classification for representation of the Arab American community in national health surveys found positive results.[10] In March 2024, the OMB revised Statistical Policy Directive 15 to combine the 2 race/ethnicity questions and add a separate checkbox for MENA Americans.[11] Federal agencies and other entities that receive government funds have until September 2025 to submit plans for how they will make the changes, which should include plans to address nonresponse bias. March 2029 is the deadline for implementing the changes.[11]

The MENA region includes Arab and non-Arab countries and transnational communities in the Middle East and North Africa. Although the MENA population has been defined as part of the White racial group for many decades, research demonstrates that MENA Americans are not perceived by others as White and experience institutional and interpersonal discrimination. Events such as wars and government policies like travel bans result from and contribute to this discrimination, affecting their mental and physical health across the life course.[12] Previous studies have shown that most MENA individuals self-identify as MENA or MENA and White when given these options.[12]

MENA individuals who experience more discrimination because of external factors, such as their appearance, name, and religion, and second-generation immigrants are more likely to self-identify as MENA than White.[12] Furthermore, stress from lifetime discrimination has been associated with increased cognitive difficulties in other minoritized populations (e.g., Black Americans) that experience discrimination that is more similar to the cognitive difficulties of MENA Americans than those of Whites.[13]

There is limited research on cognitive difficulties among persons of MENA descent in the United States. Kindratt et al. found that the prevalence of cognitive difficulties among Arab Americans was 6.5%.[14] Studies have found that foreign-born Arab Americans have a higher prevalence of cognitive difficulties than do their US-born counterparts, with estimates ranging from 6.0% to 8.0% for foreign-born individuals and 4.0% to 5.8% for US-born individuals.[14,15] Previous studies on Arab Americans that include both US- and foreign-born populations have been limited to adults aged 45 or 50 years and older who reported an ancestry in 1 or more of the 22 countries that make up the Arab League. Other studies on cognitive difficulties have compared foreign-born MENA to US-born White adults.

Dallo et al. found that the prevalence of cognitive difficulties among foreign-born MENA adults was 9.7%, compared with 7.4% among US-born Whites, but there was no statistically significant difference after adjusting for covariates.[16] Other national studies have looked at cognitive difficulties and underdiagnosis of Alzheimer's disease and related dementias among older adults (aged ≥ 65 years), but samples were limited to foreign-born MENA adults. Results demonstrated that the prevalence of cognitive difficulties and undiagnosed Alzheimer's disease and related dementias was higher among foreign-born older MENA adults (17.3% and 15.8%, respectively) than among older US-born (9.6% and 8.1%, respectively) and foreign-born White (13.6% and 11.8%, respectively) adults.[17,18]

Previous studies on the cognitive health of MENA Americans have been limited in 3 ways. First, studies have reported on only the national, not the state, level. The only nationally representative health survey that provides state-based estimates is the Behavioral Risk Factor Surveillance System (BRFSS), which does not have a racial/ethnic identifier for MENA individuals.[4] Second, previously reported estimates are limited to either Arab Americans only[14] or foreign-born MENA participants.[16–18] Third, comparisons in previous studies have been made only to White adults and do not fully capture all racial/ethnic groups that are part of the minimum reporting categories[6] or those approved by the OMB in March 2024.[8] A more comprehensive assessment that captures all groups is needed.

To advance the science, we sought to estimate and compare the (1) age- and sex-adjusted prevalence, and (2) odds of cognitive difficulties among MENA adults (aged ≥ 45 years) compared with White, Black, Hispanic/Latino, Asian, AI/AN, and NH/OPI adults in the United States and the 4 states with the largest

MENA American populations (California, New York, Michigan, and Texas) after adjusting for covariates.

METHODS

We downloaded and combined data from the 2017–2021 American Community Survey (ACS) 5-year public use microdata samples. The ACS collects monthly samples from US households to produce annual national estimates of demographic and socioeconomic factors.[19] The ACS includes questions on demographics (e.g., sex, age, race/ethnicity, ancestry, nativity) and socioeconomic status (e.g., housing, employment, education). The ACS also measures 6 categories of disability by asking all household members about sensory, physical, and mental abilities and about difficulties with self-care, going outside the home, and employment.[1] The ACS does not ask any other questions on health behaviors or conditions. More details are provided on their website.[20]

Inclusion Criteria

Our sample included adults aged 45 years and older. We selected this age as the lower limit based on previous research indicating that cognitive difficulties begin to emerge during midlife (45–64 years)[21] and its use in other studies for assessing cognitive difficulties among minoritized groups.[4,22] To determine sample sizes for the MENA population by state, we used variables for birth country and for first ancestry and second ancestry. The ACS allows participants to provide two ancestries in response to a question on their ancestry or ethnic origin. The first line on the form is designated as "first ancestry" and the second line is designated as "second ancestry." This method has been used in previous studies to estimate the population using ACS data for Arab Americans.[14,15,23–27] We expanded the list of ancestries and birth countries to be more inclusive by adding non-Arab countries and transnational communities in the Middle East and North Africa based on US Census content testing,[28] OMB's March 2024 approved standards (e.g., Assyrian, Chaldean, Egyptian, Iranian, Israeli, Lebanese),[8] and additional countries (e.g., Armenia) listed in public comments regarding the addition of the MENA checkbox.[9] We grouped individuals who listed a MENA ancestry or birthplace in the MENA category, which includes individuals who selected White or any other racial groups on the survey. The expanded list is provided in Table A (available as a supplement to the online version of this article at http://www.ajph.org).

After creating the MENA racial/ethnic group, we created a sampling frame by calculating weighted frequencies and percentages of the MENA population in each state and ranked them by population size. National and state samples for all ages are provided in Table B (available as a supplement to the online version of this article at http://www.ajph.org). We calculated the total MENA population in the United States as 3 837 872 people, which constitutes 1.2% of the entire US population. This was larger than the AI/AN (1 951 917; 0.6%) and NH/OPI (550 122; 0.2%) populations combined. The 4 largest MENA populations lived in California (912 787; 2.4%), New York (341 361; 1.8%), Michigan (262 918; 2.7%), and Texas (258 395; 0.9%).

Participants

We further limited the sample to adults in racial/ethnic groups based on the OMB's approved March 2024 categories.[8] The final US sample included 7 284 988 adults, which corresponded to 134 690 325 adults (aged ≥ 45 years) when weighted. Sample sizes for racial/ethnic groups in the United States, California, New York, Michigan, and Texas are provided in Table 1.

Variables

The independent variable was race/ethnicity based on the OMB's March 2024 approved categories used to limit the sample.[11] In addition to the MENA category created using ancestry and birthplace, we combined questions on race/ethnicity. Ethnicity was measured by asking whether the participant was "of Hispanic, Latino, or Spanish origin." We included those who reported "yes" in the Hispanic group. We evaluated those who selected "no" to determine whether they indicated a first or second MENA ancestry or birthplace as part of the inclusion criteria.

The dependent variable was cognitive disability. The ACS has measured cognitive disability since the 1990s.[1] The most recent measure was implemented in 2008, which asked (yes/no), "because of a physical, mental, or emotional condition, does this person have serious difficulty concentrating, remembering, or making decisions?"

Covariates

Covariates included age in years (mean), sex (male/female), nativity status (US-born/foreign-born), level of education (less than high school, high school diploma/general equivalency diploma, some college or associate's degree, bachelor's degree or higher), income based on the federal poverty level (< 200%/200% or higher) based on the

TABLE 1— Unweighted Sample Sizes (Weighted Percentages) for Racially/Ethnically Diverse Adults Aged ≥45 Years: American Community Survey; United States, California, New York, Michigan, and Texas; 2017–2021

	United States, No. (%)	California, No. (%)	New York, No. (%)	Michigan, No. (%)	Texas, No. (%)
Total sample	7 284 988	798 143	449 697	248 185	536 995
Non-Hispanic MENA	67 213 (1.08)	19 311 (2.71)	6 066 (1.52)	3 887 (2.17)	3 595 (0.77)
Non-Hispanic White	5 446 242 (69.59)	394 963 (45.43)	314 024 (62.07)	213 090 (80.49)	324 428 (52.52)
Non-Hispanic Black	643 935 (10.91)	39 847 (5.66)	47 789 (13.28)	20 023 (11.62)	49 694 (11.18)
Hispanic	707 922 (12.50)	203 648 (29.27)	45 805 (14.89)	5 360 (2.86)	134 783 (30.42)
Non-Hispanic Asian	354 756 (5.26)	133 968 (16.21)	34 866 (8.01)	4 376 (2.42)	22 334 (4.79)
Non-Hispanic AI/AN	56 020 (0.53)	4 158 (0.37)	1 044 (0.20)	1 398 (0.41)	1 876 (0.25)
Non-Hispanic NH/OPI	8 900 (0.13)	2 248 (0.35)	103 (0.02)	51 (0.02)	285 (0.06)

Note. AI/AN = American Indian or Alaska Native; MENA = Middle Eastern and North African; NH/OPI = Native Hawaiian or other Pacific Islander.

US Census Bureau's Current Population Survey Annual Social and Economic Supplement, and any health insurance (yes/no) based on previous studies.[14,24]

Statistical Analysis

We used the bivariate χ^2 test to determine statistically significant differences for each covariate and race/ethnicity for the United States and the 4 states with the largest MENA populations (i.e., California, New York, Michigan, and Texas). We conducted an overall test to compare all groups. Because all comparisons were statistically significant, we conducted 2 group comparisons to compare each racial/ethnic group with MENA adults. We calculated age and sex and adjusted prevalence of cognitive difficulties with 2-group comparisons to MENA adults after conducting an overall test to compare all groups. We used multivariable logistic models to determine associations between race/ethnicity and cognitive difficulty after adjusting for age, sex, nativity status, education, income, and health insurance. We compared MENA adults with White, Black, Hispanic/Latino, Asian, AI/AN, and NH/OPI adults.

We conducted 2 sensitivity analyses. First, we removed adults who reported "Israeli" as a first or second ancestry and those who reported "Israel" as their birthplace (n = 4731) because of concerns about including this population as part of the broad MENA category.[28] Second, we limited our sample to adults aged 65 years and older based on previous research.[16] We conducted statistical analysis with the SVYSET command in Stata version 17.0 (StataCorp LP, College Station, TX).

RESULTS

Selected characteristics of national and state samples (aged ≥45 years) are provided in Table 2. On a national level, the mean age of MENA adults was 60.5 years, which was younger than the mean age of White adults (63.2; $P<.001$) but not different from other racial/ethnic groups. The MENA sample included fewer women (47.4%) than did the White (52.0%), Black (55.1%), Hispanic (51.5%), Asian (54.7%), and AI/AN (53.5%) adults ($P<.05$). MENA adults had the highest levels of education, with 46.5% reporting a bachelor's degree or higher compared with 33.9% White, 21.4% Black, 15.9% Hispanic, 46.2% Asian, 15.9% AI/AN, and 17.3% NH/OPI adults ($P<.05$).

Age- and sex-adjusted national and state prevalence estimates for cognitive difficulties are presented in Table 3. The prevalence among MENA adults in the United States was 6.1%, which was significantly higher than those of White (5.7%) and Asian (4.4%) adults but lower than those of AI/AN (10.6%), Black (8.8%), NH/OPI (7.9%), and Hispanic (7.0%) adults ($P<.05$). By state, the prevalence among MENA adults was highest in Michigan (8.3%), followed by California (7.0%).

Multivariable logistic regression results are presented in Table 4 (Table C [available as a supplement to the online version of this article at http://www.ajph.org] includes covariates). In logistic regression models adjusted for age, sex, nativity status, education, income, and health insurance, MENA adults in the United States had greater odds of reporting cognitive difficulties than did White (odds ratio [OR] = 1.49; 95% confidence interval [CI] = 1.42, 1.56), Black (OR = 1.20; 95% CI = 1.14, 1.26), Hispanic (OR = 1.46; 95% CI = 1.39, 1.53),

TABLE 2— Selected Characteristics of Adult Population Aged ≥45 Years: American Community Survey; United States, California, New York, Michigan, and Texas; 2017–2021

	Non-Hispanic MENA	Non-Hispanic White	Non-Hispanic Black	Hispanic/ Latino	Non-Hispanic Asian	Non-Hispanic AI/AN	Non-Hispanic NH/OPI
United States							
Sample size, no.	67 213	5 446 242	643 935	707 922	354 756	56 020	8 900
Age, mean, y	60.46	63.19*	60.61	58.84	60.59	60.75	60.09
Woman, %	47.42	51.96*	55.10*	51.48*	54.65*	53.35*	53.18
US-born	27.85	95.87*	87.70*	42.73*	11.87*	98.30*	65.17*
Highest level of education							
<high school	12.03	7.18*	15.11*	35.78*	17.94*	17.78*	14.47*
High school/general equivalency diploma	19.64	29.40*	32.66*	26.62*	17.60*	32.33*	36.08*
Some college/associate's degree	21.85	29.52*	30.82*	21.74*	18.29*	33.98*	32.19*
Bachelor's degree or higher	46.48	33.90*	21.40*	15.86*	46.17*	15.90*	17.26*
Income <200% federal poverty level[a]	28.19	19.88*	35.28*	34.56*	21.83*	40.40*	26.06*
Health insurance coverage	92.90	95.68*	91.90*	83.41*	93.34*	85.00*	92.29
California							
Sample size, no.	19 311	394 963	39 847	203 648	133 968	4 158	2 248
Age, mean, y	62.01	63.65*	61.14*	58.81*	61.54	61.89	59.84*
Woman	50.09	51.20*	52.59*	51.39*	55.01*	53.99*	53.51*
US-born	15.69	92.11*	91.09*	35.58*	13.10*	96.96*	51.12*
Highest level of education							
<high school	12.22	4.83*	10.11*	43.55*	16.64*	16.57*	17.30*
High school/general equivalency diploma	20.30	19.23*	23.83*	23.81*	16.33*	29.18*	31.55*
Some college/associate's degree	23.39	33.64*	39.90*	21.19*	21.08*	38.36*	33.88*
Bachelor's degree or higher	44.12	42.30*	26.16*	11.45*	45.95*	15.89*	17.27*
Income <200% federal poverty level[a]	28.83	17.66*	30.35*	32.57*	21.95*	33.56*	23.54*
Health insurance coverage	95.60	97.24*	95.15	87.28*	96.35*	91.49*	92.76*
New York							
Sample size, no.	6 066	314 024	47 789	45 805	34 866	1 044	103
Age, mean, y	60.49	63.47*	61.30*	59.92*	60.58	61.69	61.82
Woman	46.26	52.37*	57.06*	53.90*	53.08*	53.17*	42.15
US-born	27.06	89.65*	58.54*	42.17*	6.41*	84.92*	54.15
Highest level of education							
<high school	11.97	7.10*	17.51*	34.72*	29.40*	17.00*	23.04*
High school/general equivalency diploma	22.20	28.35*	33.22*	28.07*	20.94*	26.21*	24.20*
Some college/associate's degree	20.03	25.71*	26.66*	20.93*	13.54*	31.90*	41.12*
Bachelor's degree or higher	45.80	38.83*	22.62*	16.28*	36.11*	24.88*	11.64*
Income <200% federal poverty level[a]	28.83	17.66*	30.35*	32.57*	21.95*	33.56*	23.54*
Health insurance coverage	95.21	97.74*	95.03	91.18*	93.90*	94.48	96.06
Michigan							
Sample size, no.	3 887	213 090	20 023	5 360	4 376	1 398	51
Age, mean, y	59.40	62.96*	61.04*	58.24	59.02	60.58	57.79
Woman	47.44	51.77*	55.58*	49.95	52.39*	52.50*	54.38
US-born	27.62	96.86*	97.65*	66.12*	7.42*	95.89*	80.31*

Continued

TABLE 2— Continued

	Non-Hispanic MENA	Non-Hispanic White	Non-Hispanic Black	Hispanic/Latino	Non-Hispanic Asian	Non-Hispanic AI/AN	Non-Hispanic NH/OPI
Highest level of education							
<high school	25.87	6.90*	14.09*	27.58*	14.63*	13.24*	8.77
High school/general equivalency diploma	21.93	31.93*	31.94*	28.58*	13.72*	34.52*	27.83
Some college/associate's degree	21.05	32.37*	34.79*	24.87*	14.79	37.04*	31.51
Bachelor's degree or higher	31.16	28.80*	19.18*	18.97*	56.86	15.21*	31.89
Income <200% federal poverty level[a]	39.04	20.69*	39.24	32.01*	18.56*	31.45*	41.93
Health insurance coverage	93.40	96.73*	94.99*	89.42*	95.14*	91.57	87.04
Texas							
Sample size, no.	3595	324428	49694	134783	22334	1876	285
Age, mean, y	58.76	62.75*	59.59	58.82	59.07	61.12*	60.22
Woman	44.60	51.67*	54.28*	51.55*	52.89*	51.79*	57.66
US-born	23.84	96.94*	91.50*	51.61*	5.91*	97.79*	66.84*
Highest level of education							
<high school	8.00	6.07*	11.47*	39.84*	17.80*	12.79*	9.99*
High school/general equivalency diploma	15.95	24.71*	30.56*	25.73*	16.66*	28.02*	32.53*
Some college/associate's degree	20.38	31.79*	33.74*	20.13*	16.33*	36.21*	33.40*
Bachelor's degree or higher	55.67	37.43*	24.23*	14.31*	49.21*	22.98*	24.08*
Income <200% federal poverty level[a]	26.03	17.58*	32.51*	37.10*	21.37*	28.93*	33.14
Health insurance coverage	85.64	92.85*	87.83*	75.31*	89.00*	85.52	88.28

Note. AI/AN = American Indian/Alaska Native; MENA = Middle Eastern and North African; NH/OPI = Native Hawaiian/other Pacific Islander.
[a]Based on the US Census Bureau's Current Population Survey Annual Social and Economic Supplement.
*$P < .05$, 2-group comparisons with MENA adults.

Asian (OR = 1.31; 95% CI = 1.25, 1.38), and AI/AN (OR = 1.07; 95% CI = 1.01, 1.14) adults, but there was no difference when compared with NH/OPI (OR = 1.08; 95% CI = 0.96, 1.23) adults.

In California, MENA adults had higher odds of cognitive difficulties than did White, Black, Hispanic/Latino, Asian, and NH/OPI adults, but there was no difference when compared with AI/AN adults. In New York, there was no statistically significant differences in cognitive difficulties between MENA and White adults; however, MENA adults had greater odds than did Asian adults but

TABLE 3— Age- and Sex-Adjusted Prevalence of Cognitive Difficulties Among Adults Aged ≥45 Years: American Community Survey; United States, California, New York, Michigan, and Texas; 2017–2021

	United States (n = 67 213), No. (%)	California (n = 19 311), No. (%)	New York (n = 6 066), No. (%)	Michigan (n = 3 887), No. (%)	Texas (n = 3 595), No. (%)
Non-Hispanic MENA	6.05	6.96	3.96	8.30	4.44
Non-Hispanic White	5.70*	4.80*	4.82*	6.25*	4.77
Non-Hispanic Black	8.77*	9.00*	6.91*	11.32*	8.41*
Hispanic/Latino	6.68*	5.44*	7.96*	7.60	6.28*
Non-Hispanic Asian	4.43*	4.35*	3.84	3.28*	3.33
Non-Hispanic AI/AN	10.59*	10.08*	8.94*	10.37	8.41*
Non-Hispanic NH/OPI	7.92*	7.31	12.96*	11.56	8.51

Note. AI/AN = American Indian/Alaska Native; MENA = Middle Eastern and North African; NH/OPI = Native Hawaiian/other Pacific Islander.
*$P < .05$, 2-group comparisons with MENA adults.

TABLE 4— Odds of Cognitive Difficulties Among Adults Aged ≥45 Years: American Community Survey; United States, California, New York, Michigan, and Texas; 2017–2021

	United States, OR (95% CI)	California, OR (95% CI)	New York, OR (95% CI)	Michigan, OR (95% CI)	Texas, OR (95% CI)
Non-Hispanic MENA vs					
Non-Hispanic White	1.49 (1.42, 1.56)	1.83 (1.69, 1.99)	0.98 (0.82, 1.17)	1.18 (0.98, 1.42)	1.58 (1.25, 2.00)
Non-Hispanic Black	1.20 (1.14, 1.26)	1.19 (1.09, 1.31)	0.79 (0.66, 0.95)	0.81 (0.67, 0.98)	1.10 (0.87, 1.39)
Hispanic/Latino	1.46 (1.39, 1.53)	1.12 (1.96, 2.30)	0.79 (0.66, 0.95)	1.25 (1.01, 1.56)	1.46 (1.15, 1.84)
Non-Hispanic Asian	1.31 (1.26, 1.38)	1.61 (1.48, 1.74)	1.26 (1.04, 1.52)	1.75 (1.32, 2.33)	1.33 (1.03, 1.74)
Non-Hispanic AI/AN	1.07 (1.01, 1.14)	1.20 (0.99, 1.44)	0.65 (0.46, 0.94)	0.84 (0.61, 1.15)	1.05 (0.76, 1.45)
Non-Hispanic NH/OPI	1.08 (0.96, 1.23)	1.30 (1.05, 1.61)	0.41 (0.20, 0.83)	0.70 (0.22, 2.24)	0.86 (0.48, 1.55)

Note. AI/AN = American Indian/Alaska Native; CI = confidence interval; MENA = Middle Eastern and North African; NH/OPI = Native Hawaiian/other Pacific Islander; OR = odds ratio. Multivariable logistic regression models adjusted for age, sex, nativity status, highest level of education, income, and health insurance coverage.

lower odds than did Black, Hispanic/Latino, and AI/AN adults. In Michigan, there was no statistically significant difference in cognitive difficulties compared with White, AI/AN, or NH/OPI adults. MENA adults had lower odds than did Black adults but higher odds than did Hispanic/Latino and Asian adults in Michigan. In Texas, MENA adults had higher odds of having cognitive difficulties than did White, Hispanic/Latino, and Asian adults. There was no difference when compared with Black, AI/AN, or NH/OPI adults. Results from the sensitivity analysis that excluded persons of Israeli descent are presented in Table D (available as a supplement to the online version of this article at http://www.ajph.org). All point estimates and 95% CIs were largely unchanged, and all CIs overlapped with those in the initial findings. Results from the sensitivity analysis limited to adults aged 65 years and older are presented in Table E (available as a supplement to the online version of this article at http://www.ajph.org). All CIs overlapped except in 1 comparison. Older MENA adults had 1.24 times higher odds (95% CI = 1.17, 1.33) of cognitive difficulty compared with older Hispanic/Latino adults, which was greater than that for adults aged 45 years and older (OR = 1.46; 95% CI = 1.39, 1.53).

DISCUSSION

Our first main finding pertains to MENA population health on a national level. MENA adults (aged ≥45 years) had a higher burden of cognitive difficulties than did White, Black, Hispanic, Asian, and AI/AN adults after adjusting for demographic and socioeconomic factors. Our findings in comparison with all White adults were similar to those of previous studies that compared foreign-born MENA to US-born White adults,[16] but a direct comparison cannot be made because, to our knowledge, this is the first study to evaluate both US- and foreign-born MENA Americans collectively in alignment with OMB's March 2024 approved racial/ethnic groups.[8]

Although the literature on MENA health has grown substantially since the last update to Statistical Policy Directive 15 in 1997, there are not enough studies that have made statistical comparisons to other racial/ethnic groups. Our study advances the science by making direct comparisons to Black, Hispanic, Asian, AI/AN, and NH/OPI populations. Our results highlight that the cognitive health of MENA Americans is worse than not only White individuals but also Black, Hispanic, Asian, and AI/AN individuals. We hypothesize that some of the disparities may be attributable to racial discrimination and trauma from immigration from war-torn countries and modifiable risk factors.

An interesting finding in our comparison with Black Americans was that MENA Americans were less likely to report cognitive difficulty after adjusting for age and sex, but in our fully adjusted model, MENA Americans had 1.20 times greater odds than those of Black Americans. Previous research has shown that the stress of lifetime discrimination is associated with increased cognitive difficulties among Black Americans, whose experiences of discrimination more closely resemble those of MENA Americans than those of White Americans.[13] The change in the direction of our results occurred when we added both nativity status and highest level of education, which is a potentially modifiable risk factor,[29] in the model.

Only 27.8% of the MENA population in our sample was US-born (compared with 87.7% of the Black population). More MENA Americans in the national sample reported a bachelor's degree or higher (46.5%) than did Black Americans (21.4%). The ACS does not include questions on lifetime discrimination or systemic racism. Our sensitivity analysis shows an interesting finding. Compared with Hispanic/Latino older adults in the national sample, MENA adults aged 65 years and older had 1.24 times higher odds of cognitive difficulties. This differs from the comparison when we limit the samples to those aged 45 years and older. MENA adults had 1.46 times higher odds of cognitive difficulties than did Hispanic/Latino adults in this age group. This demonstrates that cognitive difficulties may be emerging earlier among MENA adults. Future research is needed to explore how lifetime discrimination and systemic racism interact with age to influence the burden of cognitive difficulty in these minoritized populations.

Our second main finding pertains to MENA population health at the state level. The prevalence of cognitive difficulties was highest in Michigan (8.3%) and then California (7.0%)—the states with the largest percentage (Michigan = 2.7%) and size (California n = 912 787) of MENA residents from our sampling frame. California and Michigan have state health surveys that include identifiers for MENA Americans. The California Health Interview Survey includes ways to identify Arab Americans for statewide health research, including ways to identify foreign-born Arab respondents, individuals with foreign-born Arab parents, and individuals who speak Arabic at home.[30]

The Michigan Department of Health and Human Services conducts a special report on Arab American health that is similar to the national BRFSS, allowing the analysis of health outcomes by state. However, the survey is conducted only periodically (most recently in 2016) and does not measure cognitive difficulties or Alzheimer's disease and related dementias.[31] These statewide health surveys have laid the groundwork for advocacy efforts for representation of this population on a national level. Our study addresses a need to broaden existing efforts and expand research on the MENA population to other states with large and growing populations of MENA residents because fewer studies on MENA health have been conducted in New York and Texas.

Strengths and Limitations

A strength of our study was the use of a nationally representative data source that has a large sample size. The ACS 5-year samples are used to represent the total population when weighted. In our sampling frame, the total weighted US sample was 318 209 446, which is approximately 4% lower than the total population size reported by the US Census in 2021 (n = 331 893 745).[32] With this smaller population, we may have underestimated the total MENA population (along with other racial/ethnic groups) and the burden of cognitive difficulties among adults aged 45 years and older.

Similar to previous research on Arab Americans,[14,15,24,27] we used questions on ancestry to create a unique identifier for MENA Americans in alignment with OMB's new March 2024 racial/ethnic categories. We acknowledge that this variable is limited because it does not capture self-identification of a MENA racial/ethnic category. If participants were able to self-identify as MENA and White, this would reduce our sample size for both singular racial/ethnic groups and potentially inflate our results for cognitive difficulty. Once the latest guidelines for Statistical Policy Directive 15 have been implemented, we will be able to provide more accurate assessments of cognitive difficulties among those who identify as MENA alone and as MENA and White.

Our study was limited to cognitive difficulty. The ACS includes only health-related questions on disability.[1] The ACS does not measure any additional health behaviors or conditions. Future studies using this data source as the only current method to provide nationally representative estimates for both US- and foreign-born persons of MENA descent in the United States should explore ways to link this data source with others (e.g., Centers for Medicare & Medicaid Services) to obtain a broader assessment of health outcomes.

Another limitation is that the written form of the ACS is available in English and Spanish only. The US Census Bureau has made many efforts to offer telephone support services and in-person interviewing with approximately 30 different languages, including Arabic.[33] However, households with limited English proficiency may not understand how to access those languages resources. Previous studies have shown that cognitive testing using English and Arabic showed similar results, so we expect that if Arabic was available as an option, the estimates would be higher.[34]

Our dependent variable of cognitive difficulties was self-reported. Because of the high likelihood of underdiagnosed Alzheimer's disease and related dementias among MENA Americans,[18] this measure may be more valid than diagnostic testing.

Public Health Implications

Our findings expand on previous research uncovering cognitive difficulties by using the OMB's approved March 2024 racial/ethnic categories to include MENA as a checkbox as part of the minimum reporting standards. Furthermore, our findings support calls from MENA researchers and community leaders to remove MENA from the White race group to advance the science on health disparities for all racial/ethnic groups.[35] Our study also provides the first, to our knowledge, state-based estimates of cognitive difficulties among MENA adults living in California, New York, Michigan, and Texas. Results emphasize the urgent need for a separate checkbox for MENA Americans so that health outcomes, beyond the limited outcomes on disability collected by the ACS, can be studied in more detail and funds can be allocated more appropriately for research and community needs at the state and national levels. AJPH

ABOUT THE AUTHORS

Both authors are with the Department of Kinesiology, University of Texas at Arlington.

CORRESPONDENCE

Correspondence should be sent to Tiffany B. Kindratt, 500 West Nedderman Dr, Maverick Activities Center, University of Texas at Arlington, Arlington, TX 76019 (e-mail: tiffany.kindratt@uta.edu). Reprints can be ordered at https://www.ajph.org by clicking the "Reprints" link.

PUBLICATION INFORMATION

Full Citation: Kindratt TB, Smith A. Cognitive difficulty in Middle Eastern and North African adults living in the United States compared with other racial and ethnic categories, 2017–2021. *Am J Public Health*. 2024;114(11):1265–1274.

Acceptance Date: July 9, 2024.

DOI: https://doi.org/10.2105/AJPH.2024.307803

ORCID iDs:

Tiffany B. Kindratt https://orcid.org/0000-0003-3513-5290

Alexandra Smith https://orcid.org/0009-0007-9770-802X

CONTRIBUTORS

Tiffany B. Kindratt performed the investigation and the formal analysis, acquired study resources and funding, wrote the first draft of the article, supervised the study, and administered the project. Alexandra Smith curated the data, edited the article, and contributed to the writing. Both authors conceptualized and visualized the study, validated the data, and contributed to the methodology.

ACKNOWLEDGMENTS

Research reported in this article was supported by the Center to Accelerate Population Research in Alzheimer's, which is funded by the National Institute of Aging, National Institutes of Health (NIH; award P30AG066582).

Note. The content of this article is solely the responsibility of the authors and does not necessarily represent the official views of the NIH.

CONFLICTS OF INTEREST

The authors have no conflicts of interest to declare.

HUMAN PARTICIPANT PROTECTION

Institutional review board approval was not required because we used publicly available data from the US Census website; therefore, the study was not considered human participant research.

REFERENCES

1. US Census Bureau. How disability data are collected from the American Community Survey. 2021. Available at: https://www.census.gov/topics/health/disability/guidance/data-collection-acs.html. Accessed July 2, 2021.
2. Centers for Disease Control and Prevention. Disability and Health Data System (DHDS). Available at: https://dhds.cdc.gov/SP. Accessed December 13, 2023.
3. Centers for Disease Control and Prevention. Prevalence of disabilities and health care access by disability status and type among adults—United States, 2016. *MMWR Morb Mortal Wkly Rep*. 2018;67(32):882–887. https://doi.org/10.15585/mmwr.mm6732a3
4. Centers for Disease Control and Prevention. Racial and ethnic differences in subjective cognitive decline—United States, 2015–2020. *MMWR Morb Mortal Wkly Rep*. 2023;72(10):249–255. https://doi.org/10.15585/mmwr.mm7210a1
5. US Census Bureau. US decennial census measurement of race and ethnicity across the decades: 1790–2020. August 3, 2021. Available at: https://www.census.gov/library/visualizations/interactive/decennial-census-measurement-of-race-and-ethnicity-across-the-decades-1790-2020.html. Accessed December 27, 2023.
6. Office of Management and Budget. Revisions to the standards for the classification of federal data on race and ethnicity. 1997. Available at: https://obamawhitehouse.archives.gov/omb/fedreg_1997standards. Accessed March 14, 2023.
7. Kindratt TB, Moncriffe B, Ajrouch KJ, Zahodne LB, Dallo FJ. Diabetes among racial and ethnically diverse older adults in the United States with cognitive limitations. *J Racial Ethn Health Disparities*. 2023;11(1):238–247. https://doi.org/10.1007/s40615-023-01514-8
8. Office of Management and Budget. Initial proposals for updating OMB's race and ethnicity statistical standards. *Fed Regist*. 2023;88(18):5375–5384. Available at: https://www.federalregister.gov/documents/2023/01/27/2023-01635/initial-proposals-for-updating-ombs-race-and-ethnicity-statistical-standards. Accessed March 14, 2023.
9. Kindratt TB. Improving the collection of national health data: the case for the Middle Eastern and North African checkbox for communities in the USA. *J Racial Ethn Health Disparities*. 2023; Epub ahead of print. https://doi.org/10.1007/s40615-023-01759-3
10. Dallo FJ, Kindratt TB, Ajrouch KJ. Suitability of Middle Eastern and North African immigrant minimal reporting category for Arab immigrant health research in the National Health Interview Survey. *Soc Sci Med*. 2023;336:116260. https://doi.org/10.1016/j.socscimed.2023.116260
11. Office of Management and Budget. Revisions to OMB's Statistical Policy Directive No. 15: standards for maintaining, collecting, and presenting federal data on race and ethnicity. March 29, 2024. Available at: https://www.federalregister.gov/documents/2024/03/29/2024-06469/revisions-to-ombs-statistical-policy-directive-no-15-standards-for-maintaining-collecting-and. Accessed April 11, 2024.
12. Maghbouleh N, Schachter A, Flores RD. Middle Eastern and North African Americans may not be perceived, nor perceive themselves, to be White. *Proc Natl Acad Sci U S A*. 2022;119(7):e2117940119. https://doi.org/10.1073/pnas.2117940119
13. Zahodne LB, Sharifian N, Kraal AZ, et al. Longitudinal associations between racial discrimination and hippocampal and white matter hyperintensity volumes among older Black adults. *Soc Sci Med*. 2023;316:114789. https://doi.org/10.1016/j.socscimed.2022.114789
14. Kindratt TB, Dallo FJ, Zahodne LB. Cognitive disability among Arab Americans by nativity status and arrival year: lack of evidence for the healthy migrant effect. *J Racial Ethn Health Disparities*. 2022;9(5):2056–2062. https://doi.org/10.1007/s40615-021-01144-y
15. Al-Rousan T, Kamalyan L, Bernstein Sideman A, et al. Migration and cognitive health disparities: the Arab American and refugee case. *J Gerontol B Psychol Sci Soc Sci*. 2023;78(1):111–123. https://doi.org/10.1093/geronb/gbac129
16. Dallo FJ, Kindratt TB, Zahodne L. Prevalence of self-reported cognitive impairment among Arab American immigrants in the United States. *Innov Aging*. 2021;5(1):igaa058. https://doi.org/10.1093/geroni/igaa058
17. Kindratt TB, Dallo FJ, Zahodne LB, Ajrouch KJ. Cognitive limitations among Middle Eastern and North African immigrants. *J Aging Health*. 2022;34(9–10):1244–1253. https://doi.org/10.1177/08982643221103712
18. Kindratt TB, Ajrouch KJ, Zahodne LB, Dallo FJ. Suspected undiagnosed ADRD among Middle Eastern and North African Americans. *J Immigr Minor Health*. 2023;25(5):1098–1107. https://doi.org/10.1007/s10903-023-01509-x
19. US Census Bureau. Understanding and using American Community Survey data: what all data

users need to know. 2020. Available at: https://www.census.gov/content/dam/Census/library/publications/2020/acs/acs_general_handbook_2020.pdf. Accessed August 21, 2024.

20. US Census Bureau. American Community Survey (ACS). Available at: https://www.census.gov/programs-surveys/acs. Accessed December 6, 2023.
21. Hersi M, Irvine B, Gupta P, Gomes J, Birkett N, Krewski D. Risk factors associated with the onset and progression of Alzheimer's disease: a systematic review of the evidence. *Neurotoxicology*. 2017;61:143–187. https://doi.org/10.1016/j.neuro.2017.03.006
22. Kindratt T, Dallo F, Zahodne L. Cognitive disability among Arab Americans by nativity status: lack of evidence for the healthy migrant effect. *Innov Aging*. 2020;4(suppl 1):613. https://doi.org/10.1093/geroni/igaa057.2078
23. Dallo FJ, Kindratt TB, Seaton R, Ruterbusch JJ. The disproportionate burden of COVID-19 cases among Arab Americans. *J Racial Ethn Health Disparities*. 2023;10(3):1108–1114. https://doi.org/10.1007/s40615-022-01298-3
24. Dallo FJ, Booza J, Nguyen ND. Functional limitations and nativity status among older Arab, Asian, Black, Hispanic, and White Americans. *J Immigr Minor Health*. 2015;17(2):535–542. https://doi.org/10.1007/s10903-013-9943-0
25. Read JG, West JS, Kamis C. Immigration and health among non-Hispanic Whites: the impact of arrival cohort and region of birth. *Soc Sci Med*. 2020;246:112754. https://doi.org/10.1016/j.socscimed.2019.112754
26. Read JG, Lynch SM, West JS. Disaggregating heterogeneity among non-Hispanic Whites: evidence and implications for U.S. racial/ethnic health disparities. *Popul Res Policy Rev*. 2021;40(1):9–31. https://doi.org/10.1007/s11113-020-09632-5
27. Read JG, Ajrouch KJ, West JS. Disparities in functional disability among Arab Americans by nativity, immigrant arrival cohort, and country of birth. *SSM Popul Health*. 2019;7:100325. [Erratum in: Erratum regarding missing declaration of competing interest statements in previously published articles. *SSM Popul Health*. 2020;12:100715. https://doi.org/10.1016/j.ssmph.2020.100715]. https://doi.org/10.1016/j.ssmph.2020.100715
28. Matthews K, Phelan J, Jones N, et al. 2015 National content test race and ethnicity analysis report: a new design for the 21st century. 2017. Available at: https://www2.census.gov/programs-surveys/decennial/2020/program-management/final-analysis-reports/2015nct-race-ethnicity-analysis.pdf. Accessed August 21, 2024.
29. Livingston G, Huntley J, Sommerlad A, et al. Dementia prevention, intervention, and care: 2020 report of the Lancet Commission. *Lancet*. 2020;396(10248):413–446. [Erratum in Department of error. Lancet. 2023;402(10408):1132. https://doi.org/10.1016/S0140 6736(23)02043-3]. https://doi.org/10.1016/S0140-6736(20)30367-6
30. Abuelezam NN, El-Sayed AM, Galea S. Relevance of the "immigrant health paradox" for the health of Arab Americans in California. *Am J Public Health*. 2019;109(12):1733–1738. https://doi.org/10.2105/AJPH.2019.305308
31. Neumayer H, Weir S, Fussman C, McKane P. *Health Risk Behaviors Among Arab Adults Within the State of Michigan: 2016 Arab Behavioral Risk Factor Survey*. Lansing, MI: Michigan Department of Health and Human Services; 2017.
32. US Census Bureau. New vintage 2021 population estimates available for the nation, states and Puerto Rico. Available at: https://www.census.gov/newsroom/press-releases/2021/2021-population-estimates.html. Accessed December 29, 2023.
33. US Census Bureau. Design and methodology report. Available at: https://www.census.gov/programs-surveys/acs/methodology/design-and-methodology.html. Accessed December 29, 2023.
34. Zahodne LB, Brauer S, Tarraf W, Morris EP, Antonucci TC, Ajrouch KJ. Measurement and structural invariance of a neuropsychological battery among Middle Eastern/North African, Black, and White older adults. *Neuropsychology*. 2023;37(8):975–984. https://doi.org/10.1037/neu0000902
35. Awad GH, Abuelezam NN, Ajrouch KJ, Stiffler MJ. Lack of Arab or Middle Eastern and North African health data undermines assessment of health disparities. *Am J Public Health*. 2022;112(2):209–212. https://doi.org/10.2105/AJPH.2021.306590

Role of Doulas in Improving Maternal Health and Health Equity Among Medicaid Enrollees, 2014–2023

April M. Falconi, PhD, Leah Ramirez, MS, Rebecca Cobb, MS, Carrie Levin, PhD, Michelle Nguyen, MPH, and Tiffany Inglis, MD

See also Horan, p. 1161, and Marshall and Kozhimannil, p. 1164.

Objectives. To assess the relationship between doula utilization and health outcomes of females enrolled in Medicaid-affiliated plans in the United States.

Methods. In this retrospective, observational cohort study, we used Medicaid claims data from a national health insurer to compare health outcomes between females who used and who did not use a doula (2014–2023). We conducted propensity score matching using a 1:1 case–control match, without replacement, and fit logistic regressions to analyze the relative risks for maternal health outcomes.

Results. The study population included 722 matched pairs with and without a doula. Results indicate females with doulas had a 47% lower risk of cesarean delivery and a 29% lower risk of preterm birth, and were 46% more likely to attend a postpartum checkup (all differences $P < .05$).

Conclusions. Doula care is associated with improved health outcomes among Medicaid enrollees.

Public Health Implications. Doulas have garnered increasing interest from policymakers as a strategy to address increasing trends in maternal morbidity and persistent health disparities. This study provides evidence from Medicaid enrollees across the United States that doula care can improve maternal health.
(*Am J Public Health*. 2024;114(11):1275–1285. https://doi.org/10.2105/AJPH.2024.307805)

AJPH November 2024, Vol. 114, No. 11

Health insurance coverage for birth doulas in the United States has recently gained traction at the federal level as a strategy for improving persistent challenges in maternal health, such as increasing trends in maternal morbidity and mortality and maternal health disparities.[1–3] The Surgeon General recommended in their 2020 Call to Action coverage of doulas to help broaden access to quality care.[4] Similarly, the White House recommended coverage for doula services to help expand the perinatal workforce to address provider shortages and increase provider diversity in its 2022 Blueprint for Addressing the Maternal Health Crisis.[5]

According to DONA International, a doula is "a trained [nonclinical] professional who provides continuous physical, emotional, and informational support . . . before, during, and shortly after childbirth to help them achieve the healthiest, most satisfying experience possible."[6] Evidence thus far links doulas with decreased rates of cesarean deliveries, birth complications, postpartum depression and anxiety, low birth weight, and preterm birth.[7–9]

Some research suggests that integrating doulas into maternal health care could also help reduce maternal health disparities.[10] Black women have 3 to 4 times higher risk of maternal mortality, relative to White women, and are more than twice as likely to experience severe maternal morbidity, regardless of the amount of prenatal care received, socioeconomic status, insurance type, or preexisting conditions.[10,11] Doulas may help mitigate maternal health disparities by facilitating the delivery of culturally relevant care and helping empower their patients to advocate for themselves.[11–13]

Although research linking doulas to improved maternal health appears promising, the evidence base on doulas in the United States is just being developed. Data collected through administrative claims has only recently become available because of the passage of legislation in several states allowing for health insurance coverage of doulas through Medicaid. In 2018, for example, only Minnesota and Oregon provided Medicaid coverage for doula care. As of May 2024, however, 14 states and Washington, DC, provide coverage for doula services through Medicaid.[14]

Most previous evaluations of doula care, therefore, come from a single hospital or within a single state, affecting the broader generalizability of study findings. Other methodological challenges include self-reported data, which introduce self-reporting bias into analyses; small sample sizes, which can impede the ability to discern statistical significance on maternal health outcomes that are not highly prevalent; and a lack of standardization of how or whether a doula was trained and certified, which impacts the validity of inferences made about doulas.[10]

The objective of this study was to provide insight on the relationship between doula care covered through Medicaid managed care and health outcomes. This study addresses limitations of previous studies by using an adjudicated source of clinical claims and doula data, including into analysis only certified doulas, and analyzing a geographically diverse, multistate study population. This study also provides insight into how doula care affects race disparities in maternal health through race-specific analysis on the relationship between doula utilization and maternal health.

A unique contribution of this study is the analysis of area-level measures, including number of hospitals in a county providing obstetric care (a measure of health care access), neighborhood-level socioeconomic status (an indicator of socioeconomic disadvantage), and infant mortality rate (a sensitive measure of the overall health of a population).[15,16] Integration of these area-level measures into analyses is important because maternal health is affected not only by individual-level factors but also through area-level influences.[17] The relationship between doula care and maternal health outcomes, accordingly, is impacted by the community in which someone lives. These area-level factors, however, have been minimally addressed in earlier studies.

METHODS

In this retrospective cohort study, we used administrative claims data from the Healthcare Integrated Research Database, a proprietary repository of medical and pharmacy claims data from more than 88 million individuals enrolled in health plans across the United States.[18] A limited data set was used that was stripped of individual member identifiers to comply with the laws and regulations included in the Health Insurance Portability and Accountability Act (HIPAA) and HIPAA Privacy Rule (45 CFR 164.514[e][3]i).

The study population included self-reported females with at least 1 pregnancy outcome diagnosis or procedure code (*International Classification of Diseases, Ninth Revision* [*ICD-9*; Geneva, Switzerland: World Health Organization; 1980] and *International Classification of Disease, Tenth Revision* [*ICD-10*; Geneva, Switzerland: World Health Organization; 1992]) and at least 1 day of Medicaid eligibility between January 1, 2014, and June 30, 2023. (See Table A, available as a supplement to the online version of this article at https://ajph.org, for definitions and lists of relevant *ICD-9*, *ICD-10*, Current Procedural Terminology, and Healthcare Common Procedure Coding System codes.) These years were selected based on data availability (doula utilization data were available in at least 1 state starting in 2014).

We excluded members who were not of reproductive ages (15 to 49 years) from the study. The study population was further restricted to members in 9 states (California, New Jersey, Missouri, Texas, Wisconsin, and 4 other states located in different US regions) where doula care was provided (either as a legislated benefit or alternatively funded via pilots, grants, etc.; Figure 1). Some states could not be specified because of compliance rules that prohibit us from identifying specific states without their approval (these states were contacted, but they did respond to our request).

Health plan members received access to doula care through a few different approaches. Some individuals requested a doula of their own volition, while others received access because they were identified as high risk through their health plan's care management teams. Alternatively, some individuals were connected to doulas as a result of community outreach. Specific communities outreached to about doulas varied by state. Programs in some states, for example, focused outreach on Black women, while programs in other states focused outreach on orthodox Jewish women, adolescent pregnancies, women in rural settings, or women experiencing substance use disorder.

Health plan members who received doula care were identified in claims through 3 strategies. In states with Medicaid coverage of doulas, doula

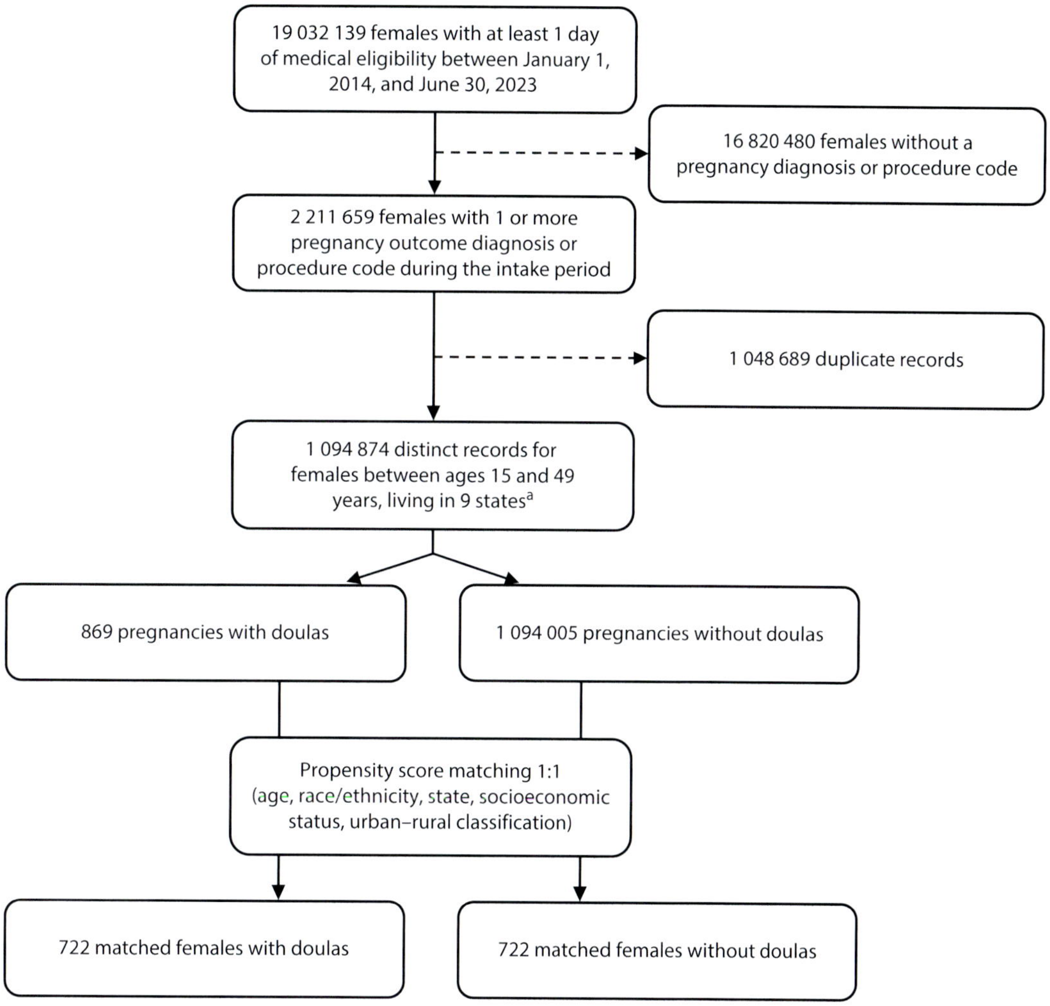

FIGURE 1— Study Population Attrition of Women Enrolled in Medicaid-Affiliated Plans in the United States: 2014–2023

[a]The study population was restricted to members in 9 states (CA, NJ, MO, TX, WI, and 4 other states located in different US regions; some states could not be named because of health plan compliance rules that prohibit us from identifying specific states without their approval.) where doula care was provided (either as a legislated benefit or alternatively funded via pilots, grants, etc.).

utilization was identified through the Centers for Medicare & Medicaid Services taxonomy code for doula services (374J00000X). Unique National Provider Identifier codes for doulas also were used to identify members who used doulas. In states where Medicaid does not yet cover doulas, we received masked identifier codes of members who received doula care from Elevance Health–affiliated health plans. Representatives from all affiliated health plans confirmed that the number of members identified as receiving doula care was consistent with their knowledge of doula utilization in their state. All doulas were required to be trained and certified, although states varied on who provided the certification.

Outcomes

Maternal health characteristics and outcomes were evaluated during pregnancy (from estimated start of pregnancy until the day before delivery), at delivery, and during the postpartum period—from the day after birth through 84 days following birth (i.e., 12 weeks postpartum or the "fourth trimester")—when many physiological and psychological changes occur as individuals recover from childbirth).[19] The start of pregnancy was estimated by subtracting the gestational age (identified from *ICD-10* Z3A codes) from the date of the pregnancy outcome. In rare instances when no Z3A codes were identified on the date of the pregnancy outcome, the last or closest Z3A code was used.

Health outcomes included cesarean delivery, vaginal birth after cesarean delivery, preterm birth, emergency department (ED) visit within 30 days of delivery, inpatient admission within 30 days of delivery, attendance at a postpartum visit between 7 and 84 days after delivery, prevalence of postpartum depression and anxiety, and prevalence of severe maternal morbidity, which is unintended outcomes of labor and delivery that can significantly impact women's health. These outcomes were selected because they are relatively more prevalent indicators of maternal morbidity and because of previous evidence suggesting their association with doula care. We did not evaluate maternal mortality, because we lacked statistical power to evaluate the small number of maternal deaths that occurred. We also did not assess the relationship between doula care and prenatal visit adherence given that many women did not learn about the availability of doula services until after they had attended a prenatal visit.

Statistical Analysis

We used propensity score matching (PSM) because it allows an observational, unrandomized study to simulate a randomized control trial to enable causal inference.[20] The advantages of PSM include that it helps reduce the potential impact of selection bias,[21] and it is an effective methodology when the study population has a large pool of "unexposed" individuals (without doulas) compared with those "exposed" (with doulas).[22]

We estimated the propensity score for members receiving doula care with a multivariable logistic regression model that incorporated the following sociodemographic and clinical variables: age at the time of pregnancy outcome, race/ethnicity (identified through self-report in either electronic health records or patient enrollment files or derived from the RAND imputation algorithm),[23] state of residence, neighborhood socioeconomic status (Agency for Healthcare Research and Quality–validated socioeconomic status index),[24] National Center for Health Statistics Urban–Rural Classification Scheme for Counties (developed to assess associations between urbanization level of residence and health),[25] and the presence of any one of the following commonly occurring pregnancy complications: gestational diabetes, gestational hypertension, pre-eclampsia or eclampsia, anemia, placental abruption, thrombocytopenia, placenta previa accreta spectrum disorder, short cervix, or infection. Cases (with doula) were matched to the controls (without doulas) using a 1:1 case–control match greedy algorithm, without replacement. Only 1 pregnancy per female (their most recent was selected for consistency purposes) was included into the matching algorithm so that an individual could not be matched more than once. Given the large pool of controls, this method tends to result in estimates with minimal bias and less variance relative to other matching approaches.[26]

We assessed the quality of the match by analyzing the standardized mean differences between the baseline characteristics of the cases and controls. The 2 groups were considered appropriately balanced with standardized differences less than 0.10. The models were further adjusted by year of delivery outcome and the number of hospitals providing obstetric care in a county. The models were not adjusted for individual comorbid conditions (which in some cases had standardized differences > 0.10) because the overall composite pregnancy complication measure was well balanced.

Subgroup Analyses

We conducted a series of subgroup analyses on the significant findings from the full PSM analyses. Specifically, PSM analyses were stratified by race (Black vs White), because of well-established maternal health disparities among Black women. Low sample sizes of other race/ethnicity groups prohibited further analyses. PSM analyses also were conducted by area-level infant mortality rate (IMR; counties in the highest quartile of IMR vs lowest quartile). Results were stratified by IMR because it is an indicator of maternal and infant health and of the socioeconomic and environmental conditions where people live.[15] Similar PSM methods were used for the subgroup analysis as for the whole study population, except the PSM models stratified for Black females and White females did not match on race.

RESULTS

We identified 1 094 874 pregnancies insured through an affiliated Medicaid plan between January 2014 and June 2023. Of these pregnancies, 869 were assisted by doula, most (69%) of which occurred between 2020 and 2023. The majority of doula-supported pregnancies occurred during this window because state legislation enabling Medicaid reimbursement for doulas in most states occurred after 2020.[27]

Recipients of doula services resided in more than 350 different zip codes in 9 states, although some states had more doula recipients than others. In 2 states, for example, we identified fewer than 10 members who received doula care, while in 3 states, we identified more than 100 members who received doula care (Table 1). Variance in the distribution of doula recipients was largely attributable to differences in the length of time doula care has been available to Medicaid enrollees in those states.

The doula group differed from the non-doula group on several characteristics. The mean age was higher in the doula group (28.0 vs 27.2); a larger proportion of members reported their race as Black (43.7% vs 22.4%); a larger proportion lived in urban settings (66.2% vs 52.5%); and individuals with doulas delivered in counties with relatively fewer available hospitals with obstetric units (mean number 4.3 vs 6.6). All differences were statistically significant at $P < .01$ and standardized mean differences greater than 0.1. Some of these differences were expected. Females who were at greater risk for adverse maternal health outcomes were more likely to be contacted about doula services through care management because of their potential for benefiting from doula services (Table 1).

Propensity Score–Matched Baseline Characteristics

A total of 722 females who received doula care were matched to females who did not receive doula care. Each matched pair included unique individuals whose most recent pregnancy was included in analysis. Therefore, we excluded 147 pregnancies from the total sample that received doula care because they represented multiple pregnancies

TABLE 1— Baseline Characteristics of Women Enrolled in Medicaid-Affiliated Plans in 9 States Across the United States, Unmatched Sample: 2014–2023

	Unmatched Sample			
	Doula (n = 869), Mean ±SD or No. (%)	No Doula (n = 1 094 005), Mean ±SD or No. (%)	P[a]	Standardized Bias[b]
Age, y	28.0 ±5.4	27.2 ±6.1	< .01	0.1
State[c]				
1	74 (8.5)	236 316 (21.6)	< .01	0.4
2	7 (0.8)	53 460 (4.9)	< .01	0.3
3	130 (15.0)	103 450 (9.5)	< .01	0.9
4	35 (4.0)	27 419 (2.5)	< .01	0.1
5	401 (46.1)	103 450 (9.5)	< .01	0.9
6	70 (8.1)	318 956 (29.2)	< .01	0.6
7	28 (3.2)	47 944 (4.4)	.1	0.1
8	122 (14.0)	122 623 (11.2)	< .01	0.1
9	2 (0.2)	97 466 (8.9)	.004	0.1
Urbanicity				
Urban	575 (66.2)	574 474 (52.5)	< .01	0.3
Suburban	223 (25.7)	374 627 (34.2)	< .01	0.2
Rural	9 (1.0)	85 178 (7.8)	< .01	0.3
Unspecified	62 (7.1)	59 726 (5.5)	.03	0.7
Patient's race/ethnicity				
Asian/Pacific Islander	36 (4.1)	65 896 (6.0)	.02	0.1
Black	379 (43.7)	244 835 (22.4)	< .01	0.5
Hispanic/Latino	148 (17.0)	405 088 (37.0)	< .01	0.5
White	261 (30.0)	306 771 (28.0)	.19	0.0
Other	33 (3.8)	68 415 (6.3)	.7	0.0
Socioeconomic status index				
Q1 (worst)	210 (26.5)	228 682 (22.4)	.006	0.1
Q2	185 (21.3)	208 373 (19.0)	.09	0.1
Q3	190 (21.9)	248 831 (22.7)	.54	0.0
Q4 (best)	208 (23.9)	335 771 (30.7)	< .01	0.2
Missing or unknown	76 (8.7)	72 348 (6.6)	.011	0.1
No. of hospitals with obstetric units in county	4.3 ±3.1	6.6 ±7.8	< .01	0.2

Continued

TABLE 1— Continued

	Unmatched Sample			
	Doula (n = 869), Mean ±SD or No. (%)	No Doula (n = 1 094 005), Mean ±SD or No. (%)	P[a]	Standardized Bias[b]
Comorbid conditions[d]				
Obesity	178 (20.5)	180 039 (16.5)	< .01	0.1
Gestational hypertension	125 (14.4)	104 126 (9.5)	< .01	0.2
Substance use disorder	44 (5.1)	64 926 (5.9)	.28	0.0
Pregnancy anemia	59 (6.8)	40 470 (3.7)	< .01	0.1
Gestational diabetes	55 (6.3)	84 024 (7.7)	.14	0.1
Any pregnancy complication[e]	303 (34.9)	290 404 (26.5)	< .01	0.2

[a]We used the χ^2 test and 2-sample *t* test to calculate *P* values.

[b]Standardized bias for continuous variables (where treatment = doula and control = non-doula):

$$d = \frac{(\bar{x}_{\text{treatment}} - \bar{x}_{\text{control}})}{\sqrt{\frac{s^2_{\text{treatment}} + s^2_{\text{control}}}{2}}}$$

Standardized bias for categorical variables (where treatment = doula and control = non-doula):

$$d = \frac{(\hat{p}_{\text{treatment}} - \hat{p}_{\text{control}})}{\sqrt{\frac{\hat{p}_{\text{treatment}}(1-\hat{p}_{\text{treatment}}) + \hat{p}_{\text{control}}(1-\hat{p}_{\text{control}})}{2}}}$$

[c]Some states could not be named because of health plan compliance rules that prohibit us from identifying specific states without their approval. All states are listed as state number to prevent identification of any particular state.

[d]Conditions are defined using *International Classification of Diseases, Ninth Revision,* and *International Classification of Diseases, Tenth Revision*, codes, which are included in Appendix Table A (available as a supplement to the online version of this article at https://ajph.org).

[e]Any pregnancy complication is defined as the presence of at least 1 of the following conditions: gestational diabetes; gestational hypertension, preeclampsia, or eclampsia; anemia; placental abruption; thrombocytopenia; placenta previa accreta spectrum disorder; short cervix; or infection.

associated with the same woman. Upon matching by propensity score for baseline sociodemographic characteristics, results indicated balance between the doula and nondoula females, with standardized mean differences less than 0.1 (Table 1).

Maternal Health Outcomes

The clinical characteristics of females with doulas compared very similarly to females with no doulas in the propensity score–matched sample. The only significant differences were that females with doulas had a lower prevalence of gestational diabetes (6.4% vs 10.3%; $P < .01$) and a lower prevalence of substance use disorder during pregnancy (5.1% vs 10.3%; $P < .01$). The doula and nondoula groups were not matched on these individual conditions and instead were matched on the presence of any pregnancy complication, for which the groups showed strong balance (Table 2).

In adjusted analyses, doula care was associated with a 47% lower risk of cesarean delivery (relative risk [RR] = 0.53; 95% CI = 0.43, 0.66) and 29% lower risk of preterm birth (RR = 0.71; 95% CI = 0.51, 0.98). Doula recipients also were 116% more likely to have a vaginal birth after cesarean delivery (RR = 2.16; 95% CI = 1.10, 4.24) and 46% more likely to have timely attendance at a postpartum visit (RR = 1.46; 95% CI = 1.31, 1.61). We observed no significant differences between doula care and ED visits, inpatient admissions, prevalence of postpartum depression and anxiety, or prevalence of severe maternal morbidity within 30 days of delivery (Table 3).

Subgroup Analyses

Results indicate both White and Black recipients of doula care were more likely to have timely attendance at a postpartum visit, although the RR was greater for White females (RR = 1.54; 95% CI = 1.23, 1.92) than Black females (RR = 1.33; 95% CI = 1.12, 1.58). No other differences observed between Black and White females were statistically significant. In counties with high IMR, doula care was associated with a 57% lower risk of cesarean delivery (RR = 0.43; 95% CI = 0.23, 0.81) but was not statistically significant among counties with low IMR (Table 3).

DISCUSSION

Results from this analysis of propensity score–matched pairs of females enrolled in Medicaid show doula care was associated with a 47% lower risk of cesarean delivery and 29% lower risk for preterm birth. These findings are consistent in effect size with other studies showing similar associations between doulas and decreased risk of cesarean delivery (~41%) and preterm birth (~22%).[10,13,28]

This study contributes unique evidence on the relationship between doula care and attendance at a postpartum visit, demonstrating that females supported by doulas were 46% more likely to have timely attendance at a postpartum visit. Other novel findings from this study include how the effects of doula care on RR of cesarean

TABLE 2— Baseline Characteristics of Women Enrolled in Medicaid-Affiliated Plans in 9 States Across the United States, Matched Sample: 2014–2023

	Matched Sample			
	Doula (n = 722), Mean ±SD or No. (%)	No Doula (n = 722), Mean ±SD or No. (%)	P[a]	Standardized Bias[b]
Age, y	28.4 ±5.4	28.4 ±5.5	.97	0.0
State[c]				
1	62 (8.7)	62 (8.6)	.99	0.0
2	7 (1.0)	6 (1.0)	.78	0.0
3	113 (16.4)	118 (15.7)	.7	0.0
4	18 (2.5)	18 (2.5)	.99	0.0
5	346 (47.8)	344 (47.8)	.96	0.0
6	49 (6.8)	49 (6.8)	.99	0.0
7	27 (3.8)	26 (3.6)	.88	0.0
8	96 (13.1)	94 (13.3)	.89	0.0
9	2 (0.3)	3 (0.4)	.66	0.0
Urbanicity				
Urban	463 (64.2)	465 (64.4)	.93	0.0
Suburban	202 (27.9)	199 (27.6)	.88	0.0
Rural	6 (0.8)	7 (1.0)	.78	0.0
Unspecified	51 (14.2)	51 (14.2)	.99	0.0
Patient's race/ethnicity				
Asian/Pacific Islander	28 (3.9)	28 (3.9)	.99	0.0
Black	294 (40.8)	295 (40.9)	.99	0.0
Hispanic/Latino	126 (17.5)	126 (17.5)	.98	0.0
White	233 (32.3)	232 (32.3)	.98	0.0
Other	41 (5.7)	41 (5.7)	.99	0.0
Socioeconomic status index				
Q1 (worst)	171 (23.6)	170 (40.2)	.99	0.0
Q2	155 (21.5)	157 (21.8)	.92	0.0
Q3	160 (22.2)	162 (22.4)	.92	0.0
Q4 (best)	172 (23.9)	171 (23.7)	.94	0.0
Missing or unknown	64 (8.9)	62 (8.6)	.67	0.0
No. of hospitals with obstetric units in county	4.2 ±2.9	4.8 ±3.8	<.01	0.1

Continued

TABLE 2— Continued

	Matched Sample			
	Doula (n = 722), Mean ±SD or No. (%)	No Doula (n = 722), Mean ±SD or No. (%)	P[a]	Standardized Bias[b]
Comorbid conditions[d]				
Obesity	150 (20.8)	124 (17.2)	.08	0.1
Gestational hypertension	104 (14.4)	86 (11.9)	.15	0.1
Substance use disorder	37 (5.1)	74 (10.3)	< .001	0.2
Pregnancy anemia	52 (7.2)	46 (6.4)	.52	0.0
Gestational diabetes	46 (6.3)	74 (10.3)	.008	0.1
Any pregnancy complication[e]	255 (35.4)	255 (35.4)	.99	0.0

[a]We used the χ^2 test and 2-sample *t* test to calculate *P* values.
[b]Standardized bias for continuous variables (where treatment = doula and control = non-doula):

$$d = \frac{(\overline{X}_{\text{treatment}} - \overline{X}_{\text{control}})}{\sqrt{\frac{s^2_{\text{treatment}} + s^2_{\text{control}}}{2}}}$$

Standardized bias for categorical variables (where treatment = doula and control = non-doula):

$$d = \frac{(\hat{p}_{\text{treatment}} - \hat{p}_{\text{control}})}{\sqrt{\frac{\hat{p}_{\text{treatment}}(1 - \hat{p}_{\text{treatment}}) + \hat{p}_{\text{control}}(1 - \hat{p}_{\text{control}})}{2}}}$$

[c]Some states could not be named because of health plan compliance rules that prohibit us from identifying specific states without their approval. All states are listed as state number to prevent identification of any particular state.
[d]Conditions are defined using *International Classification of Diseases, Ninth Revision*, and *International Classification of Diseases, Tenth Revision*, codes, which are included in Appendix Table A (available as a supplement to the online version of this article at https://ajph.org).
[e]Any pregnancy complication is defined as the presence of at least 1 of the following conditions: gestational diabetes; gestational hypertension, preeclampsia, or eclampsia; anemia; placental abruption; thrombocytopenia; placenta previa accreta spectrum disorder; short cervix; or infection.

delivery varies by county-level IMR. Cesarean deliveries, while sometimes necessary, are associated with increased risk of maternal morbidity.[29] This study's finding that doulas were linked with a 57% reduction in cesarean delivery risk among counties with high IMR suggest that utilization of doulas could be an effective strategy for mitigating disparities (and their sequelae of maternal morbidity risk).

Other findings from this study's subgroup analyses that may be considered for addressing maternal health disparities include the lack of significant differences in cesarean deliveries and preterm births between Black and White doula recipients. Previous studies have reported worse outcomes for Black women—even after adjusting for maternal characteristics such as age, education, insurance status, and clinical conditions.[30,31] In addition, the finding that doula care was positively correlated with postpartum visits for Black females is important because most incidences of maternal morbidity and mortality occur in the weeks following birth. Attendance at postpartum visits is critical, therefore, for identifying potential health problems before their onset or increase in severity occurs.[32]

Results, of course, are contingent on who receives doula care. Individuals who received doula care in this study, for example, were at higher risk for adverse maternal health outcomes based on sociodemographic and clinical characteristics. As doula utilization in the Medicaid population grows, further research may consider exploring the relationship between doula care and maternal health outcomes among populations that are at relatively lower risk for adverse outcomes.

Results may also depend upon when doula care is initiated and utilized. Previous research, for example, indicates lower odds of a postpartum depression or anxiety diagnosis when doula care is utilized during labor and delivery, specifically.[8] As doula programs mature in currently covered states and legislation enabling Medicaid coverage of doulas expands to new states, a more nuanced analysis of the timing of doula utilization and the relationship with maternal outcomes using medical claims data may be more feasible.

TABLE 3— Relative Risk of Health Outcomes by Receipt of Doula Care Among Propensity Score–Matched (PSM) Women Enrolled in Medicaid-Affiliated Plans: United States, 2014–2023

	Doula (n = 722) No. (%)	No Doula (n = 722) No. (%)	PSM RR (95% CI) All Women With Doula	Black Women With Doula	White Women With Doula	Women With Doula in Counties With Low IMR	Women With Doula in Counties With High IMR
Cesarean delivery	172 (23.9)	316 (43.9)	0.53 (0.43, 0.66)	0.74 (0.51, 1.1)	0.79 (0.48, 1.30)	0.56 (0.27, 1.19)	0.43 (0.23, 0.81)
Vaginal birth after cesarean section	27 (3.8)	12 (1.4)	2.48 (1.29, 4.76)	. . .[a]	. . .[a]	. . .[a]	. . .[a]
Preterm birth	61 (8.5)	83 (11.5)	0.71 (0.51, 0.98)	0.70 (0.43, 1.14)	0.70 (0.28, 1.77)	0.67 (0.19, 2.36)	0.71 (0.34, 1.48)
ED visit within 30 d postpartum	42 (5.8)	42 (5.8)	0.85 (0.55, 1.31)	. . .[a]	. . .[a]	. . .[a]	. . .[a]
Inpatient admission within 30 d postpartum	38 (5.3)	35 (4.9)	1.04 (0.65, 1.66)	. . .[a]	. . .[a]	. . .[a]	. . .[a]
Severe maternal morbidity or mortality	24 (3.3)	20 (2.8)	1.25 (0.70, 2.24)	. . .[a]	. . .[a]	. . .[a]	. . .[a]
Postpartum anxiety or postpartum depression	82 (11.4)	74 (10.3)	1.12 (0.82, 1.53)	. . .[a]	. . .[a]	. . .[a]	. . .[a]
Postpartum visit within 7–84 d of birth	465 (64.6)	322 (44.6)	1.46 (1.31, 1.61)	1.33 (1.12, 1.58)	1.54 (1.23, 1.92)	1.54 (0.99, 2.38)	1.71 (0.95, 1.44)

Note. CI = confidence interval; ED = emergency department; IMR = infant mortality rate; RR = relative risk. PSM models were matched on maternal age, race/ethnicity, state of residence, socioeconomic status quartile, and urban–rural classification. PSM models were additionally adjusted for year of pregnancy outcome and the number of hospitals in the county providing obstetric care. Separate PSM models were run on health outcomes with significant results and sufficient sample size for stratified categories (i.e., Black vs White, low IMR vs high IMR). The PSM models stratified by race/ethnicity were not matched on race/ethnicity. Conditions are defined using *International Classification of Diseases, Ninth Revision*; *International Classification of Diseases, Tenth Revision*; and Healthcare Common Procedure Coding System codes, which are included in Appendix Table A (available as a supplement to the online version of this article at https://ajph.org).
[a]Outcomes that were not statistically significant in the overall (nonstratified) PSM model and were not evaluated in the stratified models.

Limitations

The following limitations should be considered when interpreting this study's findings. First, while this study offers one of the most geographically diverse study populations on doula care in the United States, doula-assisted pregnancies represent a very small (< 1%) proportion of the total number of births covered by Medicaid. We have used a robust methodology to reduce the effects of potential selection bias, but unmeasured confounders could remain. The primary study findings, however, are consistent with results previously reported.

Second, because we do not have the complete medical histories of any member in the study, we do not know which pregnancy (e.g., first, second, third) was assessed. The direction of effect of pregnancy number on health outcomes is unclear, however, because risk could increase or decrease depending on the outcome. The way in which pregnancy number affects the relationship between doula utilization and maternal health outcomes should be explored in future research.

Lastly, results from this study generalize only to the Medicaid-insured population. The relationship between doula care and health outcomes may differ in commercially insured populations, which account for more than half of all births in the United States.[33]

Public Health Implications

As part of the blueprint for addressing the maternal health crisis in the United States, the federal government is actively making efforts to grow and diversify the doula workforce.[34] Results from this study provide evidence to support this endeavor, by showing the positive impact doulas can make toward decreasing maternal health risks. This study demonstrates how partnership with doulas was associated with reductions in cesarean deliveries and preterm births, and improved adherence to postpartum care recommendations. This study's stratified analyses further provide support for how doula care may reduce maternal health disparities between Black and White females and may be an especially effective strategy for reducing cesarean deliveries in communities at greatest risk for poor maternal and infant health outcomes.

Because doula services are an optional benefit through Medicaid, however, it is at the discretion of the state to reimburse doulas for providing services to Medicaid enrollees. Access to doula care, therefore, varies substantially among Medicaid programs, with some states operating a fully funded Medicaid doula benefit, some states offering small doula programs not widely available to all Medicaid beneficiaries, and some states where the only option for individuals is to self-pay for doula services. As more states begin to operationalize a Medicaid doula benefit and uptake of doula services increases, future research will be able to evaluate how the differences in these state policies affect the relationship between doula care and maternal health outcomes. Causal mechanisms will be able to be explored through analysis of, for example, timing and frequency of doula utilization and how it relates to maternal health. In addition, there is growing momentum for doula coverage mandates through private and commercial insurance coverage, and more employer groups are adding doula coverage to their health plans. This growth in doula coverage will allow for a better understanding of the relationship between doula care and maternal health across lines of business and a broader, more diverse population. AJPH

ABOUT THE AUTHORS

April M. Falconi, Leah Ramirez, Rebecca Cobb, Carrie Levin, and Michelle Nguyen are with the Public Policy Institute, Elevance Health, Washington, DC. Tiffany Inglis is with Carelon Health, Indianapolis, IN.

CORRESPONDENCE

Correspondence may be sent to April M. Falconi, Public Policy Institute, Elevance Health, 1001 Pennsylvania Ave NW, Suite 710, Washington, DC 20004 (e-mail: april.falconi@elevancehealth.com). Reprints can be ordered at https://www.ajph.org by clicking the "Reprints" link.

PUBLICATION INFORMATION

Full Citation: Falconi AM, Ramirez L, Cobb R, Levin C, Nguyen M, Inglis T. Role of doulas in improving maternal health and health equity among Medicaid enrollees, 2014–2023. *Am J Public Health*. 2024; 114(11):1275–1285.

Acceptance Date: July 10, 2024.

DOI: https://doi.org/10.2105/AJPH.2024.307805

ORCID iDs:

Leah Ramirez https://orcid.org/0009-0008-1682-7965

Carrie Levin https://orcid.org/0009-0000-1893-0167

CONTRIBUTORS

A. M. Falconi and L. Ramirez conceptualized the study. A. M. Falconi and C. Levin collected data. A. M. Falconi and R. Cobb analyzed the data. T. Inglis supervised the study and provided subject matter and program expertise. All authors wrote and edited the article.

ACKNOWLEDGMENTS

We are grateful to the individuals we corresponded with from the various state health plans about the doula programs in their states. These individuals helped support us with data and provided us with a rich context about the people, challenges, and successes associated with these programs.

CONFLICTS OF INTEREST

All authors were employed by Elevance Health or its subsidiary, Carelon Research, at the time of study and writing of the article.

HUMAN PARTICIPANT PROTECTION

This observational study, conducted under the research exception provisions of Privacy Rule 45 CFR 164.514(e), was exempt from institutional board review because researchers accessed a limited data set for analysis that was devoid of individual patient identifiers and complied with all relevant provisions of the Health Insurance Portability and Accountability Act. Institutional review board exemption was not necessary because the study was an analysis of the managed care organization's membership data for the purposes of health plan treatment, planning, and operations. All data were anonymized before being used.

REFERENCES

1. Declercq E, Zephyrin LC. *Severe Maternal Morbidity in the United States: A Primer*. New York, NY: The Commonwealth Fund; 2021.
2. Fink DA, Kilday D, Cao Z, et al. Trends in maternal mortality and severe maternal morbidity during delivery-related hospitalization in the United States, 2008 to 2021. *JAMA Netw Open*. 2023;6(6): e2317641. https://doi.org/10.1001/jamanetworkopen.2023.17641
3. Gunja MZ, Gumas ED, Williams RD II. *US Health Care From a Global Perspective, 2022: Accelerating Spending, Worsening Outcomes*. New York, NY: The Commonwealth Fund; 2023.
4. Office of the Surgeon General. *The Surgeon General's Call to Action to Improve Maternal Health*. Washington, DC: US Department of Health and Human Services; 2020.
5. White House. Fact sheet: President Biden's and Vice President Harris's maternal health blueprint delivers for women, mothers, and families. June 24, 2022 Available at: https://www.whitehouse.gov/briefing-room/statements-releases/2022/06/24/fact-sheet-president-bidens-maternal-health-blueprint-delivers-for-women-mothers-and-families. Accessed February 6, 2024.
6. DONA International. What is a doula? Available at: https://www.dona.org/what-is-a-doula-2. Accessed June 6, 2024.
7. Kozhimannil KB, Attanasio LB, Jou J, Joarnt LK, Johnson PJ, Gjerdingen DK. Potential benefits of increased access to doula support during childbirth. *Am J Manag Care*. 2014;20(8):e340–e352.
8. Falconi AM, Bromfield SG, Tang T, et al. Doula care across the maternity care continuum and impact on maternal health: evaluation of doula programs across three states using propensity score matching. *EClinicalMedicine*. 2022;50: 101531. https://doi.org/10.1016/j.eclinm.2022.101531
9. Knocke K. Chappel A, Sugar S, De Lew N, Sommers BD. Doula care and maternal health: an evidence review. (Issue Brief No. HP-2022-24). Washington, DC: Office of the Assistant Secretary for Planning and Evaluation, US Department of Health and Human Services; December 2022.
10. Sobczak A, Taylor L, Solomon S, et al. The effect of doulas on maternal and birth outcomes: a scoping review. *Cureus*. 2023;15(5):e39451. https://doi.org/10.7759/cureus.39451
11. McHugh K, Martinez RM, Alper J, eds. *Advancing Maternal Health Equity and Reducing Maternal Morbidity and Mortality: Proceedings of a Workshop*. National Academies Press; 2021. Available at: https://www.ncbi.nlm.nih.gov/books/NBK575266. Accessed February 6, 2024.
12. Safon CB, McCloskey L, Ezekwesili C, Feyman Y, Gordon SH. Doula care saves lives, improves equity, and empowers mothers. State Medicaid programs should pay for it. *Health Affairs Blog*.

May 26, 2021. https://doi.org/10.1377/hblog20210525.295915.

13. Kozhimannil KB, Hardeman RR, Attanasio LB, Blauer-Peterson C, O'Brien M. Doula care, birth outcomes, and costs among Medicaid beneficiaries. *Am J Public Health.* 2013;103(4):e113–e121. https://doi.org/10.2105/AJPH.2012.301201
14. National Health Law Program. Doula Medicaid Project. Available at: https://healthlaw.org/doulamedicaidproject. Accessed May 22, 2024.
15. Reidpath DD, Allotey P. Infant mortality rate as an indicator of population health. *J Epidemiol Community Health.* 2003;57(5):344–346. https://doi.org/10.1136/jech.57.5.344
16. Bhavsar NA, Gao A, Phelan M, et al. Value of neighborhood socioeconomic status in predicting risk of outcomes in studies that use electronic health record data. *JAMA Netw Open.* 2018;1(5):e182716. https://doi.org/10.1001/jamanetworkopen.2018.2716
17. Howell EA. Reducing disparities in severe maternal morbidity and mortality. *Clin Obstet Gynecol.* 2018;61(2):387–399. https://doi.org/10.1097/GRF.0000000000000349
18. Carelon Research. Carelon Research's Healthcare Integrated Research Database (HIRD). 2023. Available at: https://lp.carelonresearch.com/rs/621-UKX-708/images/Carelon-Research-HIRD-technical-white-paper-fv.pdf. Accessed February 6, 2024.
19. Presidential Task Force on Redefining the Postpartum Visit, Committee on Obstetric Practice. Optimizing postpartum care. American College of Obstetricians and Gynecologists; May 2018; No. 736. Available at: https://www.acog.org/-/media/project/acog/acogorg/clinical/files/committee-opinion/articles/2018/05/optimizing-postpartum-care.pdf. Accessed June 6, 2024.
20. Shiba K, Kawahara T. Using propensity scores for causal inference: pitfalls and tips. *J Epidemiol.* 2021;31(8):457–463. https://doi.org/10.2188/jea.JE20210145
21. D'Agostino RB Jr. Propensity score methods for bias reduction in the comparison of a treatment to a non-randomized control group. *Stat Med.* 1998;17(19):2265–2281. https://doi.org/10.1002/(SICI)1097-0258(19981015)17:19<2265::AID-SIM918>3.0.CO;2-B
22. Ross ME, Kreider AR, Huang Y-S, Matone M, Rubin D, Localio R. Propensity score methods for analyzing observational data like randomized experiments: challenges and solutions for rare outcomes and exposures. *Am J Epidemiol.* 2015;181(12):989–995. https://doi.org/10.1093/aje/kwu469
23. Sorbero ME, Euller R, Kofner A, Elliott MN. Imputation of race and ethnicity in health insurance marketplace enrollment data, 2015–2022 open enrollment periods. RAND Corporation. 2022. Available at https://www.rand.org/pubs/research_reports//RRA1853-1.html. Accessed June 6, 2024.
24. Bonito AJ, Bann C, Eicheldinger C, Carpenter L. Creation of new race-ethnicity codes and socioeconomic status (SES) indicators for Medicare beneficiaries. Final Report, Sub-Task 2. AHRQ Publication No. 08-0029-EF. Rockville, MD: Agency for Healthcare Research and Quality; January 2008.
25. Ingram DD, Franco SJ. 2013 NCHS urban-rural classification scheme for counties. National Center for Health Statistics. *Vital Health Stat 2.* 2014;(166):1–73. Available at: https://www.cdc.gov/nchs/data/series/sr_02/sr02_166.pdf. Accessed September 9, 2024.
26. Austin PC. A comparison of 12 algorithms for matching on the propensity score. *Stat Med.* 2014;33(6):1057–1069. https://doi.org/10.1002/sim.6004
27. Ogunwole SM, Karbeah J, Bozzi DG, et al. Health equity considerations in state bills related to doula care (2015–2020). *Womens Health Issues.* 2022;32(5):440–449. https://doi.org/10.1016/j.whi.2022.04.004
28. Kozhimannil KB, Hardeman RR, Alarid-Escudero F, Vogelsang CA, Blauer-Peterson C, Howell EA. Modeling the cost-effectiveness of doula care associated with reductions in preterm birth and cesarean delivery. *Birth.* 2016;43(1):20–27. https://doi.org/10.1111/birt.12218
29. Kozhimannil KB, Law MR, Virnig BA. Cesarean delivery rates vary tenfold among US hospitals; reducing variation may address quality and cost issues. *Health Aff (Millwood).* 2013;32(3):527–535. https://doi.org/10.1377/hlthaff.2012.1030
30. Blebu BE, Waters O, Lucas CT, Ro A. Variations in maternal factors and preterm birth risk among non-Hispanic Black, White, and mixed-race Black/White women in the United States, 2017. *Womens Health Issues.* 2022;32(2):140–146. https://doi.org/10.1016/j.whi.2021.10.010
31. Debbink MP, Ugwu LG, Grobman WA, et al.; for the Eunice Kennedy Shriver National Institute of Child Health and Human Development Maternal-Fetal Medicine Units Network. Racial and ethnic inequities in cesarean birth and maternal morbidity in a low-risk, nulliparous cohort. *Obstet Gynecol.* 2022;139(1):73–82. https://doi.org/10.1097/AOG.0000000000004620
32. Dol J, Hughes B, Bonet M, et al. Timing of maternal mortality and severe morbidity during the postpartum period: a systematic review. *JBI Evid Synth.* 2022;20(9):2119–2194. https://doi.org/10.11124/JBIES-20-00578
33. Valenzuela CP, Osterman MJK. Characteristics of mothers by source of payment for the delivery: United States, 2021. NCHS Data Brief, no 468. Hyattsville, MD: National Center for Health Statistics; 2023. https://doi.org/10.15620/cdc:127266
34. White House. Blueprint for addressing the maternal health crisis. June 2022. Available at: https://www.whitehouse.gov/wp-content/uploads/2022/06/Maternal-Health-Blueprint.pdf. Accessed June 6, 2024.

Erratum In: "Control of SARS-CoV-2 Infection Rates at a Spanish University With In-Person Class Attendance"

In: Gil-Conesa M, Amer F, Carlos S, Ariño AH, Martínez-González MA, Fernandez-Montero A. Control of SARS-Cov-2 infection rates at a Spanish university with in-person class attendance. *Am J Public Health*. 2022;112(4):570–573.

When originally published, author Fares Amer's degree was listed incorrectly. The author byline should read:

Mario Gil-Conesa, MD, MPH, Fares Amer, BPharm, Silvia Carlos, PharmD, PhD, Arturo H. Ariño, PhD, Miguel A. Martínez-González, MD, MPH, PhD, and Alejandro Fernandez-Montero, MD, PhD AJPH

https://doi.org/10.2105/AJPH.2021.306682e

UNITED STATES POSTAL SERVICE® **Statement of Ownership, Management, and Circulation (All Periodicals Publications Except Requester Publications)**

1. Publication Title: American Journal of Public Health	2. Publication Number: 0090-0036	3. Filing Date: 09/30/2024
4. Issue Frequency: Monthly	5. Number of Issues Published Annually: 12	6. Annual Subscription Price: $993–$1445 Online + Print
7. Complete Mailing Address of Known Office of Publication (Not printer) (Street, city, county, state, and ZIP+4®): American Public Health Association, 800 I St., NW, Washington, DC 20001-3710		Contact Person: Brian Selzer; Telephone (Include area code): 202-777-2464

8. Complete Mailing Address of Headquarters or General Business Office of Publisher (Not printer)
American Public Health Association
800 I St., NW, Washington, DC 20001-3710

9. Full Names and Complete Mailing Addresses of Publisher, Editor, and Managing Editor (Do not leave blank)
Publisher (Name and complete mailing address)
American Public Health Association
800 I St., NW, Washington, DC 20001-3710

Editor (Name and complete mailing address)
Alfredo Morabia, MD, PhD, Barry Commoner Center for Health and the Environment, Queens College at City University of New York, Remsen #311, 65-30 Kissena Blvd, Flushing, NY 11369

Managing Editor (Name and complete mailing address)
Brian Selzer, American Public Health Association
800 I St., NW, Washington, DC 20001-3710

10. Owner (Do not leave blank. If the publication is owned by a corporation, give the name and address of the corporation immediately followed by the names and addresses of all stockholders owning or holding 1 percent or more of the total amount of stock. If not owned by a corporation, give the names and addresses of the individual owners. If owned by a partnership or other unincorporated firm, give its name and address as well as those of each individual owner. If the publication is published by a nonprofit organization, give its name and address.)

Full Name	Complete Mailing Address
American Public Health Association	800 I St., NW, Washington, DC 20001-3710

11. Known Bondholders, Mortgagees, and Other Security Holders Owning or Holding 1 Percent or More of Total Amount of Bonds, Mortgages, or Other Securities. If none, check box ☐ None

Full Name	Complete Mailing Address
District of Columbia	Washington, DC

12. Tax Status (For completion by nonprofit organizations authorized to mail at nonprofit rates) (Check one)
The purpose, function, and nonprofit status of this organization and the exempt status for federal income tax purposes:
☑ Has Not Changed During Preceding 12 Months
☐ Has Changed During Preceding 12 Months (Publisher must submit explanation of change with this statement)

13. Publication Title: American Journal of Public Health
14. Issue Date for Circulation Data Below: 09/30/2022

15. Extent and Nature of Circulation		Average No. Copies Each Issue During Preceding 12 Months	No. Copies of Single Issue Published Nearest to Filing Date
a. Total Number of Copies (Net press run)		4227	850
b. Paid Circulation (By Mail and Outside the Mail)	(1) Mailed Outside-County Paid Subscriptions Stated on PS Form 3541 (Include paid distribution above nominal rate, advertiser's proof copies, and exchange copies)	3716	564
	(2) Mailed In-County Paid Subscriptions Stated on PS Form 3541 (Include paid distribution above nominal rate, advertiser's proof copies, and exchange copies)	0	0
	(3) Paid Distribution Outside the Mails Including Sales Through Dealers and Carriers, Street Vendors, Counter Sales, and Other Paid Distribution Outside USPS®	150	170
	(4) Paid Distribution by Other Classes of Mail Through the USPS (e.g., First-Class Mail®)	0	0
c. Total Paid Distribution [Sum of 15b (1), (2), (3), and (4)]		3866	734
d. Free or Nominal Rate Distribution (By Mail and Outside the Mail)	(1) Free or Nominal Rate Outside-County Copies included on PS Form 3541	0	0
	(2) Free or Nominal Rate In-County Copies Included on PS Form 3541	0	0
	(3) Free or Nominal Rate Copies Mailed at Other Classes Through the USPS (e.g., First-Class Mail)	0	0
	(4) Free or Nominal Rate Distribution Outside the Mail (Carriers or other means)	0	0
e. Total Free or Nominal Rate Distribution (Sum of 15d (1), (2), (3) and (4))		0	0
f. Total Distribution (Sum of 15c and 15e)		3866	734
g. Copies not Distributed (See Instructions to Publishers #4 (page #3))		362	116
h. Total (Sum of 15f and g)		0	0
i. Percent Paid (15c divided by 15f times 100)		100	100

* If you are claiming electronic copies, go to line 16 on page 3. If you are not claiming electronic copies, skip to line 17 on page 3.

UNITED STATES POSTAL SERVICE® **Statement of Ownership, Management, and Circulation (All Periodicals Publications Except Requester Publications)**

16. Electronic Copy Circulation	Average No. Copies Each Issue During Preceding 12 Months	No. Copies of Single Issue Published Nearest to Filing Date
a. Paid Electronic Copies	10,542	7468
b. Total Paid Print Copies (Line 15c) + Paid Electronic Copies (Line 16a)	14,769	8202
c. Total Print Distribution (Line 15f) + Paid Electronic Copies (Line 16a)	14,769	8202
d. Percent Paid (Both Print & Electronic Copies) (16b divided by 16c × 100)	100	100

☑ I certify that 50% of all my distributed copies (electronic and print) are paid above a nominal price.

17. Publication of Statement of Ownership
☑ If the publication is a general publication, publication of this statement is required. Will be printed in the 11/01 issue of this publication. ☐ Publication not required

18. Signature and Title of Editor, Publisher, Business Manager, or Owner: [signature] Director of Publication Services
Date: 9/26/24

I certify that all information furnished on this form is true and complete. I understand that anyone who furnishes false or misleading information on this form or who omits material or information requested on the form may be subject to criminal sanctions (including fines and imprisonment) and/or civil sanctions (including civil penalties).